Recent Results
in Cancer Research 162

Managing Editors
P.M. Schlag, Berlin · H.-J. Senn, St. Gallen

Associate Editors
P. Kleihues, Lyon · F. Stiefel, Lausanne
B. Groner, Frankfurt · A. Wallgren, Göteborg

Founding Editors
P. Rentchnik, Geneva

Springer

Berlin
Heidelberg
New York
Hong Kong
London
Milan
Paris
Tokyo

H. Allgayer · M. M. Heiss
F. W. Schildberg (Eds.)

Molecular
Staging of Cancer

With 24 Figures and 25 Tables

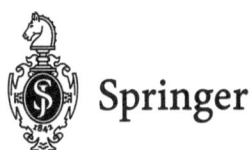 Springer

Dr. Heike Allgayer
Dr. Markus M. Heiss
Prof. Dr. Friedrich W. Schildberg

Ludwig Maximilians Universität, Dept. of Surgery,
Klinikum Großhadern, Marchioninistr. 15,
81377 München, Germany

Indexed in Current Contents and Index Medicus

ISBN-13: 978-3-642-63945-6
ISSN 0080-0015

Library of Congress Cataloging-in-Publication Data

International Meeting on Molecular Staging on Cancer (1st: 2001: Klinicum Gross-hadern). Molecular staging of cancer / H. Allgayer, M. Heiss, F. Schildberg (eds.). p.; cm. – (Recent results in cancer research, ISSN 0080-0015; 162). Proceedings of the 1st International Meeting on Molecular Staging of Cancer, held. December 6–8, 2001 at the Klinikum Grosshadern, Munich. Includes bibliographical references and index. ISBN-13: 978-3-642-63945-6 (alk. paper). 1. Tumors – Classification – Congresses. 2. Cancer – Molecular aspects – Congresses. I. Allgayer, H. (Heike), 1969– II. Heiss, M. (Markus), 1956– III. Title. IV. Series. [DNLM: 1. Neoplasms – diagnosis – Congresses. 2. Neoplasms – ultrastructure – Congresses. 3. Models, Molecular – Congresses. 4. Neoplasm Staging – Congresses. QZ 241 I595 2003]. RC258 ..I466 2003   616.99'4071–dc21

Cataloging-in-Publication Data applied for
Bibliographic information published by Die Deutsche Bibliothek
Die Deutsche Bibliothek lists this publication in the Deutsche Nationalbibliografie; detailed bibliographic data is available in the Internet at <http://dnb.ddb.de>.

Springer-Verlag Berlin · Heidelberg · New York
a member of BertelsmannSpringer Science-Business Media GmbH

http://www.springer.de

ISBN-13: 978-3-642-63945-6   e-ISBN-13: 978-3-642-59349-9
DOI: 10.1007/978-3-642-59349-9

© Springer-Verlag Berlin · Heidelberg 2003
Softcover reprint of the hardcover 1st edition 2003

Typesetting: Stürtz AG, 97080 Würzburg, Germany
Cover design: design & production GmbH, 69121 Heidelberg, Germany

Printed on acid-free paper   21/3150/ag – 5 4 3 2 1 0

Preface

Dear colleagues, honored guests, ladies and gentlemen,

It is an honor and a pleasure for me to welcome you to Munich, to our department, and to the First International Meeting on Molecular Staging of Cancer. We are happy that our meeting has attracted so many national and international speakers, well-known experts in their field, and that it can be held under the auspices of the German Society of Surgeons, its subdivision of Molecular Oncology, the Metastasis Research Society of the United States, and the Professional Board of German Surgeons.

The meeting was called because there is still a large gap between what modern research has discovered about the biology and molecular characteristics of various cancers and clinical practice. On the one hand, experimental fields such as molecular biology have been defining the biological behavior of tumor cells – e.g., regarding proliferation, immortalization, transformation, invasion, dissemination, and the process of metastasis – with an amazing rate of progressive knowledge. But on the other hand, for the definition of patient subgroups regarding individually adjusted clinical decision making on tumor surgery, neoadjuvant/adjuvant therapy, and follow-up, the clinician still uses long-established tumor staging systems which are exclusively defined by morphological criteria.

Gradually, of course, experimental medicine cannot be prevented from having an impact on clinical and surgical decisions. There are examples that already show how theoretical knowledge of individual tumor biology can define the therapeutic strategy for cancer patients. These examples include multiple endocrine neoplasia (MEN) type II, which can be diagnosed with a high specificity by a mutation in the *ret* proto-oncogene. Diagnosis of this mutation has already led to the surgical consequence of prophylactic thyroidectomy in carriers. Other examples are hereditary colorectal cancers such as familial adenomatous polyposis coli (FAP), in which a mutation in the APC tumor suppressor gene can select high-risk individuals out of a suspect family. As a surgical consequence, prophylactic colectomy is being discussed for severely affected individuals. In breast cancer, mutations of the BRCA1/2 genes can identify familial breast cancer syndromes, and the detection of

ErbB-2-receptor in individual breast cancers has led to a new adjuvant therapy concept involving treatment with Herceptin. These examples clearly show how an integration of experimental medicine into clinical thinking can benefit the cancer patient.

However, we think that these examples are only the beginning of a development which can possibly lead to a paradigm shift. The objective of our meeting is to outline what the development will be, how future molecular staging models could look, which markers are likely to become candidates, and how they can be defined. Furthermore, the meeting will ask what impact further promising molecular discoveries can or will have on the selection of patients at high risk for disease, on surgical tumor therapy, on adjuvant therapy, and on follow-up. The meeting aims to:

1. Focus on specific topics that we believe will have a high potential of becoming candidates for new molecular staging models. These topics include:

- *Tumor-associated proteolysis.* Evidence has accumulated in the past years that the process of invasion and metastasis is, at least in part, achieved by the overexpression of proteases and their inhibitors, which lead to an efficient degradation of the extracellular matrix and basement membranes of vessels. Talks on this topic will show how these proteases are upregulated in tumor cells, how they function, give an early status report on strategies to inhibit them, and suggest how they can be integrated into staging models.
- *Minimal residual disease.* There has been strong evidence that also in epithelial solid tumors a so-called minimal residual disease (MRD) component can be detected even in early tumor stages. This MRD component is postulated to contribute to tumor recurrence even after the primary tumor has been curatively surgically resected. The meeting will discuss methods of MRD detection and their limitations, give an actual status on the prognostic impact of MRD in different carcinoma types, and outline how molecular phenotyping and long-term follow-up could help to establish MRD as a clinically helpful staging marker.

2. The meeting introduces different promising markers within different clinical models and cancer types. This will involve different tumor entities such as colon, gastric, breast, pancreatic and skin cancer, and it will address hereditary cancer syndromes as well as sporadic cancer types.

3. The meeting presents methodology that can help to define new staging models, including not only new molecular technology such as microarrays or proteomics, but also biostatistical methods such

as neuronal networks. Additionally, the role and strategies of bio-tech companies in this context, in the search for and transfer of staging markers into clinical applications, will be discussed.

And finally, the meeting presents the first therapeutic concepts us-ing different molecular markers which may be integrated into sur-gical and medical tumor therapy in the future. It also introduces new technology which can serve as an efficient tool to target mo-lecular markers.

In conclusion, I hope that this meeting will illustrate that, especial-ly as clinicians, it is imperative that we get used to the increasing importance of diverse molecular markers which will clearly influ-ence our clinical decisions, including the staging of disease, the definition of precise prognostic subgroups, the planning of surgi-cal strategies in tumor surgery, neoadjuvant and adjuvant therapy, and the clinical follow-up of our patients. Ultimately, we postulate that this will result in a more and more individualized multidisci-plinary tumor therapy, combining theoretical concepts with the clinic.

It is an exciting development bearing outstanding chances, and again, ladies and gentlemen, thank you all for coming to Munich from all over the world. I wish all of us a pleasant, informative, in-teresting, and exciting meeting, and on behalf of the organizers and myself, to all of you: *Welcome.*

Klinikum Grosshadern   *Friedrich Wilhelm Schildberg*

Contents

1 Reviews

2 Original Papers

3 Summary

Reviews 1

The Urokinase Receptor (uPAR, CD87) as a Target for Tumor Therapy: uPA-Silica Particles (SP-uPA) as a New Tool for Assessing Synthetic Peptides to Interfere with uPA/uPA-Receptor Interaction

Elke Guthaus, Niko Schmiedeberg, Markus Bürgle, Viktor Magdolen, Horst Kessler, Manfred Schmitt

E. Guthaus (✉)
Klinische Forschergruppe, Frauenklinik, Technische Universität München, 81675 Munich, Germany

Abstract

Many different processes in the physiology and pathophysiology of human beings are regulated protein/protein interactions such as receptor/ligand interactions. A more detailed knowledge of the nature of receptor/ligand binding sites and mechanisms of interaction is necessary as well in order to understand the process of cancer spread and metastasis. For instance, the cell surface receptor uPAR (CD87) and its ligand, the serine protease urokinase-type plasminogen activator (uPA), facilitate tumor invasion and metastasis in solid malignant tumors. Besides its proteolytic function in activating the zymogen plasminogen into the serine protease plasmin, binding of uPA to tumor cell-associated uPAR initiates various cell responses such as tumor cell migration, adhesion, proliferation, and differentiation. Hence, the tumor-associated uPA/uPAR system is considered a potential target for cancer therapy. Here we briefly describe a new technology using micro-silica particles coated with uPA (yields SP-uPA) and reaction of SP-uPA with recombinant soluble uPAR (suPAR) to test the competitive antagonistic potential of synthetic uPA peptides by flow cytofluorometry (FACS). We discuss the data obtained with the SP-uPA system from two different points of view: (1) The enhanced potential of improved uPA-derived synthetic peptides compared to previously described peptides, and (2) comparison of the new technique to other test systems currently used to identify uPA/uPAR or other protein/protein interactions.

The Plasminogen Activation System

The plasminogen activation system with its components uPA receptor (uPAR, CD87), the serine proteases uPA and tPA (tissue-type plasminogen activator), and the uPA/tPA inhibitors plasminogen activator inhibitor type-1 and type-2 (PAI-1/-2) plays a central role in degradation and reorganization of the extracellular matrix, also in cancer (Schmitt et al. 1997; Andreasen et al. 1997; Reuning et al. 1998). In tumors, enzymatically inactive plasminogen, a liver-derived blood zymogen, is converted into the serine protease plasmin by uPA (Ellis 1996). For this, the uPAR-bound pro-enzyme form of uPA, pro-uPA (released by tumor and normal cells), is activated by plasmin and cysteine proteases cathepsin B/L to yield enzymatically active uPA (Kobayashi et al. 1991; Goretzki et al. 1992).

uPAR is a three-domain cysteine-rich glycoprotein attached to the plasma membrane via a covalent linkage of its carboxyterminus to a glycosyl-phos-phatidylinositol (GPI) anchor (Ploug et al. 1991). Its ligand uPA encompasses two main domains: the catalytic carboxy-terminal domain and the non-catalytic amino-terminal domain (Schmitt et al. 1992). The uPAR binding epitope of uPA has been assigned to an epitope encompassing amino acids (aa) 19 to 31 in the growth factor-like domain (GFD, aa 1–46) of uPA (Appella et al. 1987; Magdolen et al. 1996; Bürgle et al. 1997). Occupation of uPAR by uPA, derivatives thereof, or synthetic uPA peptides activates different signaling pathways eventually leading to cell proliferation, migration, adhesion, and differentiation (Fischer et al. 1998; Yebra et al. 1999; Waltz et al. 1994, 2000; Webb et al. 2001). Based on various clinical studies, high protein levels of uPAR, uPA, and/or PAI-1 found to be present in solid malignant tumors do correlate with an elevated risk of disease recurrence, and thus with a poor prognosis of the cancer patient. (Schmitt et al. 1997; Look et al. 2002). Consequently, in addition to directly blocking uPA protease activity, uPA/uPAR interaction represents an attractive target to reduce tumor spread and metastasis by use of small antagonistic uPA peptides (Sperl et al. 2001; Sato et al. 2002).

uPA-Derived Peptides

In 1985, the uPA receptor was detected independently on human monocytes and on mouse fibroblasts (Vassalli et al. 1985; del Rosso et al. 1985). The uPAR binding region of uPA was originally mapped to aa 18 to 32 of the growth factor-like domain of uPA using a panel of linear uPA-derived peptides (Appella et al. 1987). Since then, other uPA/uPAR-interfering synthetic peptides have been reported. For instance, using a bacteriophage library, Goodson et al. (1994) depicted a potent antagonistic 17-mer peptide (clone 20) to inhibit the uPA-uPAR interaction. This peptide sequence is different from the uPAR-binding region in uPA, but the discovered motif FXXYLW is in close order to that of the uPAR-binding ^{24}YFXXIXW^{30} within uPA (Magdolen et al. 1996; Bürgle et al. 1997). In another approach, by systematic mutational analysis with linear uPA peptides, it was revealed that amino acids Cys19, Lys23, Tyr24, Phe25, Ile28, Trp30, and Cys31 of uPA mediate effective binding of uPA to uPAR (Magdolen et al. 1996). In view of this, Bürgle et al. (1997) synthesized the linear peptide uPA$_{19-31}$ and showed its inhibitory capacity on tumor cell uPA/uPAR interaction (Schmitt et al. 1991) and also in a model uPA/uPAR binding assay (Goretzki et al. 1997). They also demonstrated that the novel cy-

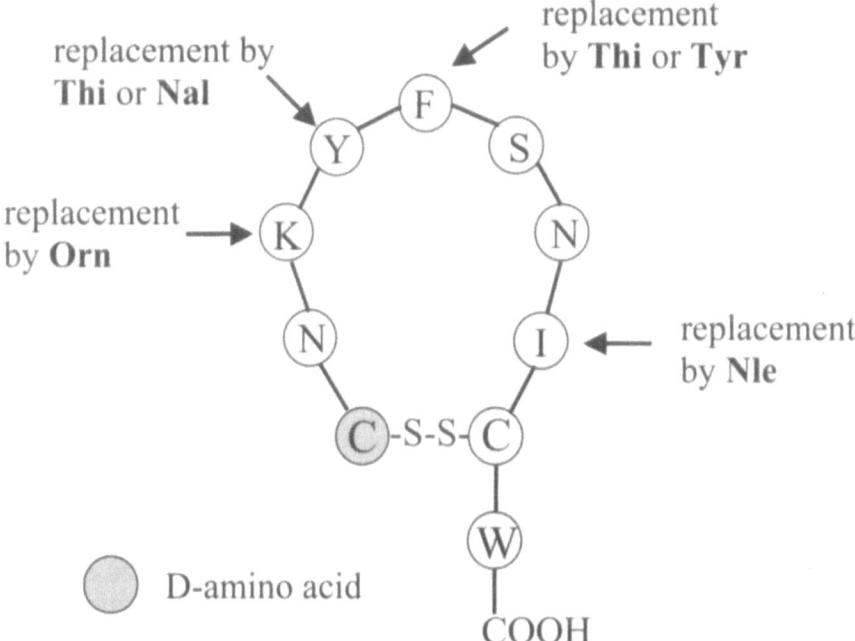

Fig. 1. Amino acid exchange in the lead peptide cyclo^{21,29} [D-Cys^{21}Cys^{29}]-uPA$_{21-30}$. Lead structure of cyclo^{21,29}[D-Cys^{21}Cys^{29}]-uPA$_{21-30}$. Replacing certain single amino acids (*arrows*) by non-proteinogenic amino acids: lysine (*Lys, K*) by ornithine (*Orn*), tyrosine (*Tyr, Y*) by 2-naphthylalanine (*2-Nal*) or β-2-thienylalanine (*Thi*), phenylalanine (*Phe, F*) by tyrosine (*Tyr*) or β-2-thienylalanine (*Thi*), and isoleucine (*Ile, I*) by norleucine (*Nle*)

clic disulfide-bridged form of uPA$_{19-31}$, cyclo^{19,31}[D-Cys^{19}]-uPA$_{19-31}$, also competes with uPA for binding to uPAR. By flow cytofluorometry (FACS) using U937 tumor cells as the source of uPAR and fluorescent uPA as the uPA ligand, for this peptide, an IC$_{50}$ value of 0.7 µM was achieved (Bürgle et al. 1997; Schmitt et al. 2000; Magdolen et al. 2001). Replacement of Cys19 in peptide cyclo^{19,31}uPA$_{19-31}$ by the corresponding D-Cys19 led to a significant increase in inhibitory capacity resulting in a decrease of the IC$_{50}$ value to 0.2 µM (Magdolen et al. 2001) and stabilized the peptides toward proteolytic attack. A shorter, cyclic uPA-peptide and a more potent variant was obtained by replacing Ser21 by D-Cys and His29 by Cys with concomitant formation of a disulfide bond (Schmiedeberg et al. 2000, 2002). This 10-mer peptide cyclo^{21,29}[D-Cys^{21}Cys^{29}]-uPA$_{21-30}$ represents an even more rigid and therefore more stable molecule towards proteolytic degradation than the uPA-peptide variants described previously. Employing cyclo^{21,29}[D-Cys^{21}Cys^{29}]-uPA$_{21-30}$ as the lead peptide, a pool of different peptides was synthesized and their inhibitory capacity tested by FACS using U937/FITC-uPA, and used in comparison, the recently established particle-based SP-uPA-system (Guthaus et al. 2002). Replacing single amino acids with the non-proteinogenic amino acids 2-naphthylalanine (2-Nal), norleucine (Nle), β-2-thienylalanine (Thi), or ornithine

(Orn) (Fig. 1) resulted in the competitive uPA-peptides cyclo^{21,29} [D-Cys^{21}2-Nal^{24}Cys^{29}]-uPA$_{21-30}$, cyclo^{21,29} [D-Cys^{21}Nle^{28}Cys^{29}]-uPA$_{21-30}$, and cyclo^{21,29} [D-Cys^{21}Orn^{23}Thi^{24}Thi^{25}Cys^{29}]-uPA$_{21-30}$. Interestingly, replacing the aromatic amino acid Phe^{25} by aromatic amino acid Tyr in cyclo^{21,29}[D-Cys^{21}Cys^{29}]-uPA$_{21-30}$ resulted in a peptide devoid of uPAR binding activity in both the SP-uPA/uPAR and the U937/FITC-uPA systems (Guthaus et al. 2002).

uPA/uPAR Interaction-Determining Methods

The ever-increasing knowledge of the importance of the plasminogen activation system in cancer cell invasion and metastasis stimulated vivid interest in fine-tuned methods for investigating uPA/uPAR interaction and testing the impact of potential uPA analogs (Crowley et al. 1993; Min et al. 1996; Kobayashi et al. 1998; Li et al. 1998; Tressler et al. 1999; Krüger et al. 2000; Schmitt et al. 2000; Lutz et al. 2001; Mazar 2001; Rabbani and Mazar 2001).

Several types of assays including test systems using cell-bound uPAR or non-cellular uPAR were established (Table 1). Enzyme-linked immunosorbent assays with suPAR immobilized to microtiter plates were established and the interaction with uPA or ATF was identified using specific primary antibodies (Rettenberger et al. 1995; De Witte et al. 1998). Goodson et al. (1994) and Min et al. (1996) described an alternative microtiter plate assay involving streptavidin-coated microtiter plates reacting with biotinylated uPAR and ^{125}I-labeled uPA or ATF. ^{125}I-labeled pro-uPA, uPA, or uPA-mutants were also used

Table 1. Test systems using cell-associated uPAR or non-cellular uPAR

Cellular system		
Cell line	Ligand	Reference
U937	^{125}I-uPA	Stoppelli et al. 1985; Vassalli et al. 1985; Picone et al. 1989
U937	FITC-uPA	Schmitt et al. 1991; Chucholowski et al. 1992; Magdolen et al. 1996 and 2001; Bürgle et al. 1997; Schmiedeberg et al. 2000; Guthaus et al. 2002
Mouse fibroblasts AA12–3T3	^{125}I-uPA	Del Rosso et al. 1985
Mouse macrophages; HeLa	^{125}I-uPA; ^{125}I-[Tyr^{22}]-uPA	Quax et al. 1998
Non-cellular system		
Assay type		
Microtiter plate		Goodson et al. 1994; Rettenberger et al. 1995; Min et al. 1996; De Witte et al. 1998
SDS-PAGE/autoradiography		Engelholm et al. 2001
SPOT-membranes/Western blot		Liang et al. 2001
BIAcore (surface plasmon resonance)		Ploug et al. 1998 and 2001; Gardsvoll et al. 1999; List et al. 1999; Mühlenweg et al. 2000

to identify uPAR in cell lysates subjected to SDS-PAGE and autoradiography (Engelholm and Behrendt 2001) or in a uPA-binding assay applying uPAR-bearing tumor cells cultured in microtiter plates (Quax et al. 1998). Western blot analyses with SPOT-membranes were performed to identify uPA-uPAR binding and to qualitatively prove inhibition of this interaction (Liang et al. 2001). For this, overlapping 15-mer peptides with a three amino acid shift, covering the entire uPAR molecule, were directly synthesized as spots on cellulose membranes (SPOT-membranes), with uPA being subsequently added.

Surface plasmon resonance (BIAcore) represents another alternative, noncellular technique to study uPA/uPAR interaction. For this, uPA, uPAR, or competitive uPA-peptides are covalently bound to a CM5 BIAcore-chip, and the specific uPA/uPAR interaction behavior is determined (Ploug et al. 1998, 2001; Gardsvoll et al. 1999; List et al. 1999; Mühlenweg et al. 2000). Direct immobilization of uPAR on the CM5 sensor chip was possible by removal of sialic acid from its N-linked carbohydrates of uPAR, applying neuraminidase and thereby reaching the required isoelectric point of uPAR necessary for covalent immobilization (Ploug et al. 1998). Those authors identified involvement of domains I and III of uPAR in binding to the antagonistic 10-mer peptide SLN-FSQYLWS, representing a shortened clone 20 peptide (Goodson et al. 1994). Different analytical methods were combined: photoaffinity labeling, matrix-assisted laser desorption and ionization (MALDI) mass spectrometry, NH_2-terminal sequence analysis, and amino acid composition analysis after enzymatic fragmentation and HPLC purification (Ploug 1998).

To determine the efficiency of linear and cyclic uPA-derived peptides to bind to cellular uPAR, Schmitt et al. (1991), Magdolen et al. (1996, 2001), Bürgle et al. (1997), Schmiedeberg et al. (2000), and Guthaus et al. (2002) bound fluorescein isothiocyanate (FITC)-labeled uPA to uPAR-bearing U937 cells and determined binding efficiency by FACS. Stimulation of this tumor cell line with phorbol ester (PMA) leads to an about 10-fold increase in the number of expressed uPAR molecules concomitant with a decrease of uPA binding capacity (Stoppelli et al. 1985; Nielsen et al. 1988). Derivitization of uPA with FITC at the NH_2-group in Lys25, located in the uPAR-binding region of the uPA molecule, however, does result in a somewhat lower binding affinity of uPA to uPAR (Schmitt et al. 1991; Chucholowski et al. 1992).

The Particle-Based SP-uPA System

A novel cytometric method to rapidly but quantitatively assess the uPA/uPAR interaction was introduced by Guthaus et al. (2002). uPA was coupled to silica particles (SP) to yield SP-uPA, and then soluble, recombinant uPAR (suPAR) added, and binding of suPAR was verified by reaction with the monoclonal antibody HD13.1 directed to uPAR, followed by a cyan dye (cy5)-labeled antibody to mouse IgG (Fig. 2). With this system the naturally occurring ligands HMW-uPA and ATF were tested, as well as the uPA-derived peptides (cyclo^{21,29} [D-Cys^{21}Cys^{29}]-uPA$_{21-30}$, cyclo^{21,29} [D-Cys^{21}2-Nal^{24}Cys^{29}]-uPA$_{21-30}$, cy-

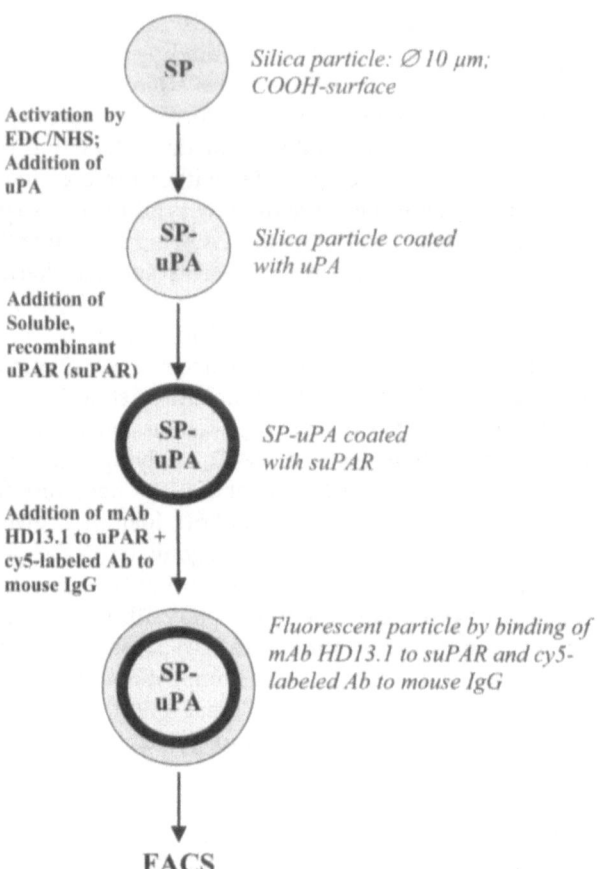

Fig. 2. Preparation of SP-uPA to screen for potential uPA competitors using FACS. uPA is coupled to silica particles (*SP*) 10 µm in diameter using the EDC/NHS method. Soluble, recombinant uPA (*suPAR*) is added and the receptor/ligand interaction verified by reaction with a monoclonal antibody (HD13.1) directed to uPAR, followed by a cyan dye (cy5)-labeled, fluorescent antibody to mouse IgG. SP-uPA/suPAR are then subjected to flow cytometry (FACS), and particle-associated fluorescence is determined as a measure of particle-bound suPAR. Reduction in fluorescence indicates an inhibitory potential of the competitive agent in question

clo^{21,29}[D-Cys^{21}Orn^{23}Thi^{24}Thi^{25}Cys^{29}]-uPA$_{21-30}$, cyclo^{21,29} [D-Cys^{21}Nle^{28}Cys^{29}]-uPA$_{21-30}$, and cyclo^{21,29} [D-Cys^{21}Tyr^{25}Cys^{29}]-uPA$_{21-30}$ (Fig. 1).

For the preparation of SP-uPA, silica particles 10 µm in diameter and with COOH-surface were activated with EDC/ NHS. After washing, uPA was added and free binding sites were blocked by incubation of the particles with ethanol amine. To evaluate binding and distribution of uPA on the silica particle surface, SP-uPA were incubated with mAb no. 3689 directed to uPA, and after a washing step with polyclonal, they were incubated with cy5-labeled rabbit antibody to mouse IgG. To verify binding of suPAR to SP-uPA, SP-uPA were incubated with suPAR first, and thereafter with mAb HD13.1 to uPAR, followed

Table 2. IC$_{50}$ values of uPA, ATF, and synthetic cyclic uPA-peptides. IC$_{50}$ values of HMW-uPA, ATF, cyclo^{21,29} [D-Cys^{21}Cys^{29}]-uPA$_{21-30}$, cyclo^{21,29} [D-Cys^{21}2-Nal^{24}Cys^{29}]-uPA$_{21-30}$, cyclo^{21,29} [D-Cys^{21}Orn^{23}-Thi^{24}Thi^{25}Cys^{29}]-uPA$_{21-30}$, cyclo^{21,29} [D-Cys^{21}Nle^{28}Cys^{29}]-uPA$_{21-30}$, and cyclo^{21,29} [D-Cys^{21}Tyr^{25}Cys^{29}]-uPA$_{21-30}$. Comparison of fluorescence mean channel obtained using both the SP-uPA system and the U937 cell system to determine the antagonistic potential of HMW-uPA, ATF, and synthetic cyclic uPA-peptides (adapted from Guthaus et al. 2002)

Competitor	IC$_{50}$ [nM]	
	SP-uPA	U937 cells
HMW-uPA	12	10
ATF	11	5
cyclo^{21,29} [D-Cys^{21}Cys^{29}] -uPA$_{21-30}$	400	150
cyclo^{21,29} [D-Cys^{21}Nle^{28}Cys^{29}] -uPA$_{21-30}$	400	200
cyclo^{21,29} [D-Cys^{21}2-Nal^{24}Cys^{29}] -uPA$_{21-30}$	400	130
cyclo^{21,29} [D-Cys^{21}Orn^{23}Thi^{24}Thi^{25}Cys^{29}] – uPA$_{21-30}$	>4,000	>4,000
cyclo^{21,29} [D-Cys^{21}Tyr^{25}Cys^{29}] -uPA$_{21-30}$	No effect	No effect

by incubation with polyclonal cy5-labeled rabbit antibody to mouse IgG. The particles were analyzed by FACS. To investigate the capacity of uPA, ATF, or synthetic peptides to interact with fluid-phase suPAR, increasing amounts of these competitive analogs were incubated simultaneously with suPAR and SP-uPA. Non-coupled (SP-COOH) and BSA-coupled particles (SP-BSA) were used in control experiments.

The results obtained with this system were highly comparable to those obtained with the FITC-uPA/U937 system (Schmitt et al. 1991; Chucholowski et al. 1992). HMW-uPA, ATF, and cyclic peptide cyclo^{21,29}[D-Cys^{21}Cys^{29}]-uPA$_{21-30}$ as well as its 2-Nal^{24}- and Nle^{28}-derivatives were highly effective in both systems (Table 2).

Other Particle-Based Analysis Methods to Screen for Protein/Protein Interaction

Flow cytofluorometry (FACS) represents a widely used and highly effective analytical method, originally established to simultaneously measure physical and biochemical parameters of single cells (e.g., tumor cells, lymphocytes, or bacteria; O'Connor et al. 2001; Wedemeyer et al. 2001). In such systems replacing cells with artificial particles led to new and interesting approaches in cytofluorometry. Additionally, a high throughput flow cytometry technique with measurement of about 100,000 samples per day (Kuckuck et al. 2001) was made available, allowing an extension of the field of application. Müller et al. (1996) established a cytometric method to identify high-affinity ligands to the SH2 domain of the glutathione S-transferase by fluorescence-activated bead sorting (FABS). In this approach, recombinant SH2 domains were incubated with a peptide library (6.4×10^6 individual peptides) displayed on beads, and the binding was determined with a specific FITC-labeled antibody. Highly fluorescent beads, representing a single high-affinity ligand, were selected. The amino acid sequence of such a peptide was determined, the peptide synthesized in bulk, and binding characteristics further evaluated using surface plasmon resonance. By another technique, beads with distinct fluorescence intensities coupled with antibodies to different cytokines – one antibody bound to one distinct fluorescent bead – were used to simultaneously quantify some 15 different cytokines (Carson and Vignali 1999). This setup is equivalent to an ELISA format: a catching antibody bound to beads, the cytokine bound to the primary antibody, biotinylated detection antibody, and streptavidin-ALEXA488. A multiplexed, bead-based method which utilizes nucleic acid hybridization on the surface of microscopic polystyrene spheres was used to identify specific sequences in heterogeneous mixtures of DNA sequences (Spiro et al. 2000). Oligonucleotides–"capture probes"–were covalently attached to the beads using the EDC/NHS method. The amount of bound, 5'-fluoresceinated cDNA was measured by flow cytometry.

Other methods involving particles to detect protein/protein interactions generally require a broad spectrum of basic techniques. To name two, the Bead ARray Counter (BARC) uses biological interactions such as DNA-DNA, antibody-antigen, or protein-ligand to link micron-sized magnetic beads to a sensor surface. After removal of non-specifically bound beads, an embedded array of giant magnetoresistive (GMR) sensors detects the specifically bound beads that remain. Patterning different receptor DNA, antibodies, or ligands above this sensor array allows the simultaneous detection of several analytes (Edelstein et al. 2000). The Origen technique enables detection of proteins in the ELISA-sandwich format on magnetic beads, whereas proteins are detected by luminescence-tagged antibodies. A magnet captures the beads on the electrode. When the magnet is removed the electrode excites the luminescence-tag and a detector measures the light, whose intensity depends on the amount of bound, labeled antibody (Abraham et al. 1996; Swanson et al. 1999).

Conclusion

The recently established SP-uPA system for rapidly screening potential competitive peptides of the uPA/uPAR interaction is superior to cell-based methods in several aspects. There is no need for rather expensive and time-consuming cell cultures to grow uPAR-bearing cells. Most important, silica particle-bound uPA (SP-uPA) and recombinant, soluble uPAR can be kept in stock, ready for instant use. Thereby, an ongoing high-quality level of the test reagents can be assured. This system adds further potential to the general advantages of flow cytofluorometry (e.g., high sample throughput, short measuring time, etc.).

Series of applications are generally envisaged for extending this system to other receptor/ligand interactions or protein/protein interactions. Proteins other than uPA can be bound to the silica particles, for example, integrins, EGF-receptors, or enzyme/inhibitor complexes, and their interaction with known or unknown binding partners can be investigated. Using fluorescent particles with different intensities would allow parallel detection of various protein/protein interactions in one sample. Another approach is to use ferro-magnetic silica particles coated with proteins. By this, reactive proteins present in body fluids, for example, blood plasma, effusion fluids, cell or tissue extracts, as well as those present in cell culture supernatants can be detected and enriched. Characterization of bound material would be performed using analytical systems such as SELDI, MALDI, PAGE, HPLC, or Western blot. The silica particle system harbors an enormous potential for other types of application.

References

Abraham R, Buxbaum S, Link J, Smith R, Venti C, Darsley M (1996) Determination of bind-ing constants of diabodies directed against prostate-specific antigen using electrochemi-luminescence-based immunoassays. J Mol Recognit 9:456–461

Andreasen PA, Kjöller L, Christensen L, Duffy MJ (1997) The urokinase-type plasminogen activator system in cancer metastasis: A review. Int J Cancer 72:1–22

Appella E, Robinson EA, Ullrich SJ, Stoppelli MP, Corti, A, Cassani G, Blasi F (1987) The re-ceptor-binding sequence of urokinase. A biological function for the growth-factor mod-ule of proteases. J Biol Chem 262:4437–4440

Bürgle M, Koppitz M, Riemer C, Kessler H, König B, Weidle UH, Kellermann J, Lottspeich F, Graeff H, Schmitt M, Goretzki L, Reuning U, Wilhelm O, Magdolen V (1997) Inhibition of the interaction of urokinase-type plasminogen activator (uPA) with its receptor (uPAR) by synthetic peptides. Biol Chem 378:231–237

Carson RT, Vignali DA (1999) Simultaneous quantitation of 15 cytokines using a multiplexed flow cytometric assay. J Immunol Methods 227:41–52

Chucholowski N, Schmitt M, Rettenberger P, Schüren E, Moniwa N, Goretzki L, Wilhelm O, Weidle U, Jänicke F, Graeff H (1992) Flow cytometric analysis of the urokinase receptor (uPA-R) on tumor cells by fluorescent uPA-ligands or monoclonal antibody #3936. Fi-brinolysis 6 [Suppl 4]:95–102

Crowley CW, Cohen RL, Lucas BK, Lui G, Shuman M, Levinson AD (1993) Prevention of me-tastasis by inhibition of the urokinase receptor. Proc Natl Acad Sci USA 90:5021–5025

Del Rosso M, Dini G, Fibbi G (1985) Receptors for plasminogen activator, urokinase, in nor-mal and Rous sarcoma virus-transformed mouse fibroblasts. Cancer Res 45:630–636

De Witte H, Sweep F, Brünner N, Heuvel J, Beex L, Grebenschikov N, Benraad T (1998) Com-plexes between urokinase-type plasminogen activator and its receptor in blood as deter-mined by enzyme-linked immunosorbent assay. Int J Cancer 77:236–242

Edelstein RL, Tamanaha CR, Sheehan PE, Miller MM, Baselt DR, Whitman LJ, Colton RJ (2000) The BARC biosensor applied to the detection of biological warfare agents. Biosens Bioelectron 14:805–813

Ellis V (1996) Functional analysis of the cellular receptor for urokinase in plasminogen acti-vation. Receptor binding has no influence on the zymogenic nature of pro-urokinase. J Biol Chem 271:14779–14784

Engelholm LH, Behrendt N (2001) Differential binding of urokinase and peptide antagonists to the urokinase receptor: Evidence from characterization of the receptor in four primate species. Biol Chem 382:435–442

Fischer K, Lutz V, Wilhelm O, Schmitt M, Graeff H, Heiss P, Nishiguchi T, Harbeck N, Kessler H, Luther T, Magdolen V, Reuning U (1998) Urokinase induces proliferation of human ovarian cancer cells: characterization of structural elements required for growth factor function. FEBS Lett 438:101–105

Gårdsvoll H, Danø K, Ploug M (1999) Mapping part of the functional epitope for ligand binding on the receptor for urokinase-type plasminogen activator by site-directed mutagenesis. J Biol Chem 274:37995–38003

Goodson RJ, Doyle MV, Kaufman SE, Rosenberg S (1994) High-affinity urokinase receptor antagonists identified with bacteriophage peptide display. Proc Natl Acad Sci USA 91:7129–7133

Goretzki L, Schmitt M, Mann K, Calvete J, Chucholowski N, Kramer M, Günzler WA, Jänicke F, Graeff H (1992) Effective activation of the proenzyme form of the urokinase-type plasminogen activator (pro-uPA) by the cysteine protease cathepsin L. FEBS Lett 297:112–118

Goretzki L, Bognacki J, Koppitz M, Rettenberger P, Magdolen V, Creutzburg S, Hammelburger J, Weidle UH, Wilhelm O, Kessler H, Graeff H, Schmitt M (1997) Quantitative assessment of interaction of urokinase-type plasminogen activator and its receptor (CD87) by use of a solid-phase uPA-ligand binding assay. Fibrinol Proteol 1:11–19

Guthaus E, Bürgle M, Schmiedeberg N, Hocke S, Eickler A, Kramer MD, Sweep CGJF, Magdolen V, Kessler H, Schmitt M (2002) uPA-Silica-Particles (SP-uPA): A novel analytical system to investigate uPA-uPAR-interaction and to test synthetic uPAR-antagonists as potential cancer therapeutics. Biol Chem

Kobayashi H, Schmitt M, Goretzki L, Chucholowski N, Calvete J, Kramer M, Günzler WA, Jänicke F, Graeff H (1991) Cathepsin B efficiently activates the soluble and the tumor cell receptor-bound form of the proenzyme urokinase-type plasminogen activator (Pro-uPA). J Biol Chem 266:5147–5152

Kobayashi H, Sugino D, She M Y, Ohi H, Hirashima Y, Sinohara H, Fujie M, Shibata K, Terao T (1998) A bi-functional hybrid molecule of the amino-terminal fragment urokinase and domain II of bikunin. Eur J Biochem 253:817–826

Krüger A, Soeltl R, Lutz V, Wilhelm OG, Magdolen V, Rojo EA, Hantzopoulos PA, Graeff H, Gänsbacher B, Schmitt M (2000) Reduction of breast carcinoma tumor growth and lung colonization by overexpression of the soluble urokinase-type plasminogen activator receptor (CD87). Cancer Gene Ther 7:292–299

Kuckuck FW, Edwards BS, Sklar LA (2001) High throughput flow cytometry. Cytometry 44:83–90

Li H, Lu H, Griscelli F, Opolon P, Sun LQ, Ragot T, Legrand Y, Belin D, Soria J, Soria C, Pericaudet M, Yeh P (1998) Adenovirus-mediated delivery of a uPA/uPAR antagonist suppresses angiogenesis-dependent tumor growth and dissemination in mice. Gene Ther 5:1105–1113

Liang OD, Chavakis T, Kanse SM, Preissner KT (2001) Ligand binding regions in the receptor for urokinase-type plasminogen activator. J Biol Chem 276:28946–28953

List K, Høyer-Hansen G, Rønne E, Danø K, Behrendt N (1998) Different mechanisms are involved in the antibody mediated inhibition of ligand binding to the urokinase receptor: a study based on biosensor technology. J Immunol Methods 222:125–133

Look MP, van Putten WLJ, Duffy MJ, Harbeck N, Christensen IJ, Thomssen C, Kates R, Spyratos F, Fernö M, Eppenberger-Castori S, Sweep CGJ, Ulm K, Peyrat JP, Martin PM, Magdelenat H, Brünner N, Duggan C, Lisboa BW, Bendahl PO, Quillien V, Daver A, Ricolleau G, Meijer-van Gelder ME, Manders P, Fiets WE, Blankenstein MA, Broet P, Romain S, Daxenbichler G, Windbichler G, Cufer T, Borstnar S, Kueng W, Beex LVAM, Klijn JGM, O'Higgins N, Eppenberger U, Jänicke F, Schmitt M, Foekens J (2002) Pooled analysis of prognostic impact of uPA and PAI-1 in 8,377 breast cancer patients. J Natl Cancer Inst

Lutz V, Reuning U, Krüger A, Luther T, Pildner von Steinburg S, Graeff H, Schmitt M, Wilhelm OG, Magdolen V (2001) High level synthesis of recombinant soluble urokinase receptor (CD87) by ovarian cancer cells reduces intraperitoneal tumor growth and spread in nude mice. Biol Chem 382:789–798

Magdolen V, Bürgle M, Arroyo de Prada N, Schmiedeberg N, Riemer C, Schroeck F, Kellermann J, Degitz K, Wilhelm OG, Schmitt M, Kessler H (2001) Cyclo ^{19,31}[D-Cys^{19}]-uPA$_{19-31}$ is a potent competitive antagonist of the interaction of urokinase-type plasminogen activator with its receptor (CD87). Biol Chem 382:1197–1205

Magdolen V, Rettenberger P, Koppitz M, Goretzki L, Kessler H, Weidle UH, König B, Graeff H, Schmitt M, Wilhelm O (1996) Systematic mutational analysis of the receptor-binding region of the human urokinase-type plasminogen activator. Eur J Biochem 237:743–751

Mazar AP (2001) The urokinase plasminogen activator receptor (uPAR) as a target for the diagnosis and therapy of cancer. Anticancer Drugs 12:387–400

Min HY, Doyle LV, Vitt CR, Zandonella CL, Stratton-Thomas JR, Shuman MA, Rosenberg S (1996) Urokinase receptor antagonists inhibit angiogenesis and primary tumor growth in syngeneic mice. Cancer Res 56:2428–2433

Mühlenweg B, Assfalg-Machleidt I, Parrado SG, Burgle M, Creutzburg S, Schmitt M, Auerswald EA, Machleidt W, Magdolen V (2000) A novel type of bifunctional inhibitor directed against proteolytic activity and receptor/ligand interaction. Cystatin with a urokinase receptor binding site. J Biol Chem 275:33562–33566

Müller K, Gombert FO, Manning U, Grossmüller F, Graff P, Zaegel H, Zuber JF, Freuler F, Tschopp C, Baumann G (1996) Rapid identification of phosphopeptide ligands for SH2 domains. Screening of peptide libraries by fluorescence-activated bead sorting. J Biol Chem 271:16500–16505

Nielsen LS, Kellerman GM, Behrendt N, Picone R, Dano K, Blasi F (1988) A 55,000–60,000 Mr receptor protein for urokinase-type plasminogen activator. Identification in human tumor cell lines and partial purification. J Biol Chem 263:2358–2363

O'Connor JE, Callaghan RC, Escudero M, Herrera G, Martinez A, Monteiro MD, Montoliu H (2001) The relevance of flow cytometry for biochemical analysis. IUBMB Life 51:231–239

Picone R, Kajtaniak EL, Nielsen LS, Behrendt N, Mastronicola MR, Cubellis MV, Stoppelli MP, Pedersen S, Dano K, Blasi F (1989) Regulation of urokinase receptors in monocytelike U937 cells by phorbol ester phorbol myristate acetate. J Cell Biol 108:693–702

Ploug M (1998) Identification of specific sites involved in ligand binding by photoaffinity labeling of the receptor for the urokinase-type plasminogen activator. Residues located at equivalent positions in uPAR domains I and III participate in the assembly of a composite ligand-binding site. Biochemistry 37:16494–16505

Ploug M, Behrendt N, Lober D, Danø K (1991) Protein structure and membrane anchorage of the cellular receptor for urokinase-type plasminogen activator. Semin Thromb Hemost 17:183–193

Ploug M, Østergaard S, Hansen LB, Holm A, Danø K (1998) Photoaffinity labeling of the human receptor for urokinase-type plasminogen activator using a decapeptide antagonist. Evidence for a composite ligand-binding site and a short interdomain separation. Biochemistry37:3612–3622

Ploug M, Østergaard S, Gårdsvoll H, Kovalski K, Holst-Hansen C, Holm A, Ossowski L, Dano K (2001) Peptide-derived antagonists of the urokinase receptor. Affinity maturation by combinatorial chemistry, identification of functional epitopes, and inhibitory effect on cancer cell intravasation. Biochemistry 40:12157–12168

Quax PH, Grimbergen JM, Lansink M, Bakker AH, Blatter MC, Belin D, van Hinsbergh VW, Verheijen JH (1998) Binding of human urokinase-type plasminogen activator to its receptor: residues involved in species specificity and binding. Thromb Vasc Biol 18:693–701

Rabbani SA and Mazar AP (2001) The role of the plasminogen activation system in angiogenesis and metastasis. Surg Oncol Clin N Am 10:393–415

Rettenberger P, Wilhelm O, Oi H, Weidle UH, Goretzki L, Koppitz M, Lottspeich F, König B, Pessara U, Kramer MD, Schmitt M, Magdolen V (1995) A competitive chromogenic assay to study the functional interaction of urokinase-type plasminogen activator with its receptor. Biol Chem 376:587–594

Reuning U, Magdolen V, Wilhelm O, Fischer K, Lutz V, Graeff H, Schmitt M (1998) Multifunctional potential of plasminogen activation system in tumor invasion and metastasis. Int J Oncol 13:893–906

Sato 2002

Schmiedeberg N, Bürgle M, Wilhelm O, Lottspeich F, Graeff, Schmitt M, Magdolen V, Kessler H (2000) Design and biological activity of new high-affinity ligands for the urokinase-type plasminogen activator receptor (CD87). In: Fields GB, Tam JP, Barany G (eds) Peptides for the New Millennium (Proc. 16th American Peptide Symposium, June 26-July

1, 1999, Minneapolis, Minnesota, USA). Kluwer Academic Publishers, Dordrecht, pp 543–545

Schmiedeberg 2002

Schmitt M, Chucholowski N, Busch E, Hellmann D, Wagner B, Goretzk, L, Jänicke F, Günzler WA, Graeff H (1991) Fluorescent probes as tools to assess the receptor for the urokinase-type plasminogen activator on tumor cells. Semin Thromb Hemost 17:291–302

Schmitt M, Harbeck N, Thomssen C, Wilhelm O, Magdolen V, Reuning U, Ulm K, Höfler H, Jänicke F, Graeff H (1997) Clinical impact of the plasminogen activation system in tumor invasion and metastasis: Prognostic relevance and target for therapy. Thromb Hemost 78:285–296

Schmitt M, Jänicke F, Graeff H (1992) Tumor-associated proteases. Fibrinolysis 6 [Suppl]4:3–26

Schmitt, M, Wilhelm OG, Reuning U, Krüger A, Harbeck N, Lengyel E, Graeff H, Gänsbacher B, Kessler H, Bürgle M, Stürzebecher J, Sperl S, Magdolen V (2000) The urokinase plasminogen activator system as a novel target for tumour therapy. Fibrinol Proteol 14:114–132

Sperl 2001

Spiro A, Lowe M, Brown D (2000) A bead-based method for multiplexed identification and quantitation of DNA sequences using flow cytometry. Appl Environ Microbiol 66:4258–4265

Stoppelli MP, Corti A, Soffientini A, Cassani G, Blasi F, Assoian RK (1985) Differentiation-enhanced binding of the amino-terminal fragment of human urokinase plasminogen activator to a specific receptor on U937 monocytes. Proc Natl Acad Sci USA 82:4939–4943

Swanson SJ, Jacobs SJ, Mytych D, Shah C, Indelicato SR, Bordens RW (1999) Applications for the new electrochemiluminescent (ECL) and biosensor technologies. Dev Biol Stand 97:135–147

Tressler RJ, Pitot PA, Stratton JR, Forrest LD, Zhuo S, Drummond RJ, Fong S, Doyle MV, Doyle LV, Min HY, Rosenberg S (1999) Urokinase receptor antagonists: discovery and application in vivo models of tumor growth. APMIS 107:168–173

Vassalli JD, Baccino D, Belin D (1985) A cellular binding site for the Mr 55,000 form of the human plasminogen activator, urokinase. J Cell Biol 100:86–92

Waltz DA, Chapman HA (1994) Reversible cellular adhesion to vitronectin linked to urokinase receptor occupancy. J Biol Chem 269:14746–14750

Waltz DA, Fujita RM, Yang X, Natkin L, Zhuo S, Gerard CJ, Rosenberg S, Chapman HA (2000) Nonproteolytic role for the urokinase receptor in cellular migration in vivo. Am J Respir Cell Mol Biol 22:316–322

Webb DJ, Thomas KS, Gonias SL (2001) Plasminogen activator inhibitor 1 functions as a urokinase response modifier at the level of cell signaling and thereby promotes MCF-7 cell growth. J Cell Biol 152:741–752

Wedemeyer N, Potter T (2001) Flow cytometry: an 'old' tool for novel applications in medical genetics. Clin Genet 60:1–8

Yebra M, Goretzki L, Pfeifer M, Mueller BM (1999) Urokinase-type plasminogen activator binding to its receptor stimulates tumor cell migration by enhancing integrin-mediated signal transduction. Exp Cell Res 250:231–240

Molecular Regulation of Urokinase-Receptor Gene Expression as One Potential Concept for Molecular Staging and Therapy

Heike Allgayer

H. Allgayer (✉)
Department of Surgery, Klinikum Grosshadern,
Ludwig Maximilians University of Munich, Marchioninistr. 15,
81377 Munich, Germany

Abstract

The urokinase-receptor (u-PAR) is a central molecule of invasion and metastasis promoting plasminogen-dependent extracellular matrix degradation in diverse carcinoma types such as gastric or colon cancer. Overexpression of u-PAR has been reported to occur mainly at the transcriptional level in malignant cells, and has been shown to indicate a poor clinical prognosis of cancer patients. This review will give an overview on experimental findings on u-PAR and its function, molecular mechanisms of its regulation, and its impact for future clinical decision planning and potential therapeutic concepts.

Introduction

During the last decade, accumulating evidence has emerged indicating that the process of invasion and metastasis in tumors involves different proteolytic enzymes and their inhibitors which achieve the degradation of the surrounding tissue ("tumor-associated proteolysis"). The phenomenon of tumor-associated proteolysis has been acknowledged as a decisive step in the progression of cancer [1]. Therefore, these proteolytic enzymes and the molecular mechanisms leading to their expression by tumor and non-tumor cells are potential attractive candidates for future therapeutic strategies in cancer. Furthermore, they could help in establishing new so-called molecular tumor staging models where new molecular parameters are integrated into established staging systems such as pTNM, not only to define subgroups of patients with an individual risk for tumor recurrence more biologically and precisely, but moreover to serve as new therapeutic targets for these subgroups at the same time, which will potentially redefine and broaden established tumor-therapy strategies such as surgery and adjuvant chemotherapy/radiation. This review (1) focuses on urokinase-receptor (u-PAR), one of the molecules mediating tumor-associated proteolysis, (2) briefly summarizes existing knowledge about u-PAR, and (3) gives an overview of our own results regarding its transcriptional regulation and potential clinical relevance, and thus its potential as a new molecular staging marker in gastrointestinal cancers.

Urokinase, Tumor-Associated Proteolysis, and Invasion

Invasion and metastasis of malignant tumor cells require the degradation of extracellular matrix elements (type IV collagen, laminin, vitronectin), allowing access of the tumor cells to the systemic circulation [2, 3]. These events can be achieved, at least in part, by a series of "tumor-associated proteases" [4] which, according to their catalytically active site, are classified into serine, aspartic, cysteine, threonine, and metalloproteinases [4]. The proteases are secreted either by the tumor cells or by cells in the surrounding stromal compartment recruited by the tumor cells.

It should be emphasized that these proteases are not restricted to cancer. Indeed, these enzymes are involved in several tissue remodelling processes such as wound healing, fibrinolysis, inflammation, embryogenesis, and angiogenesis [3, 5–9]. It is thought that their involvement in cancer invasion/metastases represents an extension of their normal biological roles in tissue remodelling.

One of the proteases which has been implicated in the invasive phenotype of tumor cells is the urokinase-type plasminogen activator (u-PA), a 55-kDa serine protease which, via activation of plasminogen to active plasmin, is able to cleave several components of the extracellular matrix including fibrin, fibronectin, proteoglycans, and, as the main molecules in basement membranes, laminin and collagen IV [10–13]. Urokinase is secreted from cells of the urogenital system, leukocytes, fibroblasts, and also some tumor cells as an inactive, single-chain proform, being proteolytically activated either in the extracellular space or bound to the urokinase-receptor (u-PAR, see next section) [12–17].

u-PAR Accelerates u-PA Activation by Specific Structural and Functional Properties

The proteolytic efficacy of the urokinase enzyme relies on its interactions with factors that, together with u-PA, comprise the "u-PA-system" according to the definition of F. Blasi [6]. Among these components of the u-PA-system, the u-PA-specific inhibitors plasminogen-activator-inhibitor (PAI)-1, PAI-2, and nexin 1, and the cell surface receptor u-PAR appear to be crucial. U-PA, as an inactive one-chain proenzyme, binds to a 55–60-kDa heavily glycosylated, disulfide-linked cell surface receptor (u-PAR) specifically and with high affinity [18]. The u-PAR binds the A-chain of the active two-chain form of u-PA, allowing activation of ubiquitously available plasminogen and initiation of the proteolytic cascade by the catalytic B-chain [19]. The receptor-bound u-PA is inactivated by PAI-1 (-2), the trimeric complex u-PAR/u-PA/PAI is internalized into the cell together with α-2-macroglobulin receptor and its ligand [20–25], the free u-PAR is recycled to the cell surface, and binding and activation of a second u-PA-molecule can occur.

The u-PAR consists of three similar repeats approximately 90 residues each, the last of which is anchored to the cell membrane via a glycosyl-phosphatidylinositol chain [26, 27]. This GPI-anchor is hypothesized to enable a high intramembrane mobility [18, 26, 29–31]. Furthermore, the u-PAR is glycosylated at N-residues of glucosamine and sialic acid within the binding site, thereby regulating its affinity (K_D of 0.1–1.0 nM) for u-PAR [26]. Receptor-bound u-PA, as compared to the fluid phase enzyme, activates plasminogen much more efficiently, this being reflected by a 40-fold decrease in K_m of urokinase for its substrate [32].

Physiological Functions of u-PAR

Physiologically, the u-PAR gene is expressed in peripheral leukocytes, inflammatory-activated monocytes [17, 21, 33, 34], the more mature forms of myeloic precursors in the bone marrow [35, 36], and endothelial cells and keratinocytes at the leading edge in re-epithelializing wounds [37, 38]. Correspondingly, u-PAR gene expression plays an important role in inflammation, tissue remodeling, and wound healing [2, 5, 6, 29, 39].

Regarding embryogenesis, studies on u-PAR knockout mice have suggested that the u-PAR is not critical for mouse development. However, granulocytes and monocytes of these mice are severely impaired in their migratory and chemotactic capacity towards inflammatory sites [40] and are characterized by a deficient in vitro plasminogen-activating potential [41]. These findings are corroborated by similar observations on granulocytes isolated from human patients with paroxysmal nocturnal hemoglobinuria, a disease in which cells are deficient of all GPI-linked surface receptors and therefore lacking in cell surface u-PAR [42].

Regarding cellular functions, the u-PAR has been implicated in chemotaxis [43]. Moreover, studies showing that the u-PAR is colocalized with integrins and acts as a coreceptor for vitronectin [40, 44–46] suggested a paradoxical role for the u-PAR in adhesion. Interestingly, the interaction of u-PAR with integrins and resulting signal transduction events have been suggested to regulate the transition of the cell to dormancy [47]. Furthermore, the u-PAR can be found localized at cellular focal contacts, lamellipodia, and in caveolae, and has been demonstrated to induce the phosphorylation of focal adhesion kinase (FAK), cytoskeletal proteins, and Src-family members [40, 45, 48–54]. Therefore, evidence supports a role for u-PAR in cell migration, dormancy, and cytoskeletal rearrangement, both via its expression at the cell surface and via modulating signal transduction pathways.

The Relevance of u-PAR Gene Expression to Invasion and Metastasis

The aforementioned studies implicate u-PAR in diverse physiological process-es. However, numerous studies have shown an overexpression of the u-PAR gene in diverse human malignant tumors compared to the corresponding nor-mal tissue and/or surrounding stromal cells [55–63] and suggest u-PAR as a characteristic of the invasive or even the malignant phenotype [64–67].

Direct evidence implicating u-PAR in tumor invasion and metastasis is as follows: Overexpression of a human u-PAR cDNA increased the ability of hu-man osteosarcoma cells to penetrate a barrier of reconstituted basement membrane [68]. Ossowski [69] demonstrated that the invasive potential of tu-mor cells into a chicken embryo chorioallantoic membrane is correlated with u-PAR-associated proteolytic activity. Another study [70] revealed that the ex-pression of an antisense u-PAR cDNA in Hep3 squamous carcinoma cells de-creased their invasiveness into a modified chorioallantoic membrane. Further-more, anti-messenger oligonucleotides inhibiting u-PAR gene expression re-duced in vitro invasion of transformed human fibroblasts [71]. In glioblasto-ma, an anti-u-PAR monoclonal antibody effectively blocked matrigel invasion of treated cells [72]. In cultured lung cancer, optimum invasiveness was seen only if u-PA, PAI-1, and u-PAR were coexpressed [73]. Moreover, Kim et al. [74] have shown elegantly that the expression of the u-PAR gene by tumor cells, besides u-PA and MMP-9, is required for the intravasation of blood ves-sels. Finally, Min et al. [75] reported that u-PAR antagonists prevent tumor growth and angiogenesis, suggesting that u-PAR gene expression is important for tumor and metastasis establishment and outgrowth. Taken together, all of these studies suggest u-PAR as a critical molecule for invasion, intravasation, and metastasis.

In colon cancer, highly invasive cell lines (in vitro) displayed tenfold more u-PAR than their poorly invasive counterparts [66], and cultivation of u-PAR-rich colon cancer cells with either an antibody to the u-PA-binding site or a peptide corresponding to the receptor-binding sequence of u-PA, both impair-ing u-PA-binding, reduced the ability of the cells to degrade laminin and in-vade an extracellular matrix-coated porous filter [66, 76]. Another study dem-onstrated that polyclonal anti-u-PAR antibodies decreased extracellular ma-trix degradation in the HT29 colon cancer cell line by 80% [77]. In in situ hy-bridization studies, Pyke et al. [57, 58] even postulated an in vivo paracrine interaction between tumor cells and surrounding stromal cells, the former overexpressing u-PAR, the latter secreting u-PA and PAIs [57, 58].

The Clinical Relevance of u-PAR as a Poor Prognostic Factor and a Potential Therapeutic Target in Cancer

The systemic spread of a local primary carcinoma resulting in metastasis is the main cause of death from solid tumors. This systemic spread is accomplished by the invasion and degradation of surrounding normal tissue, the breakdown of basement membranes to gain access to blood vessels, the systemic dissemination of clonogenic tumor cells, the extravasation at metastatic sites, and finally the establishment of distant metastases.

The u-PAR has been implicated in at least some of these steps as outlined in the previous paragraph. The clinical relevance of u-PAR and its association with invasion and metastasis has been proposed by investigators who found a higher amount of u-PAR in metastases as compared to primary tumors [78–80]. Moreover, prospective studies on diverse cancers involving large patient numbers have demonstrated a correlation of high u-PAR (and/or u-PA-/PAI-1) expression with short survival times and advanced tumor stages. Thus, the u-PAR and/or u-PA/PAI-1 have already been shown to be significant prognostic risk factors in many cancers including breast [81, 79], lung [42], colon [82, 83], esophageal, and gastric cancer [59, 60, 84–88], and some of these studies even reported an independent impact on survival probability in multivariate analysis. In a series of 203 gastric cancer patients, we showed that the u-PA system (represented by PAI-1) together with the evidence of minimal residual disease (see below) is appropriate to establish a new biological staging of gastric cancer that is able to identify new subgroups of patients who are at high risk despite having early-stage tumors according to the pTNM classification [85].

u-PAR as One Characteristic of the Metastatic Phenotype in Minimal Residual Disease

The existence of minimal residual tumor disease as single clonogenic tumor cells potentially leading to a relapse of the disease has been postulated not only for hematologic malignancies, but also for solid carcinomas. More and more, also in carcinomas, minimal residual disease (MRD) is thought to be the major cause of macroscopic tumor recurrence and therefore disease progression after curative (meaning even microscopically complete) tumor resection. Ultimately, such events are responsible for the fatal clinical outcome of cancer patients [89–91]. With immunocytochemistry for cytokeratin markers, MRD was detected by our group [80] as single disseminated tumor cells in the bone marrow compartment of diverse cancer patients and in gastric cancers. In a prospective series of 78 curatively resected patients with gastric cancers analyzed for the development over time of disseminated tumor cells in follow-up, we observed that patients who showed an increase or continuously high cell numbers of disseminated tumor cells in bone marrow suffered from early recurrence and death of the tumor in 90% of cases. However, most of the patients showing a decrease or elimination of disseminated tumor cells in follow-up remained tumor-free. With double-immunocytochemistry, we found that the detection of u-PAR on disseminated tumor cells at the time of primary surgery correlated with a later increase in numbers of disseminated tumor cells in these patients, and the percentage of tumor cells with evidence of u-PAR increased significantly over time [80, 92], indicating that the expression of u-PAR is a potential marker for a positive in vivo selection of disseminated tumor cells and a characteristic for the establishment of MRD. In addition, the evidence of u-PAR on these cells significantly correlated with poor survival of gastric cancer patients. These results suggested u-PAR as one characteristic of metastatic phenotypes of disseminated tumor cells found in the bone marrow, and thus a promising staging marker characterizing a clinically relevant minimal residual disease component [80, 36, 92]. Therefore, the downregulation of u-PAR appears to be an attractive potential tool not only as an anti-invasive therapy [71, 93], but also for preventing the establishment of a minimal residual tumor component and clinical disease progression in cancer.

The Current Status of Studies of the Transcriptional Regulation of u-PAR Gene Expression

The objective of countering u-PAR gene expression in malignant tumors necessarily involves the question of how it is regulated. The mechanisms of regulation and the causes of an upregulation of u-PAR in malignant cells remain the focus of intensive investigations. Although altered mRNA stability and receptor recycling may be involved, the amounts of u-PAR are controlled mainly at the transcriptional level in some malignancies such as colon cancer [94–99].

The u-PAR gene spans seven exons and is located on chromosome 19q13 [100] Transcription from the gene yields a 1.4-kb mRNA or an alternatively spliced variant lacking the membrane attachment peptide sequence [101, 102]. The human u-PAR promoter sequence was first described by Wang et al. [64] and Soravia et al. [103]. Like classical "housekeeping genes," it lacks TATA and CAAT boxes and contains a GC-rich proximal sequence with multiple Sp1 consensus elements. Using primer extension analysis, Soravia et al. [103] reported three potential transcriptional start sites, the most upstream of which – an A following a C – appeared to be the main transcription initiation site and revealed partial similarity to the consensus initiator sequence of the dihydrofolate reductase (DHFR) gene [103, 104]. The most proximal 135 basepairs of the human u-PAR promoter showed 68% similarity to the murine u-PAR promoter [105].

Soravia et al. [103] reported that the basal expression of the gene was regulated via Sp1 motifs proximal and upstream of the transcriptional start site. In colon cancer, both the constitutive and PMA-inducible expression of the gene required a footprinted region located at basepairs –190 to –171 of the promoter containing an AP-1 consensus motif bound with Jun-D, c-Jun, c-Fos, and Fra-1 [94], this motif mediating the induction of u-PAR gene expression via the MAPK- and the JNK-pathways [95, 106]. This AP-1 consensus motif was also required for induction of u-PAR gene expression brought about by the

K-ras oncogene (see "Molecules Inducing u-PAR Gene Expression – Induction of u-PAR Gene Expression by the *c-src* and K-*ras* Oncogenes" below).

Another region (–148 to –124) containing putative (one base pair-mismatched) Sp1, AP-2, and PEA3 binding motifs [94] was shown to be bound by an AP-2-like protein and Sp1 and Sp3 transcription factors, and the basepairs required for binding were identified as –152 to –135 [107]. Binding of the AP-2-like protein was found to be important for a constitutively high u-PAR-promoter activity in a highly invasive colon cancer cell line and for PMA-stimulated u-PAR-expression in a cell line with low constitutive u-PAR expression. Interestingly, a dominant-negative AP-2 expression construct not only reduced u-PAR promoter activity and u-PAR gene expression but also substantially inhibited u-PAR-mediated proteolysis. These results suggest that inhibition at the transcriptional level can be applied to suppress u-PAR-mediated proteolysis, thereby potentially invasion and metastasis.

The binding of Sp1 transcription factor to region –152 to –135 of the u-PAR promoter was shown to be important in part for PMA-induced u-PAR promoter activity, but, more interestingly, for the induction of u-PAR gene expression by the *c-src* oncogene in colon cancer. A more detailed overview on these results is given in the following section. In a first clinical study investigating transcription factor binding in 145 patients with colorectal or gastric cancers in primary tumors as compared to corresponding normal mucosae, we reported a tumor-specific transactivation of u-PAR gene expression by this promoter region in about 60% of the cases (preliminary results introduced in Schewe et al., Proc Am Assoc Cancer Res 42: 618, 2001). Therefore, a subgroup of patients is suggested in whom a targeting of promoter region –152 to –135 by transcriptional targeting or targeting of upstream activators would potentially enable a tumor-specific new adjuvant to eliminate highly invasive rest tumor cells.

Molecules Inducing u-PAR Gene Expression – Induction of u-PAR Gene Expression by the *c-src* and K-*ras* Oncogenes

As the u-PAR is a key molecule in promoting tumor-associated proteolysis and is correlated with advanced disease, it is not surprising that some tumor-promoting factors are inducers of u-PAR gene expression. For example, it has been shown that epidermal growth factor (EGF), basic fibroblast growth factor (FGF), vascular endothelial growth factor (VEGF), transforming growth factor β type 1 (TGF-β1), and phorbol 12-myristate 13-acetate (PMA) upregulate u-PAR [94, 97, 108–110]. Among the second messengers mediating signal transduction, protein kinase C (PKC), protein kinase A (PKA)/ c-AMP, the MAPK- and the JNK pathway have been shown to activate u-PAR gene expression in diverse cell culture models [37, 95, 106, 111, 112].

A very interesting issue is the regulation of u-PAR gene expression by certain oncogenes. The involvement of Jun/Fos family members in the regulation of the u-PAR promoter has been discussed [94]. Also, the K-*ras* oncogene induces u-PAR gene expression, as we have shown [113]. In that study, in the colon cancer cell line HCT116 which contains mutation-activated K-Ras, the mutated K-*ras* allele was deleted and the resulting knockout-clones were compared with HCT116. We observed a substantial reduction of endogenous u-PAR-protein and u-PAR-mediated proteolysis in the clones in which activated K-ras had been deleted. In gelshift- and CAT-reporter analyses, we detected a decrease of the binding of c-Jun, JunD, c-Fos, and Fra-1 in the K-Ras-knockout clones, and this was paralleled by a severe reduction of promoter activity when the upstream AP-1 consensus motif within promoter region –190 to –171 (see previous paragraph) was deleted. These results suggest that activated K-Ras regulates u-PAR and u-PAR-mediated proteolysis in colon cancer, at least in part via region –190 to –171 of the promoter bound with AP-1 transcription factors.

The c-*src* oncogene was identified as another inducer of u-PAR gene expression. In colorectal carcinomas, the specific activity of Src, a 60-kDa nonreceptor protein tyrosine kinase, was shown to be higher in distant metastases compared to the primary tumors [114–116]. Furthermore, Pories et al. [117] demonstrated that c-*src* overexpression confers invasiveness to rat colonic cells. These observations prompted us to speculate as to whether Src is regulating the invasion-related molecule u-PAR [118].

Src-stably transfected clones were generated from SW 480 colon cancer cells, which are characterized by nondetectable endogenous Src activity. In these clones stably expressing a constitutively active Src (Y-c-*src*527F), increased u-PAR protein and laminin degradation paralleling elevated Src activity was evident compared to parental cells. Nuclear run-on experiments indicated that the increased u-PAR protein was due largely to transcriptional activation. Whereas transient transfection of SW480 cells with Y-c-*src*527F induced a u-PAR-CAT reporter, mutations preventing Sp1 binding to promoter region –152 to –135 abolished this induction. Mobility shift assays revealed increased Sp1 binding to region –152 to –135 with nuclear extracts of Src-transfected SW480 cells. Finally, the amounts of endogenous u-PAR in resected colon cancers significantly correlated with Src activity. These data suggest that u-PAR gene expression and u-PAR-mediated proteolysis are regulated by Src, this requiring the promoter region (–152 to –135) bound with Sp1, thus demonstrating for the first time that transcription factor Sp1 is a downstream effector of Src.

In addition, a specific Src inhibitor was able to inhibit u-PAR promoter activity, protein amounts, and u-PAR-mediated proteolysis [118]. These results suggest Src inhibition as a potential future strategy to inhibit u-PAR-dependent invasion and metastasis.

Conclusions

As outlined above, the u-PAR is a key factor in promoting tumor-associated proteolysis. Therefore, downregulation of its expression could be a clinically promising strategy to inhibit cancer invasion and metastasis. Furthermore, the u-PAR could represent a therapeutic target to prevent the establishment of minimal residual disease, because it is one marker for the metastatic pheno-types of disseminated tumor cells, and a potent marker in first clinical molec-ular tumor staging models. Based on our own data summarized here, poten-tial strategies that may achieve a downregulation of u-PAR-mediated proteoly-sis are the inhibition of Src and K-Ras (e.g., by small molecular compounds) or even a direct targeting of transcriptional mechanisms or the promoter (e.g., as shown above with dominant-negative AP-2 transcription factor).

Other groups have described exciting strategies at the protein level, which could be for example an interruption of the u-PAR/integrin interaction to pre-vent tumor cell growth [47]. In addition to the naturally occurring uPA in-hibitors PAI-1, PAI-2, protease nexin, and protein C inhibitor, potent synthetic low-molecular-weight inhibitors directed to the proteolytic activity of uPA [119] have been developed and are currently being tested by several compa-nies as cancer drugs. Wilhelm et al. [120] designed a soluble recombinant form of uPA-R (suPA-R), lacking the GPI anchor. suPA-R acts as an efficient scavenger of uPA, leading to inhibition of tumor cell proliferation and inva-sion. suPA-R inhibits binding of uPA to the tumor cell surface-associated uPA-R. Antibodies to uPA or uPA-R have also been employed to affect tumor cell spread. In 1983, Ossowski and Reich [121] generated rabbit polyclonal anti-bodies which inhibit the catalytic activity of human uPA. Employing these an-tibodies, they were able to inhibit tumor cell spread in a chicken tumor mod-el. Since that time, several antibodies have been generated that interfere with the catalytic activity of uPA or inhibit the interaction of uPA with its receptor, uPA-R.

These and other investigations in the next few years will determine the clin-ical potential of these anti-u-PAR approaches in the treatment of cancer inva-sion and metastasis, and the potential of new tumor staging models based upon them.

Acknowledgements. I would like to thank Dr. Markus M. Heiss, Dr. W. Schildberg (Klinikum Grosshadern, Munich), Dr. K. Messmer (University of Munich), Douglas D. Boyd, Gary E Gal-lick, Heng Wang (MD Anderson Cancer Center, Houston, TX, USA), and Dr. Henner Graeff, and Dr. E.R. Lengyel (UC-San Francisco Cancer Center) for their continuous kind support. The author is supported by grants from the Deutsche Krebshilfe, Bonn, Germany, the Wilhelm Sander Stiftung, the Faculty of Medicine of the Ludwig-Maximilians-University of Munich, the MMW-Board of Editors, Munich, Germany, and the Friedrich Baur Stiftung, Munich, Germany.

References

1. Hanahan D, Weinberg RA (2000) The hallmarks of cancer. Cell 100:57–70
2. Dvorak HF (1986) Tumors: Wounds that do not heal. N Engl J Med 315:1650–1659
3. Liotta LA (1986) Tumor invasion and metastases–role of the extracellular matrix: Rhoads Memorial Award Lecture. Cancer Res 46:1–7

4. Schmitt M, Jänicke F, Graeff H (1992) Tumor-associated proteases. Fibrinolysis 6 [Suppl 4]:3–26
5. Blasi F Surface receptors for urokinase plasminogen activator. (1988) Fibrinolysis 2:73–84
6. Blasi F (1993) Urokinase and urokinase receptor: A paracrine/autocrine system regulating cell migration and invasiveness. BioEssays 15:105–111
7. Dano K, Andreasen PA, Grondahl-Hansen J, Kristensen P, Nielsen LS, Skriver L (1985) Plasminogen-activators, tissue degradation, and cancer. Adv Cancer Res 44:139–266
8. Liotta LA, Steeg PS, Stetler-Stevenson WG (v) Cancer metastasis and angiogenesis: An imbalance of positive and negative regulation. Cell 64:327–336
9. Markus G (1988) The relevance of plasminogen activators to neoplastic growth. Enzyme 40:158–172
10. Andreasen PA, Sottrup-Jensen L, Kjoller L, Nykiaer A, Moestrup SK, Petersen CM, Gliemann JAD (1994) Receptor-mediated endocytosis of plasminogen activators and activator/inhibitor complexes. FEBS Lett 338:239–245
11. Duffy MJ (1992) The role of proteolytic enzymes in cancer invasion and metastasis. Clin Exp Metastasis 10:145–155
12. Günzler WA, Steffens GJ, Ötting F, Buse G, Flohe L (1982) Structural relationship between human high and low molecular mass urokinase. Hoppe-Seyler's J Physiol Chem 363:133–141
13. Günzler WA, Steffens GJ, Ötting F, Kim SMA, Frankus E, Flohe L (1982) The primary structure of high molecular mass urokinase from human urine. The complete amino acid sequence of the A chain. Hoppe-Seyler's J Physiol Chem 363:1155–1165
14. Wun T, Ossowski L, Reich E (1982) A proenzyme form of human urokinase. J Biol Chem 257:–7268
15. Wun TC, Reich E (1982) Isolation and characterization of urokinase from human plasma. J Biol Chem 257:3276–3283
16. Gronow M, Bliem R (1983) Production of human plasminogen activators by cell culture. Trends Biotech 1:26–29
17. Vassalli JD, Dayer JM, Wohlwend A, Belin D (1984) Concomitant secretion of pro-urokinase and of a plasminogen activator-specific inhibitor by cultured human monocytes/macrophages. J Exp Med 159:1653–1668
18. Stoppelli MP, Tacchetti C, Cubellis M, Corti A, Hearing V, Cassani G, Appella E, Blasi F (1986) Autocrine saturation of pro-urokinase receptors on human A431 cells. Cell 45:675–684
19. Stoppelli MP, Corti A, Soffientini A, Cassani G, Blasi F, Assoian RK (1985) Differentiation-enhanced binding of the amino-terminal fragment of human urokinase plasminogen activator to a specific receptor on U937 monocytes. Proc Natl Acad Sci USA 82:4939–4943
20. Olson D, Pollanen J, Hoyer-Hansen G, Ronne E, Sakaguchi K, Wun T, Appella E, Dano K, Blasi F (1992) Internalization of the urokinase-plasminogen activator type-1 complex is mediated by the urokinase receptor. J Biol Chem 267:9129–9133
21. Cubellis MV, Wun TC, Blasi F (1990) Receptor-mediated internalization and degradation of urokinase is caused by its specific inhibitor PAI-1. EMBO J 9:1079–1085
22. Conese M, Olson D, Blasi FAD (1994) Protease nexin-1-urokinase complexes are internalized and degraded through a mechanism that requires both urokinase receptor and α2-macroglobulin receptor. J Biol Chem 269:17886–17892
23. Nykjaer A, Petersen CM, Moller B, Jensen PH, Moestrup SK, Holtet TL, Etzerodt M, Thogersen HC, Munch M, Andreasen PA, Gliemann J (1992) Purified α2 macroglobulin receptor/LDL receptor related protein binds urokinase-plasminogen activator inhibitor type 1 complex. Evidence that the α2-macroglobulin receptor mediates cellular degradation of urokinase receptor-bound complexes. J Biol Chem 267:14543–14546
24. Nykjaer A, Kjoller L, Cohen RL, Lawrence DA, Garni-Wagner BA, Todd RF 3rd, van Zonnefeld AJ, Gliemann J, Andreasen PAAD (1994) Regions involved in binding of urokinase-type-1 inhibitor complex and pro-urokinase to the endocytic alpha 2 macroglobulin receptor/low density lipoprotein receptor-related protein. Evidence that the uroki-

nase receptor protects pro-urokinase against binding to the endocytic receptor. J Biol Chem 269:25668–25676

25. Nykjaer A, Kjoller L, Cohen RL, Lawrence DA, Gliemann J, Andreasen PAAD (1994) Both pro-uPA and uPA: PAI-1 complex bind to the α2-macroglobulin receptor/LDL receptor-related protein. Evidence for multiple independent contacts between the ligands and receptor. Ann N Y Acad Sci 737:483–485

26. Behrendt N, Ronne E, Ploug M, Petri T, Lober D, Nielsen LS, Schleunig WD, Blasi F, Appella E, Dano K (1990) The human receptor for urokinase plasminogen activator NH_2-terminal amino acid sequence and glycosylation variants. J Biol Chem 265:6453–6460

27. Ploug M, Behrendt N, Lober D, Dano K (1991) Protein structure and membrane anchorage of the cellular receptor for urokinase-type plasminogen activator. Sem Thromb Hem 17:183–193

28. Estreicher A, Muhlhauser J, Carpentier JL, Orci L, Vassalli JD (1990) The receptor for urokinase type plasminogen activator polarizes expression of the protease to the leading edge of migrating monocytes and promotes degradation of enzyme inhibitor complexes. J Cell Biol 111:783–792

29. Moller LB (1993) Structure and function of the urokinase receptor. Blood Coagulation and Fibrinolysis 4:293–303

30. Moller LB, Ploug M, Blasi F (1992) Structural requirements for glycosyl-phosphatidyl-inositol anchor attachment in the cellular receptor for urokinase plasminogen activator. Eur J Biochem 208:493–500

31. Ploug M, Ronne E, Behrendt N, Jensen AL, Blasi F, Dano K (1991) Cellular receptor for urokinase-plasminogen activator: Carboxyl-terminal processing and membrane anchoring by glycosyl-phosphatidylinositol. J Biol Chem 266:1926–1933

32. Ellis V, Behrendt N, and Dano K (1991) Plasminogen activation by receptor-bound urokinase. J Biol Chem 266(12)752–12,758

33. Min HY, Semnani R, Mizukami IF, Watt K, Todd RF III, Liu DY (1992) cDNA for Mo3, a monocyte activation antigen, encodes the human receptor for urokinase plasminogen activator. J Immunol 148:3636–3642

34. Vassalli JD, Baccino D, Belin D (1985) A cellular binding site for the Mr 55000 form of the human plasminogen activator, urokinase. J Cell Biol 100:86–92

35. Plesner T, Ralfkiaer E, Wittrup M, Johnsen H, Pyke C, Pedersen TL, Hansen NE, Dano KAD (1994) Expression of the receptor for urokinase-type plasminogen activator in normal and neoplastic blood cells and hematopoetic tissue. Am J Clin Pathol 102:835–841

36. Allgayer H, Heiss MM, Riesenberg R, Babic R, Jauch KW, Schildberg FW (1997) Immunocytochemical phenotyping of disseminated tumor cells in bone marrow by uPA-R and CK18: Investigation of sensitivity, specificity and reproducibility of an immunogold/alcaline phosphatase double-staining protocol. J Histochem Cytochem 45:203–212

37. Langer DJ, Kuo A, Kariko K, Ahuja M, Klugherz BD, Ivanics KM, Hoxie JA, William WV, Liang BT, Cines D B, Barnathan ES (1993) Regulation of the endothelial cell urokinase-type plasminogen activator receptor–evidence for cyclic AMP-dependent and protein kinase C-dependent pathways. Circulation Research 72:330–340

38. Romer J, Lund LR, Eriksen J, Pyke C, Kristensen P, Dano KAD (1994) The receptor for urokinase-type plasminogen activator is expressed by keratinocytes at the leading edge during re-epithelialization of mouse skin wounds. Invest Dermatol 102:519–522

39. Sillaber C, Baghestanian M, Hofbauer R, Virgolini I, Bankl HC, Fureder W, Agis H, Willheim M, Leimer M, Scheiner O, Binder BR, Kiener HP, Bevec D, Fritsch G, Majdic O, Kress HG, Gadner H, Lechner K, and Valent P (1997) Molecular and functional characterization of the urokinase receptor on human mast cells. J Biol Chem 272, 7824–7832

40. May AE, Kanse SM, Lund LR, Gisler RH, Imhof BA, Preissner KT (1998) Urokinase receptor (CD 87) regulates leukocyte recruitment via β2 integrins in vivo. J Exp Med 188:1029–1037

41. Dewerchin M, Nuffelen AV, Wallays G, Bouche A, Moons L, Carmeliet P, Mulligan RC, Collen D (1996) Generation and characterization of urokinase receptor-deficient mice. J Clin Invest 97:870–878

42. Pedersen H, Grondahl-Hansen J, Francis D, Osterlind K, Hansen HH, Dano K, Brünner N (1994) Urokinase and plasminogen activator inhibitor type 1 in pulmonary adenocarcinoma. Cancer Res 54:120–123

43. Resnati M, Gutringer M, Valcamonica S, Sidenius N, Blasi F, Fazioli F (1996) Proteolytic cleavage of the urokinse receptor substitutes for the agonist-induced chemotactic effect. EMBO J 15:1572–82

44. Xue W, Mizukami I, Todd R F IIIrd, Petty HR (1997) Urokinase-type plasminogen activator receptors associate with β_1 and β_3 integrins of fibrosarcoma cells: Dependence on extracellular matrix components. Cancer Res 57:1682–1689

45. Wei Y, Waltz DA, Rao N, Drummond RJ, Rosenberg S, Chapman HA (1994) Identification of the urokinase receptor as an adhesion receptor for vitronectin. J Biol Chem 269:32380–32388

46. Wei Y, Lukashev M, Simon DI, Bodary SC, Rosenberg S, Doyle MV, Chapman HA (1996) Regulation of integrin function by the urokinase receptor. Science 273:1551–1555

47. Aguirre-Ghiso JA, Kovalski K, Ossowski L (1999) Tumor dormancy induced by downregulation of urokinase receptor in human carcinoma involves integrin-mediated adhesion and signaling. J Cell Biol 144:1285–1294

48. Busso N, Masur SK, Lazega D, Waxman S, Ossowski L (1994) Induction of cell migration by pro-urokinase to its receptor: Possible mechanism for signal transduction in human epithelial cells. J Cell Biol 126:259–270

49. Tang H, Kerina D M:, Hao Q, Inagami T, Vaughan DE (1998) The urokinase-type plasminogen activator receptor mediates tyrosine phosphorylation of focal adhesion proteins and activation of mitogen-activated protein kinase in cultured endothelial cells. J Biol Chem 273:18268–18272

50. Stahl A, Mueller BM (1995) The urokinase-type plasminogen activator receptor, a GPI-linked protein, is localized in caveolae. J Cell Biol 129:335–344

51. Pöllänen M, Hedman K, Nielsen LS, Dano K, Vaheri A (1988) Ultrastructural localization of plasma-membrane associated urokinase-type plasminogen activator at focal contacts. Cell Biol 106:87–95

52. Del Rosso M, Anichini E, Pedersen N, Blasi F, Fibbi G, Pucci M, Ruggiero M (1993) Urokinase-urokinase receptor interaction: Non-mitogenic signal transduction in human epidermal cells. Biochem Biophys Res Commun 190:347–352

53. Konakova M, Hucho F, Schleunig WD (1998) Downstream targets of urokinase-type plasminogen-activator-mediated signal transduction. Eur J Biochem 253:421–429

54. Bohuslav J, Horejsi V, Hansmann C, Stöckl J, Weidle UH, Majdic O, Bartke I, Knapp W, Stockinger H (1995) Urokinase plasminogen activator receptor, β_2-integrins, and Src kinases within a single receptor complex of human monocytes. J Exp Med 181:1381–1390

55. Jankun J, Merrick HW, Goldblatt PJ (1993) Expression and localization of elements of the plasminogen activation system in benign breast disease and breast cancers. J Cell Biochem 53:135–144

56. Sier CF M, Vespaget HW, Griffionen G, Ganesh S, Vloedgraven HJ M, Lamers CHW (1993) Plasminogen activators in normal tissue and carcinomas of the human oesophagus and stomach. Gut 34:80–85

57. Pyke C, Kristensen P, Ralfkiaer E, Eriksen J, Dano K (1991) The plasminogen activation system in human colon cancer: Messenger RNA for the inhibitor PAI-1 is located in endothelial cells in the tumor stroma. Cancer Res 51:4067–4071

58. Pyke C, Kristensen P, Ralfkiaer E, Grondahl-Hansen J, Eriksen J, Blasi F, Dano K (1991) Urokinase-type plasminogen activator is expressed in stromal cells and its receptor in cancer cells at invasive foci in human colon adenocarcinomas. Am J Pathol 138, 1059–1067

59. Heiss MM, Babic R, Allgayer H, Grützner KU, Jauch KW, Löhrs U, Schildberg FW (1995) Tumor-associated proteolysis and prognosis: New functional risk factors in gastric cancer defined by the urokinase-type plasminogen activator system. J Clin Oncol 13:2084–2093

60. Heiss MM, Babic R, Allgayer H, Grützner KU, Jauch KW, Löhrs U, Schildberg FW (1996) The prognostc impact of the urokinase-type plasminogen activator system is associated with tumor differentiation in gastric cancer. Eur J Surg Onc 22:74–77

61. Cantero D, Friess H, Deflorin J, Zimmermann A, Bründler MA, Riesle E, Korc M, Büchler MW (1997) Enhanced expression of urokinase plasminogen activator and its receptor in pancreatic carcinoma. Brit J Cancer 75:388–395

62. Romer J, Pyke C, Lund L, Eriksen J, Kristensen P, Ronne E, Hoyer-Hansen G, Dano K, Brünner N (1994) Expression of uPA and its receptor by both neoplastic and stromal cells during xenograft invasion. Int J Cancer 57:553–560

63. Morita S, Sato A, Hayakawa H, Ihara H, Urano T, Takada Y, Takada A (1998) Cancer cells overexpress mRNA of urokinase-type plasminogen activator, its receptor, and inhibitors in human non-small cell lung cancer tissue: Analysis by Northern blotting and in situ hybridization. Int J Cancer 78:286–292

64. Wang H, Skibber J, Juarez J, Boyd D (1994) Transcriptional activation of the urokinase receptor gene in invasive colon cancer. Int J Cancer 58:650–657

65. Bianchi E, Cohen RL, Thor AT III, Mizukami IF, Lawrence DA, Ljung BM, Shuman MA, Smith HS (1994) The urokinase receptor is expressed in invasive breast cancer but not in normal breast tissue. Cancer Res 54:861–866

66. Hollas W, Blasi F, Boyd D (1991) Role of the urokinase receptor in facilitating extracellular matrix invasion by cultured colon cancer. Cancer Res 51:3690–3695

67. Sliutz G, Eder H, Koelbl H, Tempfer C, Auerbach L, Schneeberger C, Kainz C, Zeillinger R (1996) Quantification of uPA receptor expression in human breast cancer cell lines by cRT-PCR. Breast Cancer Res Treat 40:257–263

68. Kariko K, Kuo A, Boyd D, Okada S, Cines D, and Barnathan E (1993) Overexpression of urokinase receptorincreases matrix invasion without altering cell migration in a human osteosarcoma cell line. Cancer Res 53, 3109–3117

69. Ossowski L (1988) In vivo invasion of modified chorioallantoic membrane by tumor cells: The role of cell surface-bound urokinase. J Cell Biol 107:2427–2445

70. Kook YH, Adamski J, Zelent A, and Ossowski L (1994) The effect of antisense inhibition of urokinase receptor in human squamous cell carcinoma on malignancy. EMBO J 13, 3983–3991

71. Quattrone A, Fibbi G, Anichini E, Pucci M, Zamperini A, Capaccioli S, DelRosso MD (1995) Reversion of the invasive phenotype of transformed human fibroblasts by antimessenger oligonucleotide inhibition of urokinase receptor gene expression. Cancer Res 55:90–95

72. Mohanam S, Sawaya R, McCutcheon I, Ali-Oshman F, Boyd D, Rao JS (1993) Modulation of in vitro invasion of human glioblastoma cells by urokinase-type plasminogen activator receptor antibody. Cancer Res 53:4143–4147

73. Liu G, Shuman MA, Cohen RL (1995) Co-expression of urokinase, urokinase receptor and PAI 1 is necessary for optimum invasiveness of cultured lung cancer cells. Int J Cancer 60:501–506

74. Kim J, Yu W, Kovalski K, Ossowski L (1998) Requirement for specific proteases in cancer cell intravasation as revealed by a novel semiquantitative PCR-based assay. Cell 94:353–362

75. Min HY, Doyle LV, Vitt CR, Zandonella CL, Stratton-Thomas JR, Shuman MA, Rosenberg S (1996) Urokinase receptor antagonists inhibit angiogenesis and primary tumor growth in syngeneic mice. Cancer Res 56:2428–2433

76. Schlechte W, Murano G, Boyd D (1989) Examination of the role of the urokinase receptor in human colon cancer mediated laminin degradation. Cancer Res 49:6064–6069

77. Reiter LS, Kruithof EK O, Cajot JF, Sordat B (1993) The role of the urokinase receptor in extracellular matrix degradation by HT29 human colon carcinoma cells. Int J Cancer 53:444–450

78. Schmalfeldt B, Kuhn W, Reuning U, Pache L, Dettmar P, Schmitt M, Jänicke F, Höfler H, Graeff H (1995) Primary tumor and metastasis in ovarian cancer differ in their content of urokinase-type plasminogen activator, its receptor, and inhibitors types 1 and 2. Cancer Res 55:3958–3963

79. Jänicke F, Schmitt M, Pache L, Ulm K, Harbeck N, Hoefler H, Graeff H (1993) Urokinase (uPA) and its inhibitor PAI-1 are strong and independent prognostic factors in node negative breast cancer. Breast Cancer Res and Treatment 24:195–208

80. Heiss MM, Allgayer H, Gruetzner KU, Funke I, Babic R, Jauch KW, Schildberg FW (1995) Individual development and uPA-receptor-expression of disseminated tumour cells in bone marrow: A reference to early systemic disease in solid cancer. Nature Med 1:1035–1039

81. Duffy MJ, Reilly D, O'Sullivan C, O'Higgins N, Fennelly JJ, Andreasen P (1990) Urokinase plasminogen activator, a new and independent prognostic marker in breast cancer. Cancer Res 50:6827–6829

82. Mulcahy HE, Duffy MJ, Gibbons D, McCarthy P, Parfrey NA, O'Donoghue DP, Sheahan K (1994) Urokinase-type plasminogen activator and outcome in Dukes' B colorectal cancer. Lancet 344:583–584

83. Ganesh S, Sier CF M, Heerding MM, Griffionen G, Lamers CB H, Vespaget HW (1994) Urokinase receptor and colorectal cancer survival. Lancet 344:401–402

84. Nekarda H, Schmitt M, Ulm K, Wenninger A, Vogelsang H, Becker K, Roder JD, Fink U, Siewert JR (1994) Prognostic impact of urokinase-type plasminogen activator and its inhibitor PAI-1 in completely resected gastric cancer. Cancer Res 54:2900–2907

85. Heiss MM, Allgayer H, Gruetzner KU, Babic R, Jauch KW, Loehrs U, Schildberg FW (1997) Clinical value of an extended biological staging by bone marrow micrometastases and tumor-associated proteases in gastric cancer. Ann Surg 226:736–744

86. Allgayer H, Heiss MM, Schildberg FW (1997) Prognostic factors in gastric cancer: A review. Brit J Surgery 84:1651–1664

87. Allgayer H, Babic R, Grützner KU, Beyer BCM, Tarabichi A, Schildberg FW, Heiss MM (1998) Tumor-associated proteases and inhibitors in gastric cancer: Analysis of prognostic impact and individual risk protease patterns. Clin Exp Metastasis 16:62–73

88. Nekarda H, Schlegel P, Schmitt M, Stark M, Mueller JD, Fink U, Siewert JR (1998) Strong prognostic impact of tumor-associated urokinase-type plasminogen activator in completely resected adenocarcinoma of the esophagus. Clin Cancer Res 4:1755–1763

89. Osborne MP, Rosen PP (1994) Detection and management of bone marrow micrometastases in breast cancer. Oncology 8:25–31

90. Riethmueller G, Johnson J (1992) Monoclonal antibodies in the detection and therapy of micrometastatic epithelial cancer. Curr Opin Immunol 4:647–655

91. Schlimok G, Funke I, Bock B, Schweiberer B, Witte J, Riethmueller G (1990) Epithelial tumor cells in bone marrow of patients with colorectal cancer: Immunocytochemical detection, phenotypic characterization, and prognostic significance. J Clin Oncol 8:831–837

92. Allgayer H, Heiss MM, Riesenberg R, Gruetzner KU, Tarabichi A, Babic R, Schildberg FW (1997) Urokinase plasminogen activator receptor (uPA-R)–a potential characteristic of metastatic phenotypes in minimal residual tumor disease. Cancer Research 57:1394–1399

93. Cavallaro U, DelVecchio A, Lappi DA, Soria MRAD (1993) A conjugate between human urokinase and saporin, a type-1-ribosome-inactivating protein, is selectively cytotoxic to urokinase receptor-expressing cells. J Biol Chem 68:23186–23190

94. Lengyel E, Wang H, Stepp E, Juarez J, Doe W, Pfarr CM, Boyd D (1996) Requirement of an upstream AP-1 motif for the constitutive and phorbol ester-inducible expression of the urokinase-type plasminogen activator receptor gene. J Biol Chem 271, 23176–23184

95. Gum R, Juarez J, Allgayer H, Mazar A, Wang Y, Boyd D (1998) Stimulation of urokinase-type plasminogen activator receptor expression by PMA requires a JNK1-dependent signaling module. Oncogene 17:213–225

96. Shetty S, Kumar A, and Idell S (1997) Posttranscriptional regulation of urokinase receptor mRNA: Identification of a novel urokinase receptor mRNA binding protein in human mesothelioma cells. Mol Cell Biol 17, 1075–1083

97. Lund LR, Ellis V, Ronne E, Pyke C, and Dano K (1995) Transcriptional and post-transcriptional regulation of the receptor for urokinase-type plasminogen activator by cy-

tokines and tumor promoters in the human lung carcinoma cell line. A549 Biochem J 310, 345–352

98. Nykjaer A, Conese M, Cremona O, Gliemann J, and Blasi F (1997) Recycling of the urokinase receptor upon internalization of the uPA: serpin complexes. EMBO J 16, 2610–2620

99. Wagner SN, Atkinson MJ, Thanner S, Wagner C, Schmitt M, Wilhelm O, Rotter M, Höfler H () Modulation of urokinase and urokinase receptor gene expression in human renal cell carcinoma. Am J Pathol 147:183–192

100. Borglum AD, Byskov A, Ragno P, Roldan AL, Tripputi P, Cassani G, Dano K, Blasi F, Bolund L, Kruse TA (1992) Assignment of the urokinase-type plasminogen activator receptor gene (PLAUR) to chromosome 19q131-q132. Am J Hum Genet 50:492–497

101. Roldan A, Cubellis M, Masucci M, Behrendt N, Lund L, Dano K, Appella E, Blasi F (1990) Cloning and expression of the receptor for human urokinase plasminogen activator, a central molecule in plasmin-dependent proteolysis. EMBO J 9, 467–474

102. Pyke C, Eriksen J, Solberg H, Schnack B, Nielsen S, Kristensen P, Lund LR, and Dano K (1993) An alternatively spliced variant of mRNA for the human receptor for urokinase plasminogen activator. FEBS 326, 69–74

103. Soravia E, Grebe A, De Luca P, Helin K, Suh TT, Degen JL (1995) A conserved TATA-less proximal promoter drives basal transcription from the urokinase-plasminogen activator receptor gene. Blood 86:624–635

104. Means AL, Farnham PJ (1990) Transcription initiation from the dihydrofolate reductase promoter is positioned by HIP1 binding at the initiation site. Mol Cell Biol 10:653–661

105. Suh T, Nerlov K, Dano K, Degen JL (1994) The murine urokinase-type plasminogen activator receptor gene. J Biol Chem 269:25992–25998

106. Lengyel E, Wang H, Gum R, Simon C, Wang Y, Boyd D (1997) Elevated urokinase-type plasminogen activator receptor expression in a colon cancer cell line is due to a constitutively activated extracellular signal-regulated kinase-1-dependent signaling cascade. Oncogene 14:2563–2573

107. Allgayer H, Wang H, Wang Y, Heiss MM, Bauer R, Nyormoi O, Boyd D (1999) Transactivation of the urokinase-type plasminogen activator receptor gene through a novel promoter motif bound with an activator-protein-2α-related factor. J Biol Chem 274:4702–4714

108. Boyd D (1989) Examination of the effects of epidermal growth factor on the production of urokinase and the expression of the plasminogen activator receptor in a human colon cancer cell line. Cancer Res 49:2427–2432

110. Mandriota SJ, Seghezzi G, Vassalli JD, Ferrara N, Wasi S, Mazzieri R, Mignatti P, Pepper MS (1995) Vascular endothelial growth factor increases urokinase receptor expression in vascular endothelial cells. J Biol Chem 270:9709–9716

111. Ando Y, Jensen PJ (1996) Protein kinase C mediates upregulation of urokinase and its receptor in the migrating keratinocytes of wounded cultures, but urokinase is not required for movement across a substratum in vitro. J Cell Physiol 167:500–511

112. Li C, Liu JN, Gurewich V (1995) Urokinase-type plasminogen activator-induced monocyte adhesion requires a carboxyl-terminal lysine and cAMP-dependent signal transduction. J Biol Chem 270:30282–30285

113. Allgayer H, Wang H, Shirasawa S, Sasazuki T, Boyd DD (1999) Targeted Disruption of K-ras oncogene in an invasive cancer cell line down-regulates urokinase receptor expression and plasminogen-dependent proteolysis. Br J Cancer 80:1884–91

114. Talamonti MS, Roh MS, Curley SA, Gallick GE (1993) Increase in activity and level of pp60^{c-src} in progressive stages of human colorectal cancer. J Clin Invest 91:53–60

115. Cartwright, CA, Meisler, AI, Eckhardt, W (1990) Activation of the pp60^{c-src} protein kinase is an early event in colonic carcinogenesis. Proc Natl Acad Sci USA 87:558–562

116. Rösen N, Bolen JB, Schwartz AM, Cohen P, DeSeau V, Israel MA (1986) Analysis of pp60^{c-src} protein kinase activity in human tumor cell lines and tissues. J Biol Chem 261:13754–13759

117. Pories SE, Hess DT, Swenson K, Lotz M, Moussa R, Steele G, Shibata D, Rieger Christ KM, Summerhayes C (1998) Overexpression of pp60^{c-src} elicits invasive behaviour in rat colon epithelial cells. Gastroenterology 114:1335–1338

118. Allgayer H, Wang H, Gallick GE, Crabtree A, Mazar A, Jones T, Kraker AJ, Boyd DD (1999) Transcriptional induction of the urokinase-receptor (u-PAR) gene by a constitutively active Src: Requirement of an upstream motif (-152/-135) bound with Sp1. J Biol Chem 274 (26), 18428–18437

119. Renatus M, Bode W, Huber R, Sturzebecher J, Stubbs MT (1998) Structural and functional analyses of benzamidine-based inhibitors in complex with trypsin: implications for the inhibition of factor Xa, tPA, and urokinase. J Med Chem 41:5445–56

119. Mignatti P, Mazzieri R, Rifkin DB (1991) Expression of the urokinase receptor in vascular endothelial cells is stimulated by basic fibroblast growth factor. J Cell Biol 113:1193–1201

120. Wilhelm O, Weidle U, Höhl S, Rettenberger P, Schmitt M, Graeff H (1994) Recombinant soluble urokinase receptor as a scavenger for urokinase-type plasminogen activator (uPA). Inhibition of proliferation and invasion of human ovarian cancer cells FEBS Lett 337:131–134

121. Ossowski L, Reich E (1983) Antibodies to plasminogen activator inhibit human tumour metastasis. Cell 35:611–619

Stromal Cell Involvement in Cancer

Kasper Almholt, Morten Johnsen

K. Almholt (✉)
The Finsen Laboratory, Rigshospitalet, Strandboulevarden 49,
2100 Copenhagen, Denmark

Abstract

Solid tumors co-opt the body's endogenous extracellular proteolytic machinery for their invasion and metastasis. This is supported by a large number of independent observations ranging from histochemical and prognostic studies of cancer patient material to animal experiments. There are several extracellular proteolytic systems that are relevant in the context of cancer, but the plasminogen activation (PA) system and the matrix metalloproteases (MMPs) remain the most thoroughly investigated. Localization studies by immunohistochemistry and in situ mRNA hybridization in tumors of common human cancers have repeatedly identified members of the PA and MMP systems in stromal cells. The cancer cells, of epithelial origin, contribute PA and MMP components in some cases, but their contribution fades in comparison with the overwhelming expression of proteolytic components by fibroblasts, macrophages, endothelial cells, and other stromal cells. Ideal animal models of human cancers should recapitulate this fundamental proteolytic aspect of tumor biology. However, in the transplantable tumor models where PA or MMP components have been studied at the cellular level in vivo, this is most often not the case. Transgenic cancer models may provide a closer parallel to the human situation, in that PA and MMP components are synthesized by the tumor stroma. The pivotal role of stromal cells has been confirmed experimentally in mouse models in which the expression pattern of proteolytic components is strongly reminiscent of human tumors. In these models it is possible to reconstitute the wild-type tumor characteristics of proteolytically deficient tumor-bearing mice by transplantation with wild-type fibroblasts or hemapoietic cells. These studies collectively show that cancer-associated proteolysis is a collaborative effort of malignant cancer cells and various stromal cells – a collaboration in which stromal cells contribute the majority of the active proteolytic components that are necessary for the invasive behavior of the tumors. This cellular division of labor positions the stromal cells as prime targets for future research and possibly therapy. Vascular endothelial cells are already the focus of intense therapeutically relevant research, but tumor-associated fibroblasts, macrophages, neutrophils, lymphendothelial cells, etc. provide additional largely unexplored territory in the ongoing search for efficient countermeasures against invasive cancer.

Introduction

Decades of molecular cancer research have resulted in a wealth of information on cell-cycle controls and apoptotic mechanisms and their dysregulation in cancer cells. However, solid tumors are relatively complex tissues, and we believe that the importance of the stromal cell compartment in malignant tumors is presently underestimated. Although it is generally acknowledged that stromal cells are strongly influenced by the cancer cells, it is not yet generally accepted that the stromal cells actively contribute to the set of processes that define the tumor's malignancy. Studies of extracellular proteolysis have convinced us that crucial aspects of cancer development cannot be extrapolated from molecular studies of cancer cells in isolation. Thus, the development of successful clinical strategies that are based on model studies may well depend on the presence of both cancer cells and stromal cells in the models.

Extracellular Proteolytic Systems in Cancer

Solid tumors depend on extracellular proteolysis at several stages of tumor development, including the breakdown of basement membranes and other extracellular matrix (ECM) components during invasion and metastasis. The ECM embeds the cells and is responsible for most of the physical characteristics of the different tissues, and is a complex network of primarily proteins and proteoglycans. Given the complexity of this matrix, it is not surprising that pericellular proteolytic activity depends on several matrix-degrading protease systems. The biological substrates and functions of the relevant proteolytic enzymes are presently largely unknown and may well be partially overlapping. Here, we will focus on two extracellular protease systems, the plasminogen activation (PA) system and the matrix metalloproteases (MMPs). Both of these systems have been implicated in malignancy in a large number of reports, using a wide range of descriptive and experimental techniques from immunohistochemistry to genetically modified animals.

The PA cascade [1] of serine proteases leads to generation of the broad-spectrum protease plasmin. The inactive zymogen plasminogen, produced mainly in the liver and present throughout the body, is converted to plasmin by specific plasminogen activators. The urokinase-type plasminogen activator (uPA), the most cancer-relevant plasminogen activator, binds with high affinity to its cell surface-bound receptor, the urokinase receptor (uPAR). Receptor binding of uPA localizes plasmin generation to cell surfaces. The PA cascade is inhibited at several levels. Fast-acting, specific PA inhibitors, notably the extracellular plasminogen activator inhibitor-1 (PAI-1), restrict plasminogen activation to defined times and microenvironments. Similarly, the specific extracellular plasmin inhibitor α_2-antiplasmin localizes plasmin activity to cell surfaces due to its preferential inhibition of circulating plasmin. Major substrates of plasmin include fibrin and other ECM proteins, latent growth factors, pro-uPA, and pro-MMPs.

The MMPs [2–5], of which there are over 25 (23 human MMPs thus far), are also activated proteolytically and blocked by specific inhibitors, the tissue inhibitors of metalloproteases (TIMPs). MMP activity can also be localized to cell surfaces, i.e., one group of MMPs is membrane-anchored, whereas some of the soluble MMPs may interact with cellular receptors. The different in vivo substrates of individual MMPs are far from fully elucidated, but collectively MMPs can degrade practically all ECM proteins. Important substrates for the MMPs as a group include the native fibrillar collagens, latent growth factors, pro-MMPs, and major basement membrane proteins such as laminin and collagen type IV.

Stromal Origin of Extracellular Proteases

The proteases, inhibitors, and related molecules of the PA and MMP systems are expressed in a wide variety of human cancers including carcinomas of the colon, breast, lung, ovary, and prostate [2, 6, 7]. In addition to the epithelial component, carcinomas consist of ECM and a variety of stromal cells: a broad term that we apply collectively to all resident nonepithelial cells, blood, and lymphatic vessels as well as various infiltrating cells. Stromal cells rather than the cancerous epithelium express the components of the PA and MMP systems found in the major human adenocarcinomas. Although some controversy remains on this issue with respect to the PA system, several independent studies clearly identify uPA, PAI-1, and uPAR mRNAs and/or proteins in stromal cells of common tumors. In both colon and mammary adenocarcinomas for instance, stromal cells contain uPA [8–13], PAI-1 [10, 14–16], and uPAR [9, 10, 17–21]. Whereas uPA and PAI-1 always seem derived from stromal cells in the adenocarcinomas studied, uPAR is consistently also found in a fraction of the epithelial cells of colon [9, 17, 18] and mammary [19–21] carcinomas. Similarly, in thorough studies of human mammary tumors, mRNA for 8 of 10 MMPs studied were found in stromal cells: these were MMP-1, -2, -3, -9, -11, -12, -13, and -14 [11, 22–26]. As reviewed, these findings have largely been confirmed by several groups, also in other cancers [2, 6]. Indeed, matrilysin (MMP-7) is the only protease among the MMPs that is consistently expressed by the cancerous epithelium in a number of different carcinomas [2, 6]. This one exception underscores the general rule that stromal cells produce the majority of the MMPs present in human adenocarcinomas. Again, epithelial contribution to extracellular proteolysis may be important to tumor progression when found (e.g., uPAR and matrilysin), but it remains an exception to the over-whelming proteolytic contribution by stromal cells.

Insight into the division of labor between cancer cells and stromal cells calls for a more detailed analysis of which cell types among the multitude of different stromal cells produce the proteases. The identification of the exact cellular source of the proteolytic components has unraveled some interesting overall similarities among major human carcinomas. For example, in colon [8, 9] and mammary [11–13] adenocarcinomas, uPA mRNA and/or protein is found in tumor-associated fibroblasts. PAI-1 is found in endothelial cells in colon [10, 14] and mammary [15, 16] adenocarcinomas, although in the latter case some PAI-1 is also found in fibroblasts. A variety of cell types in colon and mammary adenocarcinomas have been found to contain uPAR mRNA and/or protein. Among these cell types, only macrophages and a fraction of cancer cells consistently contain uPAR in both cancer types [9, 17–21]. The cellular expression patterns of MMPs are also conserved to some extent among several carcinomas. As reviewed [6], at least collagenase-1 (MMP-1) [11, 22, 23], gelatinase A (MMP-2) [11, 22, 23], stromelysin-3 (MMP-11) [11, 22, 23], and MT1-MMP (MMP-14) [22, 23, 25] are all found in fibroblastic cells of colon and mammary adenocarcinomas, whereas gelatinase B (MMP-9) is found in various inflammatory cells [11, 23, 24, 27] and matrilysin in the neoplastic epithelial cells [11, 23, 28] in these cancers.

We have previously described that the cellular expression patterns of pro-teases in certain tumors including colon and mammary cancers are quite sim-ilar to the patterns observed during nonneoplastic tissue remodeling in the same organs: processes such as shedding of epithelial cells into the intestinal lumen and postlactational mammary gland involution [29]. Here we have highlighted a clear parallel with respect to protease expression between colon and mammary adenocarcinomas. We anticipate that these similarities may ex-tend to adenocarcinomas in a number of other tissues, although we do not be-lieve that the patterns will be universally shared. However, the dissimilarities among adenocarcinomas fade in comparison with the expression differences observed between adenocarcinomas and squamous cell carcinomas (SCCs). Whereas various stromal cells express most of the PA and MMP components in the adenocarcinomas studied, the epithelial cells express almost all of the proteases and related proteins in SCCs. Thus, in SCCs of the skin, the epithe-lial cells contain protein and/or mRNAs for uPA [30, 31], PAI-1 [30], uPAR [32], gelatinase B [33], and collagenase-3 (MMP-13) [34]. At least in the case of uPA, this pattern extends also to SCCs of the oral cavity [35] and breast [12]. This major difference is consistent even when SCCs and adenocarcino-mas from the same tissue are compared using the same technique. For exam-ple, among mammary carcinomas, uPA mRNA is present in tumor-associated myofibroblasts in the common adenocarcinomas, and present in the cancer cells of the rare SCCs [12]. These findings probably reflect a fundamental dif-ference in the properties of squamous cell carcinomas and adenocarcinomas.

An ideal animal model of human cancer should recapitulate as many as-pects as possible of the human situation. With respect to cellular expression patterns of proteases and related proteins, only some of the experimental carcinoma models that are currently in use mimic the common human adenocarcinomas, if the expression patterns have been studied at all. Perhaps it is not surprising that the cellular origin of PA and MMP components varies greatly among the transplanted tumors. Depending on the cell line used for transplantation they may be exclusively cancer cell-derived, exclusively stromal cell-derived, or expressed in both. In the much studied Lewis lung carcinoma (LLC), uPA [36–38], PAI-1 [37, 38], and uPAR [39] are almost exclusively expressed by cancer cells in vivo. In xenotransplanted MDA-MB-231 tumors derived from a mammary adenocarcinoma, human uPA and uPAR mRNAs are found in the cancer cells, whereas the mouse mRNAs are found in the stromal cells [40]. Finally, tumors derived from the metastatic colorectal cancer cell lines C170HM$_2$ and SW620S5 express gelatinase B predominantly in stromal cells [41, 42]. Interestingly, C170HM$_2$ cells express gelatinase B in vitro [41], whereas SW620S5 cells do not [42]. In contrast to what is observed with the transplanted tumors, but strongly reminiscent of human carcinomas, proteases are primarily derived from stromal cells in transgenic carcinoma models in mice. Thus, in the MMTV-PymT transgenic model of mammary carcinoma, uPA, PAI-1, uPAR, and several MMPs are produced by stromal cells [43, and our unpublished results]. Similarly, infiltrating inflammatory cells express gelatinase B in both the RIP1-Tag2 transgenic model of pancreatic islet carcinoma and the K14-HPV16 transgenic skin carcinoma model [44, 45]. It is probable that transplantable cancer cell lines propagated in vitro or in vivo by serial transplantation have acquired many additional characteristics not seen in the epithelial cells of transgenic tumor models. It remains to be seen whether conclusions drawn from transgenic models rather than transplanted models are more relevant for human tumor biology. At least, it is important to consider the proteolytic expression pattern at the cellular level in any animal model when drawing conclusions regarding a given protease or related protein.

Prognostic Studies

The notion that matrix-degrading protease systems are important for cancer progression is supported by a number of reports that show significant prognostic value associated with the levels of many of the proteolytic components in cancer patients. Detailed reviews of these studies are given elsewhere [3, 7, 46, 47], and we will limit the discussion to a few examples. Importantly, these clinical studies link the PA and MMP proteins to cancer progression regardless of their cellular origin.

The prognostic potential of the PA system in particular has been widely investigated in several types of cancer. For example in breast cancer, high levels of uPA [48–50], PAI-1 [48–50], and uPAR [50, 51] in tumor tissue are all associated with an unfavorable prognosis. This is consistent with a promoting role of these molecules in breast cancer and particularly interesting in light of their stromal origin.

By comparison, thorough studies of the prognostic significance of MMPs and TIMPs in cancer are only beginning to appear. An elevated gelatinase B level is a potential indicator of unfavorable prognosis in colon cancer patients [52, 53], whereas a high stromelysin-3 [54–56] level may predict a poor outcome in breast cancer patients. TIMP-1 may become a valuable prognostic marker for both colon [57, 58] and breast [59, 60] cancer patients, with a high level associated with poor outcome in both cancers.

Experimental Proof of Stromal Contribution to Tumor-Associated Proteolysis

As described above, mRNA expression and immunohistochemical studies have long indicated that stromal cells contribute to extracellular proteolysis in human carcinomas, and molecules of these proteolytic cascades have proven to be of prognostic value in clinical cancer treatment. Obviously, none of these observations prove that the PA and MMP components derived from stromal cells are important for cancer progression. The mere presence of a mRNA or a protein is not indicative of its importance. Likewise, correlation with poor or favorable patient prognosis could be a bystander phenomenon rather than reflect a causal relationship. The experimental verification in animal models of the importance of proteolytic components derived from stromal cells is only now beginning to appear. No studies have examined transgenic overexpression of proteases specifically in stromal cells in connection with cancer initiation or progression, but other approaches have provided compelling evidence for a crucial role of proteases derived from stromal cells in regulating the proliferation, invasion, and metastasis of genetically altered epithelial cells. Several studies implicate fibroblasts in these steps of tumor progression, and a recent study has conclusively demonstrated a role for proteases derived from hemapoietic cells.

Gene-deficient mice provide a powerful tool to analyze the overall significance of a single protease in cancer progression. Plasminogen deficiency causes decreased lung metastasis formation in the transgenic MMTV-PymT mammary carcinoma model [43, and our unpublished results]. The proteins critical for regulating plasminogen activation, namely uPA, PAI-1, and uPAR, are found only in stromal cells of the MMTV-PymT tumors [43, and our unpublished results]. This strongly indicates a crucial role of stromal cells for tumor-associated proteolysis in this model. A similar observation comes from the transgenic RIP1-Tag2-induced pancreatic islet carcinoma model. Deficiency of gelatinase B impairs tumor growth in this model. As with the MMTV-PymT model, a crucial role for stromal cells in the RIP1-Tag2 model can be inferred from the observation that stromal cells – not cancer cells – express gelatinase B [44].

These examples implicate stromal involvement based on cellular expression patterns of proteases. Several studies show stromal cell involvement in extracellular proteolysis in a more direct way. Transplanted LLC cells show reduced growth in gelatinase A-deficient mice compared with littermate wild-type mice, despite the fact that the cells display gelatinase A activity themselves [61]. This may be attributed to reduced vascularization, because angiogenesis was impaired in gelatinase A-deficient mice in a parallel in vivo angiogenesis assay [61]. Similarly, the growth of syngeneic C26 colon carcinoma cells is reduced in stromelysin-3-deficient mice compared with littermate wild-type mice [62]. The effect may be attributed to increased tumor cell apoptosis. Irrespective of the mechanisms, the LLC and C26 cells rely on host (stromal) gelatinase A or stromelysin-3 for optimal growth.

The crucial role of fibroblast-derived proteolysis was demonstrated using the human MCF-7 mammary carcinoma cell line that does not spontaneously form tumors in nude mice. Co-transplanted human fibroblasts or matrigel increases the tumorigenicity of a number of carcinoma-derived epithelial cells, including MCF-7 cells [63]. Importantly, a combination of fibroblasts and matrigel has an additive effect on MCF-7 cell tumorigenesis, but fibroblasts do not enhance tumor formation in the presence of growth factor-depleted matrigel [63, 64]. The additional effect of fibroblasts is abolished by the synthetic MMP inhibitor batimastat and by overexpressing TIMP-2 in the MCF-7 cells [64]. Even stronger evidence for the role of fibroblast-derived MMPs in tumorigenesis came from substituting human fibroblasts with mouse embryonic fibroblasts (MEFs) genetically deficient for stromelysin-3. Whereas wild-type MEFs enhance tumor formation by MCF-7 cells in the presence of matrigel, stromelysin-3-deficient MEFs do not [65]. It is likely that fibroblast-produced stromelysin-3 enhances tumor growth in this assay by proteolytically releasing and/or activating growth factors from the matrigel [66].

Analogous to the role of fibroblast-derived proteolysis, a recent study demonstrates a role for gelatinase B produced by bone marrow-derived cells. In K14-HPV16 transgene-induced skin cancer, the oncogene-positive keratinocytes in gelatinase B-deficient mice show reduced proliferation, and the incidence of carcinomas is reduced compared to wild-type mice [45]. Gelatinase B immunoreactivity is found predominantly in infiltrating stromal cells of hemapoietic origin (neutrophils, macrophages, and mast cells) within the wild-type tumors. Intriguingly, wild-type bone marrow grafted to gelatinase B-deficient recipient mice restores transgene-induced keratinocyte proliferation and carcinoma incidence to wild-type levels. However, gelatinase B produced by the hemapoietic cells is not absolutely required; even in the complete absence of gelatinase B tumors still form and eventually progress to malignancy.

Conclusion

Still growing amounts of evidence support the idea that tumor stroma very often is a co-contributor to cancer progression. It seems that the complex and multi-step process of tumor progression and dissemination requires a close interplay of cancerous epithelial cells and non-malignant stromal cells such as fibroblasts, macrophages, neutrophils, and endothelial cells [67–70]. A critical rate-limiting role of stromal cells in overall cancer progression may very well be their contribution to extracellular proteolysis. Expression analyses and localization studies demonstrate that proteolytic components are in fact predominantly expressed by stromal cells rather than by cancer cells, and studies of cancer patient material correlate the proteins of several proteolytic systems with clinical outcome of the patient's disease. In addition to the compelling constellation of localization studies and clinical findings, more recent in vivo experimental data confirm that stromal cells actively contribute to tumor-associated proteolysis. Thus, cancer-associated proteolysis is a collaborative effort of cancer cells and stromal cells. In this collaboration, stromal cells contribute the majority of the active proteolytic components.

The challenge in the future will be to identify the substrates of individual proteases and to relate these to the role(s) of proteases and related proteins in tumor progression. An important key to this lies in determining which cell type provides a given proteolytic component at crucial stages of tumor progression. Such studies may allow combat of cancer from new angles: interference with stromal cells. With the distinct exception of vascular endothelial cells, little attention has until recently been awarded any non-cancer cell of solid tumors. This may have limited our understanding of tumor biology as well as our ability to restrict malignant behavior.

References

1. Andreasen PA, Egelund R, Petersen HH (2000) The plasminogen activation system in tumor growth, invasion, and metastasis. Cell Mol Life Sci 57:25–40
2. Nelson AR, Fingleton B, Rothenberg ML, Matrisian LM (2000) Matrix metalloproteinases: biologic activity and clinical implications. J Clin Oncol 18:1135–1149
3. Sternlicht MD, Bergers G (2000) Matrix metalloproteinases as emerging targets in anticancer therapy: status and prospects. Emerging Therapeutic Targets 4:609–633
4. Sternlicht MD, Werb Z (2001) How matrix metalloproteinases regulate cell behavior. Annu Rev Cell Dev Biol 17:463–516
5. Brew K, Dinakarpandian D, Nagase H (2000) Tissue inhibitors of metalloproteinases: evolution, structure and function. Biochim Biophys Acta 1477:267–283
6. Hewitt R, Danø K (1996) Stromal cell expression of components of matrix-degrading protease systems in human cancer. Enzyme Protein 49:163–173
7. Andreasen PA, Kjøller L, Christensen L, Duffy MJ (1997) The urokinase-type plasminogen activator system in cancer metastasis: a review. Int J Cancer 72:1–22
8. Grøndahl-Hansen J, Ralfkiær E, Kirkeby LT, Kristensen P, Lund LR, Danø K (1991) Localization of urokinase-type plasminogen activator in stromal cells in adenocarcinomas of the colon in humans. Am J Pathol 138:111–117
9. Pyke C, Kristensen P, Ralfkiær E, Grøndahl-Hansen J, Eriksen J, Blasi F, Danø K (1991) Urokinase-type plasminogen activator is expressed in stromal cells and its receptor in cancer cells at invasive foci in human colon adenocarcinomas. Am J Pathol 138:1059–1067
10. Delbaldo C, Cunningham M, Vassalli J-D, Sappino A-P (1995) Plasmin-catalyzed proteolysis in colorectal neoplasia. Cancer Res 55:4688–4695
11. Wolf C, Rouyer N, Lutz Y, Adida C, Loriot M, Bellocq J-P, Chambon P, Basset P (1993) Stromelysin 3 belongs to a subgroup of proteinases expressed in breast carcinoma fibro-

blastic cells and possibly implicated in tumor progression. Proc Natl Acad Sci USA 90:1843–1847

12. Nielsen BS, Sehested M, Timshel S, Pyke C, Danø, K (1996) Messenger RNA for urokinase plasminogen activator is expressed in myofibroblasts adjacent to cancer cells in human breast cancer. Lab Invest 74:168–177

13. Nielsen BS, Sehested M, Duun S, Rank F, Timshel S, Rygaard J, Johnsen M, Danø K (2001) Urokinase plasminogen activator is localized in stromal cells in ductal breast cancer. Lab Invest 81:1485–1502

14. Pyke C, Kristensen P, Ralfkiær E, Eriksen J, Danø K (1991) The plasminogen activation system in human colon cancer: messenger RNA for the inhibitor PAI-1 is located in endothelial cells in the tumor stroma. Cancer Res 51:4067–4071

15. Bianchi E, Cohen RL, Dai A, Thor AT, Shuman MA, Smith HS (1995) Immunohistochemical localization of the plasminogen activator inhibitor-1 in breast cancer. Int J Cancer 60:597–603

16. Pappot H, Gårdsvoll H, Rømer J, Pedersen AN, Grøndahl-Hansen J, Pyke C, Brünner N (1995) Plasminogen activator inhibitor type 1 in cancer: therapeutic and prognostic implications. Biol Chem Hoppe-Seyler 376:259–267

17. Pyke C, Ralfkiær E, Rønne E, Høyer-Hansen G, Kirkeby L, Danø K (1994) Immunohistochemical detection of the receptor for urokinase plasminogen activator in human colon cancer. Histopathology 24:131–138

18. Ohtani H, Pyke C, Danø K, Nagura H (1995) Expression of urokinase receptor in various stromal-cell populations in human colon cancer: immunoelectron microscopical analysis. Int J Cancer 62:691–696

19. Pyke C, Græm N, Ralfkiær E, Rønne E, Høyer-Hansen G, Brünner N, Danø K (1993) Receptor for urokinase is present in tumor-associated macrophages in ductal breast carcinoma. Cancer Res 53:1911–1915

20. Bianchi E, Cohen RL, Thor AT, Todd RF, Mizukami IF, Lawrence DA, Ljung BM, Shuman MA, Smith HS (1994) The urokinase receptor is expressed in invasive breast cancer but not in normal breast tissue. Cancer Res 54:861–866

21. Luther T, Magdolen V, Albrecht S, Kasper M, Riemer C, Kessler H, Graeff H, Müller M, Schmitt M (1997) Epitope-mapped monoclonal antibodies as tools for functional and morphological analyses of the human urokinase receptor in tumor tissue. Am J Pathol 150:1231–1244

22. Okada A, Bellocq J-P, Rouyer N, Chenard M-P, Rio M-C, Chambon P, Basset P (1995) Membrane-type matrix metalloproteinase (MT-MMP) gene is expressed in stromal cells of human colon, breast, and head and neck carcinomas. Proc Natl Acad Sci USA 92:2730–2734

23. Heppner KJ, Matrisian LM, Jensen RA, Rodgers WH (1996) Expression of most matrix metalloproteinase family members in breast cancer represents a tumor-induced host response. Am J Pathol 149:273–282

24. Nielsen BS, Sehested M, Kjeldsen L, Borregaard N, Rygaard J, Danø K (1997) Expression of matrix metalloprotease-9 in vascular pericytes in human breast cancer. Lab Invest 77:345–355

25. Chenard M-P, Lutz Y, Mechine-Neuville A, Stoll I, Bellocq J-P, Rio M-C, Basset P (1999) Presence of high levels of MT1-MMP protein in fibroblastic cells of human invasive carcinomas. Int J Cancer 82:208–212

26. Nielsen BS, Rank F, López JM, Balbin M, Vizoso F, Lund LR, Danø K, López-Otín C (2001) Collagenase-3 expression in breast myofibroblasts as a molecular marker of transition of ductal carcinoma in situ lesions to invasive ductal carcinomas. Cancer Res 61:7091–7100

27. Nielsen BS, Timshel S, Kjeldsen L, Sehested M, Pyke C, Borregaard N, Danø K (1996) 92 kDa type IV collagenase (MMP-9) is expressed in neutrophils and macrophages but not in malignant epithelial cells in human colon cancer. Int J Cancer 65:57–62

28. McDonnell S, Navre M, Coffey RJ Jr, Matrisian LM (1991) Expression and localization of the matrix metalloproteinase pump-1 (MMP-7) in human gastric and colon carcinomas. Mol Carcinog 4:527–533

29. Johnsen M, Lund LR, Rømer J, Almholt K, Danø K (1998) Cancer invasion and tissue remodeling: common themes in proteolytic matrix degradation. Curr Opin Cell Biol 10: 667–671

30. Sappino A-P, Belin D, Huarte J, Hirschel-Scholz S, Saurat J-H, Vassalli J-D (1991) Differential protease expression by cutaneous squamous and basal cell carcinomas. J Clin Invest 88:1073–1079

31. Miller SJ, Jensen PJ, Dzubow LM, Lazarus GS (1992) Urokinase plasminogen activator is immunocytochemically detectable in squamous cell but not basal cell carcinomas. J Invest Dermatol 98:351–358

32. Rømer J, Pyke C, Lund LR, Ralfkiær E, Danø K (2001) Cancer cell expression of urokinase-type plasminogen activator receptor mRNA in squamous cell carcinomas of the skin. J Invest Dermatol 116: 353–358

33. Pyke C, Ralfkiær E, Huhtala P, Hurskainen T, Danø K, Tryggvason K (1992) Localization of messenger RNA for M_r 72,000 and 92,000 type IV collagenases in human skin cancers by in situ hybridization. Cancer Res 52:1336–1341

34. Airola K, Johansson N, Kariniemi A-L, Kähäri V-M, Saarialho-Kere UK (1997) Human collagenase-3 is expressed in malignant squamous epithelium of the skin. J Invest Dermatol 109:225–231

35. Clayman G, Wang SW, Nicolson GL, El-Naggar A, Mazar A, Henkin J, Blasi F, Goepfert H, Boyd DD (1993) Regulation of urokinase-type plasminogen activator expression in squamous-cell carcinoma of the oral cavity. Int J Cancer 54:73–80

36. Skriver L, Larsson L-I, Kielberg V, Nielsen LS, Andresen PB, Kristensen P, Danø K (1984) Immunocytochemical localization of urokinase-type plasminogen activator in Lewis lung carcinoma. J Cell Biol 99:752–757

37. Kristensen P, Pyke C, Lund LR, Andreasen PA, Danø K (1990) Plasminogen activator inhibitor-type 1 in Lewis lung carcinoma. Histochemistry 93:559–566

38. Bugge TH, Kombrinck KW, Xiao Q, Holmbäck K, Daugherty CC, Witte DP, Degen JL (1997) Growth and dissemination of Lewis lung carcinoma in plasminogen-deficient mice. Blood 90:4522–4531

39. Solberg H, Ploug M, Høyer-Hansen G, Nielsen BS, Lund LR (2001) The murine receptor for urokinase-type plasminogen activator is primarily expressed in tissues actively undergoing remodeling. J Histochem Cytochem 49:237–246

40. Rømer J, Pyke C, Lund LR, Eriksen J, Kristensen P, Rønne E, Høyer-Hansen G, Danø K, Brünner N (1994) Expression of uPA and its receptor by both neoplastic and stromal cells during xenograft invasion. Int J Cancer 57:553–560

41. Collins HM, Morris TM, Watson SA (2001) Spectrum of matrix metalloproteinase expression in primary and metastatic colon cancer: relationship to the tissue inhibitors of metalloproteinases and membrane type-1-matrix metalloproteinase. Br J Cancer 84:1664–1670

42. McDonnell S, Chaudhry V, Mansilla-Soto J, Zeng Z-S, Shu W-P, Guillem JG (1999) Metastatic and non-metastatic colorectal cancer (CRC) cells induce host metalloproteinase production in vivo. Clin Exp Metastasis 17:341–349

43. Bugge TH, Lund LR, Kombrinck KK, Nielsen BS, Holmbäck K, Drew AF, Flick MJ, Witte DP, Danø K, Degen JL (1998) Reduced metastasis of Polyoma virus middle T antigen-induced mammary cancer in plasminogen-deficient mice. Oncogene 16:3097–3104

44. Bergers G, Brekken R, McMahon G, Vu TH, Itoh T, Tamaki K, Tanzawa K, Thorpe P, Itohara S, Werb Z, Hanahan D (2000) Matrix metalloproteinase-9 triggers the angiogenic switch during carcinogenesis. Nat Cell Biol 2:737–744

45. Coussens LM, Tinkle CL, Hanahan D, Werb Z (2000) MMP-9 supplied by bone marrow-derived cells contributes to skin carcinogenesis. Cell 103:481–490

46. Stephens RW, Brünner N, Jänicke F, Schmitt M (1998) The urokinase plasminogen activator system as a target for prognostic studies in breast cancer. Breast Cancer Res Treat 52:99–111

47. Curran S, Murray GI (1999) Matrix metalloproteinases in tumour invasion and metastasis. J Pathol 189:300–308

48. Grøndahl-Hansen J, Christensen IJ, Rosenquist C, Brünner N, Mouridsen HT, Danø K, Blichert-Toft M (1993) High levels of urokinase-type plasminogen activator and its inhibitor PAI-1 in cytosolic extracts of breast carcinomas are associated with poor prognosis. Cancer Res 53:2513–2521

49. Grøndahl-Hansen J, Hilsenbeck SG, Christensen IJ, Clark GM, Osborne CK, Brünner N (1997) Prognostic significance of PAI-1 and uPA in cytosolic extracts obtained from node-positive breast cancer patients. Breast Cancer Res Treat 43:153–163

50. Foekens JA, Peters HA, Look MP, Portengen H, Schmitt M, Kramer MD, Brünner N, Jänicke F, Meijer-van Gelder ME, Henzen-Logmans SC, van Putten WLJ, Klijn JGM (2000) The urokinase system of plasminogen activation and prognosis in 2780 breast cancer patients. Cancer Res 60:636–643

51. Grøndahl-Hansen J, Peters HA, van Putten WLJ, Look MP, Pappot H, Rønne E, Danø K, Klijn JGM, Brünner N, Foekens JA (1995) Prognostic significance of the receptor for urokinase plasminogen activator in breast cancer. Clin Cancer Res 1:1079–1087

52. Zeng ZS, Huang Y, Cohen AM, Guillem JG (1996) Prediction of colorectal cancer relapse and survival via tissue RNA levels of matrix metalloproteinase-9. J Clin Oncol 14:3133–3140

53. Zucker S, Hymowitz M, Conner C, Zarrabi HM, Hurewitz AN, Matrisian L, Boyd D, Nicolson G, Montana S (1999) Measurement of matrix metalloproteinases and tissue inhibitors of metalloproteinases in blood and tissues. Clinical and experimental applications. Ann NY Acad Sci 878:212–227

54. Chenard M-P, O'Siorain L, Shering S, Rouyer N, Lutz Y, Wolf C, Basset P, Bellocq J-P, Duffy MJ (1996) High levels of stromelysin-3 correlate with poor prognosis in patients with breast carcinoma. Int J Cancer 69:448–451

55. Têtu B, Brisson J, Lapointe H, Bernard P (1998) Prognostic significance of stromelysin 3, gelatinase A, and urokinase expression in breast cancer. Hum Pathol 29:979–985

56. Ahmad A, Hanby A, Dublin E, Poulsom R, Smith P, Barnes D, Rubens R, Anglard P, Hart I (1998) Stromelysin 3: an independent prognostic factor for relapse-free survival in node-positive breast cancer and demonstration of novel breast carcinoma cell expression. Am J Pathol 152:721–728

57. Zeng ZS, Cohen AM, Zhang ZF, Stetler-Stevenson W, Guillem JG (1995) Elevated tissue inhibitor of metalloproteinase 1 RNA in colorectal cancer stroma correlates with lymph node and distant metastases. Clin Cancer Res 1:899–906

58. Holten-Andersen MN, Stephens RW, Nielsen HJ, Murphy G, Christensen IJ, Stetler-Stevenson W, Brünner N (2000) High preoperative plasma tissue inhibitor of metalloproteinase-1 levels are associated with short survival of patients with colorectal cancer. Clin Cancer Res 6:4292–4299

59. Ree AH, Flørenes VA, Berg JP, Mælandsmo GM, Nesland JM, Fodstad Ø (1997) High levels of messenger RNAs for tissue inhibitors of metalloproteinases (TIMP-1 and TIMP-2) in primary breast carcinomas are associated with development of distant metastases. Clin Cancer Res 3:1623–1628

60. McCarthy K, Maguire T, McGreal G, McDermott E, O'Higgins N, Duffy MJ (1999) High levels of tissue inhibitor of metalloproteinase-1 predict poor outcome in patients with breast cancer. Int J Cancer 84:44–48

61. Itoh T, Tanioka M, Yoshida H, Yoshioka T, Nishimoto H, Itohara S (1998) Reduced angiogenesis and tumor progression in gelatinase A-deficient mice. Cancer Res 58:1048–1051

62. Boulay A, Masson R, Chenard M-P, El Fahime M, Cassard L, Bellocq J-P, Sautès-Fridman C, Basset P, Rio M-C (2001) High cancer cell death in syngeneic tumors developed in host mice deficient for the stromelysin-3 matrix metalloproteinase. Cancer Res 61:2189–2193

63. Noël A, De Pauw-Gillet M-C, Purnell G, Nusgens B, Lapiere C-M, Foidart J-M (1993) Enhancement of tumorigenicity of human breast adenocarcinoma cells in nude mice by matrigel and fibroblasts. Br. J Cancer 68:909–915

64. Noël A, Hajitou A, L'Hoir C, Maquoi E, Baramova E, Lewalle JM, Remacle A, Kebers F, Brown P, Calberg-Bacq CM, Foidart JM (1998) Inhibition of stromal matrix metalloproteases: effects on breast-tumor promotion by fibroblasts. Int J Cancer 76:267–273

65. Masson R, Lefebvre O, Noël A, El Fahime M, Chenard M-P, Wendling C, Kebers F, LeMeur M, Dierich A, Foidart J-M, Basset P, Rio M-C (1998) In vivo evidence that the stromelysin-3 metalloproteinase contributes in a paracrine manner to epithelial cell malignancy. J Cell Biol 140:1535–1541
66. Noël A, Boulay A, Kebers F, Kannan R, Hajitou A, Calberg-Bacq C-M, Basset P, Rio M-C, Foidart J-M (2000) Demonstration in vivo that stromelysin-3 functions through its proteolytic activity. Oncogene 19:1605–1612
67. Danø K, Behrendt N, Brünner N, Ellis V, Ploug M, Pyke C (1994) The urokinase receptor. Protein structure and role in plasminogen activation and cancer invasion. Fibrinolysis 8:189–203
68. Grégoire M, Lieubeau B (1995) The role of fibroblasts in tumor behavior. Cancer Metastasis Rev 14:339–350
69. Hanahan D, Weinberg RA (2000) The hallmarks of cancer. Cell 100:57–70
70. Coussens LM, Werb Z (2001) Inflammatory cells and cancer. Think different! J Exp Med 193:F23–26

Inhibition of the Tumor-Associated Urokinase-Type Plasminogen Activation System: Effects of High-Level Synthesis of Soluble Urokinase Receptor in Ovarian and Breast Cancer Cells In Vitro and In Vivo

Viktor Magdolen, Achim Krüger, Sumito Sato, Jutta Nagel, Stefan Sperl, Ute Reuning, Peter Rettenberger, Ulla Magdolen, Manfred Schmitt

V. Magdolen (✉)
Klinische Forschergruppe der Frauenklinik der TU München,
Klinikum rechts der Isar, Ismaninger Str. 22, 81675 Munich, Germany

Abstract

Tumor cell invasion and metastasis depend on the coordinated and temporal expression of proteolytic enzymes to degrade the surrounding extracellular matrix and of adhesion molecules to remodel cell-cell and/or cell-matrix attachments. The tumor cell-associated urokinase-type plasminogen activator system, consisting of the serine protease uPA, its substrate plasminogen, its membrane-bound receptor uPAR, as well as its inhibitors PAI-1 and PAI-2, plays an important role in these pericellular processes. Especially, association of the proteolytic activity of uPA with the cell surface via interaction with uPAR significantly increases the invasive capacity of tumor cells. Consequently, various approaches have been pursued to interfere with the expression or activity of uPA and/or uPAR, including antisense strategies and the development of active-site inhibitors of uPA or inhibitors of uPA/uPAR interaction. In this review, we focus on the results obtained in vitro and in vivo with tumor cells producing high levels of a recombinant soluble form of uPAR, which efficiently inhibits uPA binding to cell surface-associated uPAR and, by this, acts as a scavenger for uPA.

Introduction

The uPA/Plasmin System in Tumor Invasion and Metastasis

Invasion and metastasis of solid tumors are complex multi-step processes. The invasive behavior of tumor cells and their ability to form distant metastases are facilitated by means of different cell-associated proteolytic systems. In the host, the extracellular matrix provides a structural barrier for the tumor cells, and malignant cells are able to degrade proteins of the extracellular matrix, leading to local invasion of the tissue and to metastasis. Proteolysis is involved in all the steps of the metastatic cascade, namely detachment of tumor cells from the primary tumor site, intravasation, dissemination through the blood circulation or the lymphatic system, extravasation, and formation of metastases at distant sites (Schmitt et al. 1997). Various proteolytic systems, including the urokinase-type plasminogen activator (uPA) system, matrix metalloproteinases (MMPs), and cysteine proteases (cathepsin B, L), which partly interact and cooperate, contribute to the net proteolytic activity at the tumor-host-interface (Andreasen et al. 1997; Chapman et al. 1997; Noel et al. 1997; Schmitt et al. 2000). Not only the tumor cells but also stromal cells present within the surrounding tissue or extracellular matrix synthesize components of the different proteolytic systems, thus contributing to proteolysis on the surface of tumor cells (Dublin et al. 2000).

The uPA system consists of several components: the three-domain serine protease uPA of $M(r) \approx 55,000$; the three-domain receptor uPAR of $M(r) \approx 45$–$55,000$; plasminogen, the substrate for uPA which is converted to plasmin ($M(r) \approx 90,000$); and the two serine protease inhibitors (serpins) plasminogen activator inhibitor type 1 (PAI-1) and type-2 (PAI-2), both of $M(r) \approx 50,000$. uPA is secreted in its single-chain pro-enzyme form and is proteolytically converted into its active, two-chain form HMW-uPA. uPA activates plasminogen to plasmin, which cleaves a wide range of extracellular matrix proteins. Moreover, the serine protease plasmin can activate other proteases, such as MMP-2 (gelatinase A) and MMP-9 (gelatinase B) via activation of MMP-3 (stromelysin-1) (Mazzieri et al. 1997; Ramos-DeSimone et al. 1999). uPAR has been found to be a key molecule for pericellular proteolysis (Schmitt et al. 1995). Although membrane-anchored uPAR is not a prerequisite, the generation of plasmin from plasminogen is much more efficient when uPA is bound to its cell-bound receptor, since plasmin(ogen) is also bound to the cell surface (Ellis et al. 1991; Ellis 1996). This interdependence of different tumor-associated proteolytic systems demonstrates the importance of the uPA system as initiator of a cascade of protease activation events. In addition to its function in proteolysis, uPA/uPAR interaction triggers intracellular signaling events finally leading to induction of cell proliferation, adhesion, migration, chemotaxis, and angiogenesis (Resnati et al. 1996; Fischer et al. 1998; Reuning et al. 1998; Kroon et al. 1999). PAI-1 not only inhibits uPA but also modulates adhesive properties of tumor cells due to its binding to the extracellular matrix component vitronectin, which interferes with the binding of uPA/uPAR and integrins to vitronectin (Stefansson and Lawrence 1996). Thus, PAI-1 mediates the transition between adhesion and detachment, which is necessary for tumor cell migration (Lauffenburger 1996). PAI-1 has been found to be associated with tumor invasion and metastasis (Bajou et al. 1998; Andreasen et al. 2000; Bajou et al. 2001), which is also reflected by the clinical evidence that high PAI-1 levels detected in tumor tissue extracts are a strong marker for poor prognosis in breast, ovarian, esophageal, gastric, colorectal, and hepatocellular cancer (Foekens et al. 2000; Harbeck et al. 2000). PAI-2 is mainly localized intracellularly (80%). Unlike PAI-1, extracellular PAI-2 does not elicit multifunctional properties, and high levels of PAI-2 in tumor tissue correlate with good prognosis for breast cancer patients (Foekens et al. 1995).

The relevance of the plasminogen activation system in local invasion and metastasis, especially that of uPA/uPAR interaction, is well established. Clinical findings have linked overexpression of uPA, uPAR, and PAI-1 to poor prognosis in various types of cancer (Andreasen et al. 1997; Schmitt et al. 1997; Reuning et al. 1998; Fisher et al. 2000). Thus, inhibition of uPA/uPAR interaction is a valuable target for molecular therapy in cancer. In contrast to traditional cancer treatment by chemotherapy, this new approach is specifically directed against components of the uPA system. The main objective of this anti-cancer therapy is inhibition of tumor cell spread and metastasis.

Reviews discussing various therapeutic approaches against the uPA/uPAR system (active-site uPA inhibitors; uPA-derived inhibitors of uPA/uPAR-interaction; antisense strategies) have been published elsewhere (Mohanam et al. 1999; Rosenberg 2000; Schmitt et al. 2000; Muehlenweg et al. 2001; Mazar 2001; Sperl et al. 2001). In the present review, we focus on the structure and function of uPA and its receptor, and on a gene therapeutic approach to modulate tumor growth and metastasis by overexpression of a soluble form of the uPAR (suPAR). The efficacy of this approach in vitro and in vivo will be discussed.

Characteristics of uPA and Its Receptor

uPA specifically catalyzes the conversion of inactive plasminogen to the broad-spectrum protease plasmin. Like plasmin, uPA is produced as an enzymatically virtually inactive single chain proenzyme (pro-uPA) (Petersen et al. 1988), which is activated to a disulfide-linked two-chain form by cleavage of a single peptide bond. Several proteases including plasmin, cathepsins, kallikrein, thermolysin, some trypsin-like proteases, tryptase, and nerve growth factor-γ have been shown to be able to carry out this activation. The C-terminal B-chain of uPA resulting from this cleavage harbors the proteolytic activity, whereas a sequence of 13 amino acids in the N-terminal A-chain (uPA$_{19-31}$) confers binding to uPAR (Appella et al. 1987; Magdolen et al. 1996; Bürgle et al. 1997; Magdolen et al. 2001). This sequence resides within a domain (growth factor-like domain, GFD) structurally homologous to the epidermal growth factor, which together with the adjacent kringle domain is referred to as the aminoterminal fragment (ATF) of uPA.

Binding of uPA to uPAR not only generates a pericellular proteolytic system, but the surface-associated feedback activation of pro-uPA by plasmin does result in potentiation of proteolytic activity compared to activation in solution (Ellis et al. 1991; Ellis 1996). Thus, the uPA/uPAR-interaction generates a powerful cell surface-associated proteolytic system allowing cells to efficiently degrade the surrounding matrix. This matrix degradation enables tumor cells to separate from the primary tumor and spread to remote sites of the body (Andreasen et al. 1997; Reuning et al. 1998). Besides its action on plasminogen, uPA has been shown to activate the mitogenic factor HGF/scatter factor (Naldini et al. 1992) and to cleave its own receptor, uPAR (Høyer-Hansen et al. 1992, 2001). Furthermore, uPA induces cell proliferation (Fischer et al. 1998; Stepanova et al. 1999).

The uPA receptor (uPAR, CD87) is a heavily glycosylated protein that consists of three homologous repeats of approximately 90 amino acids each (Roldan et al. 1990; Casey et al. 1994). Due to the characteristic arrangement of the disulfide bridges of these repeats, uPAR is assigned to a family of homologous proteins, the Ly-6 family (Ploug and Ellis 1994). Unlike uPA, uPAR does not have a single, independent binding domain responsible for the uPA/uPAR interaction, but rather requires the complete three-domain molecule for high-affinity interaction (Ploug 1998). In addition to its uPA binding activity, uPAR has been identified as a receptor for the extracellular matrix protein vitronectin (Wei et al. 1994), an interaction that also requires the intact three-domain uPAR (Høyer-Hansen et al. 1997). Owing to its capacity to physically associate with integrins (Xue et al. 1994; Simon et al. 2000), uPAR represents an important link between pericellular proteolysis and cell adhesion. uPAR is attached to the outer leaflet of the plasma membrane via a glycosylphosphatidylinositol (GPI) lipid anchor (Ploug et al. 1991). Cleavage of this anchor by GPI-specific phospholipase D regulates uPAR cell surface expression (Wilhelm et al. 1999) and may lead to the soluble uPAR variant, which is present in different types of tumors (Pedersen et al. 1993; Brünner et al. 1999). Despite the lack of a transmembrane and cytoplasmic domain and thus precluding direct interaction with intracellular molecules, binding of uPA to uPAR has been shown to trigger intracellular signaling events (Dumler et al. 1993; Montuori et al. 2000; Kjoller and Hall 2001), imposing the requirement of transmembrane adaptor molecules such as integrins (Wei et al. 1996).

Furthermore, uPAR is rapidly endocytosed after complex formation with uPA inhibited by one of the serpins (serine protease inhibitors), plasminogen activator inhibitor type 1 (PAI-1), or protease nexin 1 (PN-1) (Conese et al. 1995). This clathrin-coated pit-coupled process is mediated by receptors of the low-density lipoprotein receptor (LDLR) family, α_2-macroglobulin receptor/low-density lipoprotein receptor-related protein (α2MR/LRP, CD91), gp330/megalin, or the very low-density lipoprotein receptor (VLDLR). Following endocytosis, the uPA/serpin complex follows the degradation pathway via lysosomes (Cubellis et al. 1990) whereas uPAR, at least partially, is recycled back to the cell surface (Nykjaer et al. 1997).

Another noteworthy property of uPAR is its chemotactic activity, which has been shown to be caused by an epitope located between its domains I and II (Fazioli et al. 1997). Either uPA binding or cleavage of uPAR after domain I can trigger this chemotactic effect (Resnati et al. 1996). Interestingly, uPAR is cleaved in this region by its ligand uPA in a reaction that depends on the presence of the GPI lipid anchor (Hoyer-Hansen et al. 2001). Thus, uPAR represents an extremely versatile molecule with its functions modified by interaction with several other molecules, including its ligand uPA.

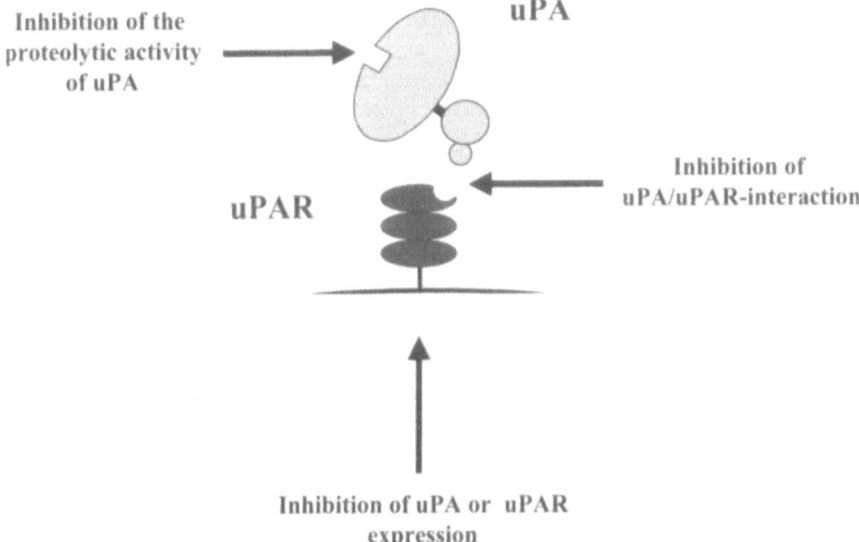

Fig. 1. Strategies to interfere with the uPA/uPAR system at the protein and mRNA/gene level. The uPA/uPAR-system serves as a novel target for the development of tumor biology-based therapeutics: (1) inhibitors of the enzymatic activity of uPA, such as naturally occurring and synthetic active-site inhibitors or antibodies to uPA; (2) inhibitors of uPA/uPAR-interaction, e.g., recombinant uPA-derivatives, synthetic peptidic or non-peptidic small molecules, and antibodies to uPA or uPAR; (3) molecules targeting the uPA or uPAR mRNA/gene such as antisense or triple helix-forming oligodeoxynucleotides, and antisense transcripts (for further details see Table 1; Muehlenweg et al. 2001; Sperl et al. 2001)

Interference with the uPA/uPAR System

Due to the complex consequences of the uPA/uPAR interaction, three targets for therapeutic intervention were identified: (1) inhibition of the catalytic activity of uPA, (2) inhibition of uPA- or uPAR expression by antisense oligodeoxynucleotides, and (3) prevention of uPA/uPAR complex formation (Fig. 1). Publications focussing on these different aspects are listed in Table 1.

Obviously, at present the main target in academia and pharmaceutical companies is the design of small molecule uPA active-site inhibitors (Rosenberg 2000; Sperl et al. 2001). Successful animal studies inhibiting tumor growth and/or metastasis employing several of these active-site uPA inhibitors have been reported. Treatment of severe combined immunodeficient (SCID) mice, inoculated with DU-145 prostate adenocarcinoma cells, with p-aminobenzamidine, a weak and rather unspecific serine protease inhibitor, significantly reduced tumor growth (Billström et al. 1995). Similar results were obtained by treatment of SCID mice with rather high doses of amiloride (200 mg/kg) (Jankun et al. 1997). The benzo[*b*]thiophen-2-carboxamidine derivative B428, which displays improved selectivity and submicromolar K_i, decreased tumor

Table 1. Selected publications describing different approaches to inhibit the uPA/uPAR-system

Inhibitors to the enzymatic activity of uPA	
Antibodies to uPA	Ossowski and Reich 1983
Substituted benzo(*b*)thiophene-2-carboxamidine	Towle et al. 1993
(B428 and B623)	Alonso et al. 1996
	Rabbani et al. 1995
	Xing et al. 1997
	Alonso et al. 1998
p-Aminobenzamidine	Billström et al. 1995
Amiloride, *p*-aminobenzamidine	Jankun et al. 1997
Amidinophenylalanine derivative (WX-UK1)	Stürzebecher et al. 1999
(4-aminomethyl)phenylguanidine derivative (WX-293)	Sperl et al. 2000
2-Naphthamidines	Nienaber et al. 2000a
Aminochinoline	Nienaber et al. 2000b
B428	Katz et al. 2000
B428, amiloride	Nienaber et al. 2000c
WX-UK1, WX-293, amiloride	Zeslawska et al. 2000
Thiophene-2-carboxamidines	Wilson et al. 2001
Indole-5-carboxamidine	Mackman et al. 2001
Antisense approaches to target the uPA/uPAR-system	
Antisense inhibition of uPA	Wilhelm et al. 1995
	Mohanam et al. 2001
Antisense inhibition of uPAR	Quattrone et al. 1995
	Mohan et al. 1999
Antisense inhibition of uPA or uPAR	Morrissey et al. 1999
Molecules interfering with uPA/uPAR interaction	
uPA-derived peptides (linear, cyclic)	Appella et al. 1987
	Magdolen et al. 1996
	Bürgle et al. 1997
	Magdolen et al. 2001; Sato et al.
	2002; Schmiedeberg et al. 2002
Peptide-derived antagonists	Goodson et al. 1994
	Ploug et al. 2001
Peptide Å6	Guo et al. 2000
	Mishima et al. 2000
Small molecules	Reviewed in Sperl et al. 2001
ATF	Rabbani et al. 1992
Inactive mutant uPA	Crowley et al. 1993
GFD-IgG conjugate	Min et al. 1996
ATF-saporin conjugate	Fabbrini et al. 2000
ATF-UTI conjugate	Kobayashi et al. 1998
ATF-albumin/adenovirus	Apparailly et al. 1998
ATF-endotoxin conjugate	Rajagopal and Kreitman 2000
Molecules interfering with uPA/uPAR interaction	
Cystatin-uPA peptide chimerae	Muehlenweg et al. 2000
Antibodies to uPA-R	Mohanam et al. 1993
	Luther et al. 1997
Recombinant uPA-R	Wilhelm et al. 1994
	Krüger et al. 2000
	Lutz et al. 2001

growth and metastasis in a syngeneic model of rat prostate cancer (Rabbani et al. 1995). These results led to growing interest in the development of more potent and selective uPA inhibitors and, in fact, modern techniques like X-ray crystallography, NMR studies, and combinatorial or parallel chemical approaches rapidly increased the number of potential lead candidates. With respect to their arginin-mimetic group, these compounds can be divided into the classes benzamidines, naphthamidines, thiophene-2-carboxamidines, amidino-benzimidazoles, phenylguanidines, guanidinoisochinolines, and aminochinolines (the latter reported to possess oral bioavailability). The amidinophenylalanine derivative WX-UK1, which, in addition to uPA also inhibits plasmin, has recently entered a phase I clinical study (www.wilex.com).

A second tumor therapy concept is targeting the expression of uPA, uPAR, or PAI-1 mRNA at the transcriptional or gene level. In an antisense approach applying an adenoviral antisense-uPAR construct (Ad-uPAR), it was reported that down-regulation of uPAR levels markedly inhibited glioma invasion in in vitro models. Injection of the Ad-uPAR construct into previously established U87-MG tumors in nude mice caused regression of these tumors, supporting the therapeutic potential of targeting the uPA/uPAR system for the treatment of gliomas and other cancers (Mohan et al. 1999).

The aminoterminal fragment of uPA (ATF) and variants thereof are effective antagonists of the uPA/uPAR interaction to prevent cell surface-directed proteolysis (Schmitt et al. 2000). In addition to ATF itself or proteolytically inactive uPA, several bifunctional chimeric protease inhibitors have been successfully tested to inhibit binding of uPA to uPAR and affect tumor growth and/or metastasis. Both a proteolytically inactive uPA variant and a uPA_{1-137}/ IgG chimera suppressed the metastatic capacity of human PC3 prostate carcinoma cells in nude mice (Crowley et al. 1993). Kobayashi et al. (1998) described a fusion protein consisting of uPA_{1-134} and domain II of the urinary trypsin inhibitor (UTI) that reduces experimental tumor invasion and metastasis. Furthermore, several cyclic peptides were derived from the uPA amino acid sequence 19–31 (Bürgle et al. 1997; Magdolen et al. 2001). The binding affinity of these peptides was further improved by substitution of a certain L-cysteine by D-cysteine and reduction of the ring size to $cyclo^{21,29}$[D-Cys^{21}]u-PA$_{21-30}$[S21C;H29C] (WX-360; Patent, WO 98/46632). Other potent uPAR-antagonizing peptides have been identified by a bacteriophage display approach and were further optimized (Goodson et al. 1994; Ploug et al. 2001). The Å6-peptide, which is derived from the non-receptor binding region of $uPA_{136-143}$ and represents a non-competitive antagonist, was recently reported to significantly inhibit tumor growth and metastasis in syngeneic and xenogeneic tumor model systems (Guo et al. 2000; Mishima et al. 2000). Beside these peptidic antagonists, other small molecules have been identified (Table 1). No in vivo data referring to these substances have been published to date, to our knowledge.

Soluble uPA Receptor

Recombinant Human uPAR From Chinese Hamster Ovary Cells

Recombinant soluble human uPAR [Chinese hamster ovary (CHO)-suPAR$_{1-277}$, comprising amino acids 1–277] has been expressed in eukaryotic CHO cells and purified from culture supernatants by ligand affinity chromatography on immobilized uPA (Wilhelm et al. 1994b; Magdolen et al. 1995). Soluble, truncated versions of uPAR have also been recombinantly produced in baculovirus-infected Sf9 insect cells (Goodson et al. 1994; Dumler et al. 1993) and display similar characteristics as CHO-suPAR$_{1-277}$ (for a summary of suPAR-characteristics and suPAR-mediated effects, see Table 2).

Soluble uPAR lacks the GPI anchor and efficiently blocks binding of uPA to cell surface-associated GPI-uPAR (Wilhelm et al. 1994b; Krüger et al. 2000; Lutz et al. 2001). It has been demonstrated that major determinants for uPA binding are located in the N-terminal domain I of uPAR: a fragment encompassing uPAR$_{1-87}$ – which results from limited digestion of uPAR – can still be cross-linked to ATF (Behrendt et al. 1991). However, uPAR$_{1-87}$ does not efficiently compete with uPA for binding to GPI-uPAR (Wilhelm et al. 1994a). In fact, high-affinity interaction with uPA is dependent on the multidomain structure of uPAR, indicating that all three protein domains are involved in the formation of a composite ligand binding site (Ploug 1998; Gårdsvoll et al. 1999; Bdeir et al. 2000; Liang et al. 2001). Therefore, in contrast to uPA-derived peptides as antagonists of uPAR (Schmitt et al. 2000; Sperl et al. 2001), it is not possible to develop uPAR-derived peptides corresponding to a continuous peptide sequence within the N-terminal domain of uPAR as an uPA-antagonist (Luther et al. 1997).

Addition of CHO-suPAR$_{1-277}$ to ovarian cancer cells, grown on fibrin gels in the presence of plasminogen, resulted in a drastic reduction of fibrin degra-

Table 2. Effects of soluble uPAR in vitro[a]

suPAR binds with high affinity to uPA
suPAR interferes with uPA binding to cell surface-associated GPI-uPAR
suPAR inhibits uPA-mediated stimulation of cell proliferation in ovarian cancer cells; no effects on cell proliferation in breast cancer cells
suPAR inhibits cell-surface-associated plasminogen activation and fibrinolytic activity
suPAR reduces the invasive capacity of cancer cells, using Matrigel as the extracellular matrix
High-level synthesis of suPAR by tumor cells does not affect endogenous GPI-uPAR or uPA synthesis, nor that of other proteolytic factors such as PAI-1 (plasminogen activator inhibitor type-1), TF (tissue factor), MMP-2, or MMP-9 (matrix metalloproteinase 2 or 9)
High-level synthesis of suPAR by tumor cells not only affects plasmin-mediated fibrin degradation but also reduces the collagenolytic activity of the tumor cells

[a] The above-described effects of suPAR were analyzed in detail by Wilhelm et al. 1994a,b; Rettenberger et al. 1995; Magdolen et al. 1995, 1996; Fischer et al. 1998; Krüger et al. 2000; Lutz et al. 2001.

dation (Lutz et al. 2001). This is very likely due to the fact that CHO-suPAR$_{1-277}$ acts as a scavenger for uPA, leading to a distinct reduction of uPA-binding to the cell surface of tumor cells and, consequently, to reduced plasminogen activation and cell surface-associated fibrinolytic capacity. Similar results have been obtained with uPA-derived peptides interfering with uPA/uPAR-interaction (Magdolen et al. 2001). In in vitro assays, using Matrigel as the extracellular matrix, the addition of CHO-suPAR$_{1-277}$ reduced the invasive capacity of these tumor cells (Wilhelm et al. 1994b). Recombinant CHO-suPAR$_{1-277}$ was also applied in an in vivo tumor model (Wilhelm et al. 1994a). For this, ovarian cancer cells (OV-MZ-6; 2×10^7 per mouse) were injected intraperitoneally together with CHO-suPAR$_{1-277}$ (200 µg/mouse). Injection of CHO-suPAR$_{1-277}$ was repeated four times (once weekly), and control mice received tumor cells only. After 5 weeks, the mice were sacrificed, tumors surgically removed, and the weight of the tumors determined. In this setting, no difference in tumor growth between treated and untreated mice was observed (Wilhelm et al. 1994a). One reason for the lack of an effect after treatment with recombinant CHO-suPAR$_{1-277}$ may be the rather large intervals between the injections of CHO-suPAR$_{1-277}$. The half-life of CHO-suPAR$_{1-277}$ in the peritoneum of nude mice has not been determined.

In addition to its effect on proteolysis, interference with uPA activation can also affect tumor cell proliferation. There is considerable evidence that uPA is a protease with growth factor-like function. However, its mitogenic activity appears to be highly cell-type restricted and cell-type specific regarding the requirement of structural elements within the uPA molecule. Whereas, for example, in epidermal, melanoma, leukemia, or breast cancer cells, both enzymatic activity of uPA and uPAR binding capacity (i.e., active full-length HMW-uPA) were required to induce a mitogenic response, in other cell systems, uPA fragments spanning the uPAR binding region may be sufficient to serve as growth-promoting molecules (Reuning et al. 1998). In fact, with ovarian cancer cells it was demonstrated that HMW-uPA (independent of its enzymatic activity) as well as ATF induced cell proliferation (Fischer et al. 1998). This uPA-mediated mitogenic effect was abrogated by CHO-suPAR$_{1-277}$ as well as by a monoclonal antibody, mAb IIIF10 (Luther et al. 1997), which efficiently blocks uPA/uPAR interaction. The role of uPA as a mitogen, mediated via binding to uPAR, makes the interference with uPA/uPAR interaction a potential target not only for the development of anti-invasive but also for anti-proliferative cancer therapy (Reuning et al. 1998).

In Vitro and In Vivo Effects of High-Level Synthesis of Recombinant suPAR in Ovarian Cancer Cells

In addition to the analysis of the effects of exogenously added recombinant purified CHO-suPAR$_{1-277}$ to human tumor cells, we also sought to test the impact of high-level synthesis of soluble uPAR (suPAR) – in addition to naturally

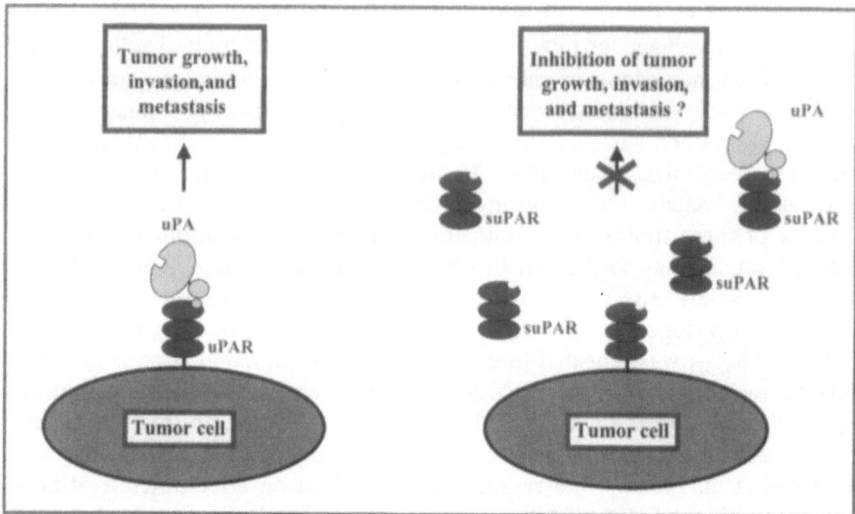

Fig. 2. Perception of the effects by high-level synthesis of suPAR by tumor cells. Focussing of active uPA to the tumor cell surface via interaction with cell membrane-anchored uPAR represents a crucial step for tumor cell proliferation, invasion, and metastasis. In in vitro and in vivo experiments, we tested whether high levels of suPAR in the tumor cell vicinity can act as a potent scavenger for uPA, thereby reducing tumor cell growth and metastasis. (Modified from Bürgle et al. 2001)

Table 3. Design of nude mouse experiments: in vivo effects of high-level synthesis of soluble uPAR by tumor cells

Ovarian cancer cell line OV-MZ-6#8	Breast cancer cell line MDA-MB-231 BAG
(Lutz et al. 2001)	(Krüger et al. 2000)
Stably transfected with an expression plasmid encoding soluble uPAR	Stably transfected with an expression plasmid encoding soluble uPAR and the bacterial *lacZ* gene
500- to 2,500-fold excess of suPAR over parental cell line	200- to 500-fold excess of suPAR over parental cell line
Injection of 4×10^7 cells into the peritoneum of nude mice	Injection of 2×10^6 cells into the mammary fat pad of nude mice
Up to 86% reduction of primary tumor growth after 42 days compared to vector-transfected parental cells	Reduction in tumor growth, reaching up to 39% after 52 days compared to parental cell-induced tumors
Smaller (and fewer) tumor cell colonies spreading across the peritoneal cavity	Injection of 2×10^6 cells into the tail vein of nude mice: suPAR-expressing tumor cells produce lower number of lung foci

expressed GPI-linked uPAR – on the malignant phenotype of the ovarian cancer cell line OV-MZ-6#8 (Fischer et al. 1998; Lutz et al. 2001) (Fig. 2; Table 3). For this, OV-MZ-6#8 cells were stably transfected with pRcRSV-derived expression plasmids encoding suPAR (amino acids 1–283), which resulted in the secretion of up to 1.6 μg of suPAR antigen per 10^6 cells into cell culture supernatants per 48 h of incubation. This corresponds to a ≈2,500-fold increase of suPAR compared to the parental cell line, which sheds small amounts of uPAR from the cell surface. In order to control for alterations in protein expression of other proteolytic factors upon transfection, the antigen contents of uPA, PAI-1, and tissue factor (the transmembrane receptor and co-factor for clotting factor VII/VIIa) were determined: no significant change in the expression levels of these proteins was detected upon transfection when compared to the parental cells. By flow cytofluorometry, we also proved that endogenous expression of GPI-anchored uPAR remained unaltered post-transfection (Table 2).

Recombinant suPAR synthesized by ovarian cancer cells was functionally active in binding uPA, since pre-incubation of suPAR-containing cell culture supernatants prevented binding of fluorescently labeled (FITC-)uPA to human uPAR-expressing U937 cells, whereas cell culture supernatants from vector-transfected clones did not. This strongly suggests the formation of a suPAR/FITC-uPA complex. In fact, the inhibitory effect of suPAR in cell culture supernatants was comparable to that elicited by purified CHO-suPAR$_{1-277}$ (Lutz et al. 2001). In line with the results obtained with CHO-suPAR$_{1-277}$, proliferation rates of ovarian cancer cell clones producing high amounts of suPAR in addition to their normal GPI-uPAR expression were significantly decreased compared to the parental cells. Furthermore, again very similar to the situation of exogenously added CHO-suPAR$_{1-277}$ to (untransfected) cancer cells, high-level synthesis of suPAR by the ovarian cancer cells provoked a drastic reduction of plasminogen activation and, in consequence, fibrin degradation when grown on a fibrin-containing matrix.

To test the effects of suPAR expression in vivo (Table 3), nude mice were inoculated intraperitoneally with suPAR-expressing (OV-suPAR) or vector control (OV-RSV) ovarian cancer cells. Injection of OV-suPAR clones resulted in a significantly reduced tumor burden compared to mice xenografted with OV-RSV cells. Regarding the tumor spread within the peritoneum, a different pattern was noted in mice inoculated with OV-suPAR and OV-RSV cells, respectively. OV-RSV cells produced a large primary tumor located below the liver and numerous clearly visible tumor cell colonies spreading over the peritoneum, mesenterium, and the diaphragm. In the case of the OV-suPAR clones, we found a significantly smaller primary tumor (reduction compared to OV-RSV-induced tumors in three different experiments (mean values, 45%, 69%, 86%) and a distinct reduction in number and size of tumor cell colonies spreading within the peritoneal cavity. Tumor tissue and blood were obtained from sacrificed mice and the uPAR antigen content was determined. High amounts of suPAR were detected in tumor tissues as well as in blood originating from mice inoculated with OV-suPAR cells, demonstrating the efficient expression of suPAR by the in vivo grafts. In mice inoculated with OV-RSV clones, very little suPAR was detected in tumor tissue (corresponding to the uPAR shed from the tumor cell-surface); no antigen was detected in blood.

In Vitro and In Vivo Effects of High-Level Synthesis of Recombinant suPAR in Breast Cancer Cells

In a parallel study on a tumor of different origin and pathogenesis, we analyzed human breast cancer cells, transfected with an expression plasmid encoding human recombinant suPAR, for primary tumor growth and experimental metastasis in vivo (Krüger et al. 2000; Fig. 2, Table 3). MDA-MB-231 BAG parental cells (which are tagged with the bacterial *lacZ*-gene) were transfected with a pcDNA3.1/hygro-derived expression plasmid encoding $suPAR_{1-283}$, and individual cell clones were isolated and tested by ELISA for suPAR secretion into cell culture supernatants. The cell clones produced variable amounts of suPAR, ranging from a 7-fold to a >500-fold excess over the parental line (clone MDA-MB-suPAR3 expressed the highest suPAR levels and secreted ≈ 1.8 µg suPAR antigen per 10^6 cells into cell culture supernatants per 24h of incubation). Secretion of uPA and gelatinases MMP-2 and MMP-9 by parental and MDA-MB-suPAR3 cells was determined by ELISA and by zymography, respectively. The levels of these proteolytic factors did not differ in the suPAR-synthesizing cells from those of the parental cell line (Table 2).

Applying a solid-phase uPA ligand-binding assay (Goretzki et al. 1997), we proved that MDA-MB-suPAR cells produced and secreted suPAR as an active, uPA-binding receptor. In contrast to the findings with stably transfected ovarian cancer cells, high-level synthesis of suPAR did not alter the cell doubling rates compared to the parental cell line. suPAR expression distinctly reduced the proteolytic activity of the breast cancer cells in vitro. Using fluorescently labeled DQ^{TM}-casein as a substrate for plasmin, an $\approx 60\%$ inhibition of the proteolytic activity of the MDA-MB-suPAR3 cells was observed in the presence of plasminogen, compared to parental cells. Interestingly, when we tested for the consequences of affecting the plasminogen activation system with suPAR on the collagenolytic activity (incubation of fluorescently labeled DQ^{TM}-collagen type IV in the presence of plasminogen), we observed an $\approx 30\%$ decrease of the collagenolytic activity of the MDA-MB-suPAR3 cells versus parental cells. This observation may be explained by the inhibition of cell surface-associated uPA-mediated plasmin generation, which results in a reduced collagen type IV-degradation by plasmin itself and/or in a reduced (direct or indirect plasmin-mediated) activation of MMP-2 and MMP-9 (Mazzieri et al. 1997).

The effect of high-level synthesis of suPAR by MDA-MB-231 BAG cells on primary tumor growth was investigated in an experimental animal model in which parental or suPAR-expressing cell lines were orthotopically injected into the mammary fat pads of nude mice (Table 3). In all cases, high-level synthesis of suPAR inhibited the orthotopic primary tumor growth. The growth

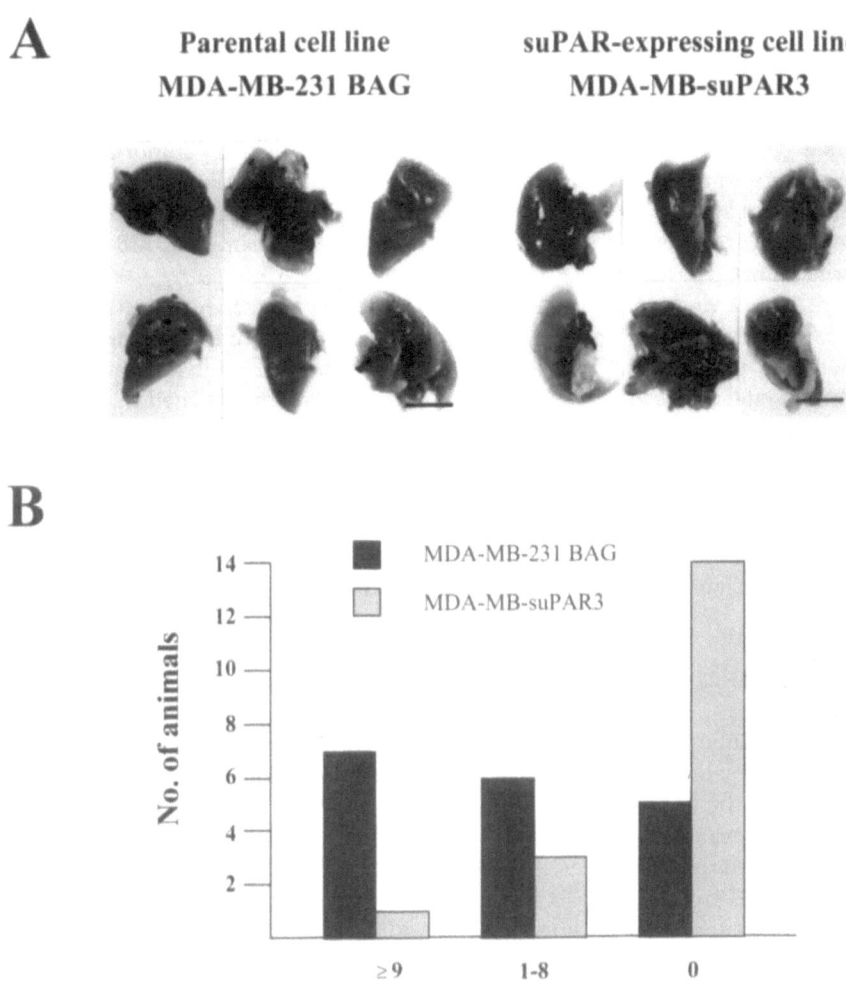

Fig. 3A, B. Effects of suPAR high-level synthesis on experimental lung metastasis.10^6 MDA-MB-231 BAG or suPAR-expressing MDA-MB-suPAR3 tumor cells were inoculated into the tail vein of nude mice to generate lung metastases (MDA-MB-231 BAG: n=18; MDA-MB-suPAR3: n=17). Fifty-two days post-inoculation, lungs were isolated and stained with X-Gal to visualize the *lacZ*-tagged tumor cells, and the metastases counted. suPAR-overexpressing tumor cells colonized the lung significantly less often than the parental cells (4/17 versus 13/18; $p<0.05$). (Krüger et al. 2000). **A** Examples of X-Gal-stained lungs of nude mice inoculated with tumor cells. Human tumor cell colonies are visible as small dark blue *spots* on the surface of some lungs. Bar, 0.5 cm. **B** Comparison of MDA-MB-suPAR3-induced lung colonization with the parental cell-line MDA-MB-231 BAG

kinetic in one of the experiments performed with MDA-MB-231 BAG and MDA-MB-suPAR3 cells was as follows: (1) after a latency period of 10 days, small tumors were palpable in all injected mice; (2) differences in primary tumor growth were visible starting at day 21 (13% reduction MDA-MB-suPAR3 versus parental cell line), reaching 30% reduction of primary tumor at day 35; (3) at the end of the experiment at day 52, MDA-MB-suPAR3-induced tumors were on the average 39% smaller compared to the MDA-MB-231 BAG-induced tumors. Highly elevated suPAR-expression was verified in MDA-MB-suPAR3-derived tumor tissue by uPAR ELISA.

In the above-described animal experiment, no spontaneous metastasis of either the parental or the suPAR-expressing cells occurred in the lung or liver. Therefore, the effect of high-level synthesis of suPAR was investigated in an experimental metastasis assay, where tumor cells were inoculated into the tail vein to generate lung colonization. Fifty-two days post-inoculation, the lungs were isolated, stained with X-Gal (to visualize the *lacZ*-tagged breast cancer cells; Fig. 3A), and metastases counted. As exemplarily depicted in Fig. 3B, MDA-MB-suPAR3 cells colonized the lung significantly less often compared to parental cells. This shows that the uPA/uPAR system is not only involved in tumor-associated proteolysis but also in cell/matrix or cell/cell interaction.

Final Remarks

The pericellular uPA/uPAR system is associated with the malignant features of a variety of solid tumors. In particular, the uPAR-mediated localization of active uPA to the tumor cell surface represents a crucial step for tumor cell proliferation, invasion, and metastasis as is evident by the inhibitory action of a series of different therapeutic molecules targeted to uPA or uPAR at the protein or mRNA/gene level. To further test the impact of tumor cell-associated uPA/uPAR-interaction on tumor progression, we sought to interfere with the uPA/uPAR-dependent tumor biological effects in human ovarian or breast cancer cells by using high-level synthesis of recombinant suPAR as a scavenger for uPA. In both model systems, we observed profound effects of suPAR not only in vitro but also in vivo, leading to a significant reduction of primary tumor growth as well as tumor spread or experimental metastasis.

In patients afflicted with cancer, a soluble form of uPAR is present in increased concentrations in plasma/serum (and tumor ascites) and is even of prognostic relevance: a significant correlation between elevated suPAR levels in blood and shorter overall survival in patients has been reported for some tumor types (Brünner et al. 2000). At first sight, this seems to be contradictory to the results obtained in the animal experiments. However, one has to take into account that increased expression of cell surface-associated, GPI-linked uPAR by tumor cells may lead to shedding of suPAR at higher frequency. This has, in fact, been observed in the blood (and ascites) of nude mice harboring uPAR-overexpressing tumors (Lutz et al. 2001). Therefore, the increase of suPAR in blood (and ascites) in patients afflicted with cancer is most likely an indirect measure for an increased GPI-uPAR expression in the tumors (and both suPAR and GPI-uPAR are increased proportionally in these patients). In contrast, in the gene therapeutical approach (Lutz et al. 2001), endogenous GPI-uPAR expression remained unaltered, i.e., the ratio of suPAR in the vicinity of the tumor cells to cell-surface GPI-uPAR was drastically increased.

The inhibitory effects of high-level synthesis of suPAR on ovarian or breast cancer cell growth and spread as well as experimental metastasis in nude mice underline the central role of the uPA/uPAR system in these tumor biological events. The therapeutic use of suPAR as a scavenger for uPA (e.g., by in vivo gene transfer by viral or non-viral delivery systems into primary tumors, tumor-adjacent stroma cells, or target organs of metastasis) may be a promising strategy for inhibiting uPA/uPAR-mediated effects in cancer.

Acknowledgements. We want to thank all of the colleagues who were involved in the studies concerning soluble uPAR, especially Rita Soeltl, Verena Lutz, and Olaf G. Wilhelm. The excellent technical assistance of Sabine Creutzburg and Katja Honert is gratefully acknowledged. Part of this work was supported by grants from the Sonderforschungsbereich 469 of the Deutsche Forschungsgemeinschaft, the Deutsche Krebshilfe (Dr. Mildred Scheel-Stiftung), and the Bundesministerium für Bildung, Wissenschaft, Forschung und Technologie/Deutsche Forschungsanstalt für Luft- und Raumfahrt e.V. (Somatic Gene Therapy).

References

Alonso DF, Farias EF, Ladeda V, Davel L, Puricelli L, Joffe EBD (1996) Effects of synthetic urokinase inhibitors on local invasion and metastasis in a murine mammary tumor model. Breast Cancer Res Tr 40:209–223

Alonso DF, Tejera AM, Farias EF, Joffe EBD, Gomez DE (1998) Inhibition of mammary tumor cell adhesion, migration, and invasion by the selective synthetic urokinase inhibitor B428. Anticancer Res 18:4499–4504

Andreasen PA, Egelund R, Petersen HH (2000) The plasminogen activation system in tumor growth, invasion, and metastasis. Cell Mol Life Sci 57:25–40

Andreasen PA, Kjøller L, Christensen L, Duffy MJ (1997) The urokinase-type plasminogen activator system in cancer metastasis, a review. Int J Cancer 72:1–22

Apparailly F, Bouquet C, Millet V, Noel D, Jacquet C, Opolon P, Perricaudet M, Sany J, Yeh P, Jorgensen C (2002) Adenovirus-mediated gene transfer of urokinase plasminogen inhibitor inhibits angiogenesis in experimental arthritis. Gene Ther 9:192–200

Appella E, Robinson EA, Ullrich SJ, Stoppelli MP, Corti A, Cassani G, Blasi F (1987) The receptor-binding sequence of urokinase. A biological function for the growth-factor module of proteases. J Biol Chem 262:4437–4440

Bajou K, Masson V, Gerard RD, Schmitt PM, Albert V, Praus M, Lund LR, Frandsen TL, Brünner N, Danø K, Fusenig NE, Weidle U, Carmeliet G, Loskutoff D, Collen D, Carmeliet P, Foidart JM, Noel A (2001) The plasminogen activator inhibitor PAI-1 controls in vivo tumor vascularization by interaction with proteases, not vitronectin. Implications for antiangiogenic strategies. J Cell Biol 152:777–784

Bajou K, Noel A, Gerard RD, Masson V, Brünner N, Holst-Hansen C, Skobe M, Fusenig NE, Carmeliet P, Collen D, Foidart JM (1998) Absence of host plasminogen activator inhibitor 1 prevents cancer invasion and vascularization. Nat Med 4:923–928

Bdeir K, Kuo A, Mazar A, Sachais BS, Xiao W, Gawlak S, Harris S, Higazi AA-R, Cines DB (2000) A region in domain II of the urokinase receptor required for urokinase binding. J Biol Chem 275:28532–28538

Behrendt N, Ploug M, Patthy L, Houen G, Blasi F, Danø K (1991) The ligand-binding domain of the cell surface receptor for urokinase-type plasminogen activator. J Biol Chem 266:7842–7847

Billström A, Hartley-Asp B, Lecander I, Batra S, Åstedt B (1995) The urokinase inhibitor p-aminobenzamidine inhibits growth of a human prostate tumor in SCID mice. Int J Cancer 61:542–547

Brünner N, Nielsen HJ, Hamers M, Cristensen IJ, Thorlacius-Ussing O, Stephens RW (1999) The urokinase plasminogen activator receptor in blood from healthy individuals and patients with cancer. APMIS 107:160–167

Bürgle M, Sperl S, Stürzebecher J, Krüger A, Schmalix W, Kessler H, Moroder L, Magdolen V, Wilhelm OG, Schmitt M (2002) The urokinase-type plasminogen activator system – a new target for tumor therapy. In: Smith HJ, Simons C (eds) Proteinase and peptidase inhibition: recent potential targets for drug development. Taylor & Francis, London and New York, pp. 231–248

Bürgle M, Koppitz M, Riemer C, Kessler H, König B, Weidle UH, Kellermann J, Lottspeich F, Graeff H, Schmitt M, Goretzki L, Reuning U, Wilhelm O, Magdolen V (1997) Inhibition of the interaction of urokinase (uPA) with its receptor (uPAR, CD87) by synthetic peptides. Biol Chem 378:231–237

Casey JR, Petranka JG, Kottra J, Fleenor DE, Rosse WF (1994) The structure of the urokinase-type plasminogen· activator receptor gene. Blood 84:1151–1156

Chapman HA, Riese RJ, Shi GP (1997) Emerging roles for cysteine proteases in human biology. Annu Rev Physiol 59:63–88

Conese M, Nykjaer A, Petersen CM, Cremona O, Pardi R, Andreasen PA, Gliemann J, Christensen EI, Blasi F (1995) Alpha-2 macroglobulin receptor/LDL receptor-related protein (LRP)-dependent internalization of the urokinase receptor. J Cell Biol 131:1609–1622

Crowley CW, Cohen RL, Lucas BK, Liu G, Shuman MA, Levinson AD (1993) Prevention of metastasis by inhibition of the urokinase receptor. Proc Natl Acad Sci USA 90:5021–5025

Cubellis MV, Wun TC, Blasi F (1990) Receptor-mediated internalization and degradation of urokinase is caused by its specific inhibitor PAI-1. EMBO J 9:1079–1085

Dublin E, Hanby A, Patel NK, Liebman R, Barnes D (2000) Immunohistochemical expression of uPA, uPAR, and PAI-1 in breast carcinoma. Fibroblastic expression has strong associations with tumor pathology. Am J Pathol 157:1219–1227

Dumler I, Petri T, Schleuning WD (1993) Interaction of urokinase-type plasminogen activator (u-PA) with its cellular receptor (u-PAR) induces phosphorylation on tyrosine of a 38 kDa protein. FEBS Lett 322:37–40

Ellis V (1996) Functional analysis of the cellular receptor for urokinase in plasminogen activation. Receptor binding has no influence on the zymogenic nature of pro-urokinase. J Biol Chem 271:14779–14784

Ellis V, Behrendt N, Danø K (1991) Plasminogen activation by receptor-bound urokinase. A kinetic study with both cell-associated and isolated receptor. J Biol Chem 266:12752–12758

Fabbrini MS, Carpani D, Soria MR, Ceriotti A (2000) Cytosolic immunization allows the expression of preATF-saporin chimeric toxin in eukaryotic cells. FASEB J 14:391–398

Fazioli F, Resnati M, Sidenius N, Higashimoto Y, Appella E, Blasi F (1997) A urokinase-sensitive region of the human urokinase receptor is responsible for its chemotactic activity. EMBO J 16:7279–7286

Fischer K, Lutz V, Wilhelm O, Schmitt M, Graeff H, Heiss P, Nishiguchi T, Harbeck N, Kessler H, Luther T, Magdolen V, Reuning U (1998) Urokinase induces proliferation of human ovarian cancer cells, characterization of structural elements required for growth factor function. FEBS Lett 438:101–105

Fisher JL, Field CL, Zhou H, Harris TL, Henderson MA, Choong PF (2000) Urokinase plasminogen activator system gene expression is increased in human breast carcinoma and its bone metastases – a comparison of normal breast tissue, non-invasive and invasive carcinoma and osseous metastases. Breast Cancer Res Treat 61:1–12

Foekens JA, Peters HA, Look MP, Portengen H, Schmitt M, Kramer MD, Brünner N, Janicke F, Meijer-van Gelder ME, Henzen-Logmans SC, van Putten WL, Klijn JG (2000) The urokinase system of plasminogen activation and prognosis in 2780 breast cancer patients. Cancer Res 60:636–643

Foekens JA, Buessecker F, Peters HA, Krainick U, van Putten WL, Look MP, Klijn JG, Kramer MD (1995) Plasminogen activator inhibitor-2, prognostic relevance in 1012 patients with primary breast cancer. Cancer Res 55:1423–1427

Gårdsvoll H, Danø K, Ploug M (1999) Mapping part of the functional epitope for ligand binding on the receptor for urokinase-type plasminogen activator by site-directed mutagenesis. J Biol Chem 274:37995–38003

Goodson RJ, Doyle MV, Kaufman SE, Rosenberg S (1994) High-affinity urokinase receptor antagonists identified with bacteriophage peptide display. Proc Natl Acad Sci USA 91:7129-71-33

Goretzki L, Bognacki J, Koppitz M, Rettenberger P, Magdolen V, Creutzburg S, Hammelburger J, Weidle UH, Wilhelm O, Kessler H, Graeff H, Schmitt M (1997) Quantitative assessment of interaction of urokinase-type plasminogen activator (uPA) and its receptor (CD87) by use of a solid-phase uPA-ligand binding assay. Fibrinol Proteol 11:11–19

Guo Y, Higazi AA, Arakelian A, Sachais BS, Cines D, Goldfarb RH, Jones TR, Kwaan H, Mazar AP, Rabbani SA (2000) A peptide derived from the nonreceptor binding region of urokinase plasminogen activator (uPA) inhibits tumor progression and angiogenesis and induces tumor cell death in vivo. FASEB J 14:1400–1410

Harbeck N, Alt U, Berger U, Kates R, Krüger A, Thomssen C, Jänicke F, Graeff H, Schmitt M (2000) Long-term follow-up with prognostic impact of PAI-1 and cathepsin D and L in primary breast cancer. Int J Biol Markers 15:79–83

Høyer-Hansen G, Pessara U, Holm A, Pass J, Weidle U, Danø K, Behrendt N (2001) Urokinase-catalysed cleavage of the urokinase receptor requires an intact glycolipid anchor. Biochem J 358:673–679

Høyer-Hansen G, Behrendt N, Ploug M, Danø K, Preissner KT (1997) The intact urokinase receptor is required for efficient vitronectin binding, receptor cleavage prevents ligand interaction. FEBS Lett 420:79–85

Høyer-Hansen G, Rønne E, Solberg H, Behrendt N, Ploug M, Lund LR, Ellis V, Danø K (1992) Urokinase plasminogen activator cleaves its cell surface receptor releasing the ligand-binding domain. J Biol Chem 267:18224–18229

Jankun J, Keck RW, Skrzypczak-Jankun E, Swiercz R (1997) Inhibitors of urokinase reduce size of prostate cancer xenografts in severe combined immunodeficient mice. Cancer Res 57:559–563

Katz BA, Mackman R, Luong C, Radika K, Martelli A, Sprengeler PA, Wang J, Chan H, Wong L (2000) Structural basis for selectivity of a small molecule, S1-binding, submicromolar inhibitor of urokinase-type plasminogen activator. Chem Biol 7:299–312

Kjøller L, Hall A (2001) Rac mediates cytoskeletal rearrangements and increased cell motility induced by urokinase-type plasminogen activator receptor binding to vitronectin. J Cell Biol 152:1145–1157

Kobayashi H, Sugino D, She MY, Ohi H, Hirashima Y, Shinohara H, Fujie M, Shibata K, Terao T (1998) A bifunctional hybrid molecule of the amino-terminal fragment of urokinase and domain II of bikunin efficiently inhibits tumor cell invasion and metastasis. Eur J Biochem 253:817–826

Kroon ME, Koolwijk P, van Goor H, Weidle UH, Collen A, van der Pluijm G, van Hinsbergh VW (1999) Role and localization of urokinase receptor in the formation of new microvascular structures in fibrin matrices. Am J Pathol 154:1731–1742

Krüger A, Soeltl R, Lutz V, Wilhelm OG, Magdolen V, Rojo EE, Hantzopoulos PA, Graeff H, Gänsbacher B, Schmitt M (2000) Reduction of breast carcinoma tumor growth and lung colonization by overexpression of the soluble urokinase-type plasminogen activator receptor (CD87). Cancer Gene Ther 7:292–299

Lauffenburger DA (1996) Cell motility. Making connections count. Nature 383:390–391

Liang OD, Chavakis T, Kanse SM, Preissner KT (2001) Ligand binding regions in the receptor for urokinase-type plasminogen activator. J Biol Chem 276:28946–28953

Luther T, Magdolen V, Albrecht S, Kasper M, Riemer C, Kessler H, Graeff H, Müller M, Schmitt M (1997) Epitope-mapped monoclonal antibodies as tools for functional and morphological analyses of the human urokinase receptor in tumor tissue. Am J Pathol 150:1231–1244

Lutz V, Reuning U, Krüger A, Luther T, Pildner von Steinburg S, Graeff H, Schmitt M, Wilhelm OG, Magdolen V. (2001) High level synthesis of recombinant soluble urokinase receptor (CD87) by ovarian cancer cells reduces intraperitoneal tumor growth and spread in nude mice. Biol Chem 382:789–798

Mackman RL, Katz BA, Breitenbucher JG, Hui HC, Verner E, Luong C, Liu L, Sprengeler PA (2001) Exploiting subsite S1 of trypsin-like serine proteases for selectivity: potent and selective inhibitors of urokinase-type plasminogen activator. J Med Chem 44:3856–3871

Magdolen V, Bürgle M, Arroyo de Prada N, Schmiedeberg N, Riemer C, Schroeck F, Kellermann J, Degitz K, Wilhelm OG, Schmitt M, Kessler H (2001) Cyclo^{19,31}[D-Cys19]-uPA$_{19-31}$ is a potent competitive antagonist of the interaction of urokinase-type plasminogen activator with its receptor (CD87). Biol Chem 382:1197–1205

Magdolen V, Rettenberger P, Koppitz M, Goretzki L, Kessler H, Weidle UH, König B, Graeff H, Schmitt M, Wilhelm O (1996) Systematic mutational analysis of the receptor-binding region of the human urokinase-type plasminogen activator. Eur J Biochem 237:743–751

Magdolen V, Rettenberger P, Lopens A, Ohi H, Lottspeich F, Kellermann J, Creutzburg S, Goretzki L, Weidle UH, Wilhelm O, Schmitt M, Graeff H (1995) Expression of the human urokinase-type plasminogen activator receptor in E. coli and Chinese hamster ovary cells: purification of the recombinant proteins and generation of polyclonal antibodies in chicken. Electrophoresis 16:813–816

Mazar AP (2001) The urokinase plasminogen activator receptor (uPAR) as a target for the diagnosis and therapy of cancer. Anticancer Drugs 12:387–400

Mazzieri R, Masiero L, Zanetta L, Monea S, Onisto M, Garbisa S, Mignatti P (1997) Control of type IV collagenase activity by components of the urokinase-plasmin system, a regulatory mechanism with cell-bound reactants. EMBO J 16:2319–2332

Min HY, Doyle LV, Vitt CR, Zandonella CL, Stratton–Thomas JR, Shuman MA, Rosenberg S (1996) Urokinase receptor antagonists inhibit angiogenesis and primary tumor growth in syngeneic mice. Cancer Res 56:2428–2433

Mishima K, Mazar AP, Gown A, Skelly M, Ji XD, Wang XD, Jones TR, Cavenee WK, Huang HJ (2000) A peptide derived from the non-receptor-binding region of urokinase plasminogen activator inhibits glioblastoma growth and angiogenesis in vivo in combination with cisplatin. Proc Natl Acad Sci USA 97:8484–849

Mohan PM, Chintala SK, Mohanam S, Kin Y, Sawaya R, Kyritsis AP, Nicolson GL, Rao JS (1999) Adenovirus-mediated delivery of antisense gene to urokinase-type plasminogen activator receptor suppresses glioma invasion and tumor growth. Cancer Res 59:3369–3373

Mohanam S, Gladson CL, Rao CN, Rao JS (1999) Biological significance of the expression of urokinase-type plasminogen activator receptors (uPARs) in brain tumors. Front Biosci 4:178–187

Mohanam S, Jasti SL, Kondraganti SR, Chandrasekar N, Kin Y, Fuller GN, Lakka SS, Kyritsis AP, Dinh DH, Olivero WC, Gujrati M, Yung WK, Rao JS (2001) Stable transfection of urokinase–type plasminogen activator antisense constructmodulates invasion of human glioblastoma cells. Clin Cancer Res 7:2519–2526

Montuori N, Salzano S, Rossi G, Ragno P (2000) Urokinase-type plasminogen activator upregulates the expression of its cellular receptor. FEBS Lett 476:166–170

Morrissey D, O'Connell J, Lynch D, O'Sullivan GC, Shanahan F, Collins JK (1999) Invasion by esophageal cancer cells: functional contribution of the urokinase plasminogen activation system, and inhibition by antisense oligonucleotides to urokinase or urokinase receptor. Clin Exp Metastasis 17:77–85

Muehlenweg B, Assfalg-Machleidt I, Parrado SG, Bürgle M, Creutzburg S, Schmitt M, Auerswald EA, Machleidt W, Magdolen V (2000). A novel type of bifunctional inhibitor directed against proteolytic activity and receptor/ligand interaction. Cystatin with a urokinase receptor binding site. J Biol Chem 275:3562–3566

Muehlenweg B, Sperl S, Magdolen V Schmitt M, Harbeck N (2001) Interference with the uro-kinase plasminogen activator system: a promising therapy concept for solid tumors. Expert Opin Biol Ther 1:683–691

Naldini L, Tamagnone L, Vigna E, Sachs M, Hartmann G, Birchmeier W, Daikuhara Y, Tsubouchi H, Blasi F, Comoglio PM (1992) Extracellular proteolytic cleavage by urokinase is required for activation of hepatocyte growth factor/scatter factor. EMBO J 11:4825–4833

Nienaber VL, Davidson D, Edalji R, Giranda VL, Klinghofer V, Henkin J, Magdalinos P, Mantei R, Merrick S, Severin JM, Smith RA, Stewart K, Walter K, Wang J, Wendt M, Weitzberg M, Zhao X, Rockway T (2000a) Structure-directed discovery of potent non-peptidic inhibitors of human urokinase that access a novel binding subsite. Struct Fold Des 8:553–563

Nienaber VL, Richardson PL, Klinghofer V, Bouska JJ, Giranda VL, Greer J (2000b) Discovering novel ligands for macromolecules using X-ray crystallographic screening. Nature Biotech 18:1105–1108

Nienaber V, Wang J, Davidson D, Henkin J (2000c) Re-engineering of human urokinase provides a system for structure-based drug design at high resolution and reveals a novel structural subsite. J Biol Chem 275:7239–7248

Noel A, Gilles C, Bajou K, Devy L, Kebers F, Lewalle JM, Maquoi E, Munaut C, Remacle A, Foidart JM (1997) Emerging roles for proteinases in cancer. Invasion Metast 17:221–239

Nykjaer A, Conese M, Christensen EI, Olson D, Cremona O, Gliemann J, Blasi F (1997) Recycling of the urokinase receptor upon internalization of the uPA/serpin complexes. EMBO J 16:2610–2620

Ossowski L, Reich E (1983) Antibodies to plasminogen activator inhibit human tumor metastasis. Cell 35:611–619

Pedersen N, Schmitt M, Ronne E, Nicoletti MI, Høyer-Hansen G, Conese M, Giavazzi R, Danø K, Kuhn W, Jänicke F, Blasi F (1993) A ligand-free, soluble urokinase receptor is present in the ascitic fluid from patients with ovarian cancer. J Clin Invest 92:2160–2167

Petersen LC, Lund LR, Nielsen LS, Danø K, Skriver L (1988) One-chain urokinase-type plasminogen activator from human sarcoma cells is a proenzyme with little or no intrinsic activity. J Biol Chem 263:11189–11195

Ploug M, Ostergaard S, Gårdsvoll H, Kovalski K, Holst-Hansen C, Holm A, Ossowski L, Danø K (2001) Peptide-derived antagonists of the urokinase receptor. Affinity maturation by combinatorial chemistry, identification of functional epitopes, and inhibitory effect on cancer cell intravasation. Biochemistry 40:12157–12168

Ploug M (1998) Identification of specific sites involved in ligand binding by photoaffinity labeling of the receptor for the urokinase-type plasminogen activator. Residues located at equivalent positions in uPAR domains I and III participate in the assembly of a composite ligand-binding site. Biochemistry 37:16494–16505

Ploug M, Ellis V (1994) Structure-function relationships in the receptor for urokinase-type plasminogen activator. Comparison to other members of the Ly-6 family and snake venom alpha-neurotoxins. FEBS Lett 349:163–168

Ploug M, Rønne E, Behrendt N, Jensen AL, Blasi F, Danø K (1991) Cellular receptor for urokinase plasminogen activator. Carboxyl-terminal processing and membrane anchoring by glycosyl-phosphatidylinositol. J Biol Chem 266:1926–1933

Quattrone A, Fibbi G, Anichini E, Pucci M, Zamperini A, Capaccioli S, Del Rosso M (1995) Reversion of the invasive phenotype of transformed human fibroblasts by anti-messenger oligonucleotide inhibition of urokinase receptor gene expression. Cancer Res 55:90–95

Rabbani SA, Mazar AP, Bernier SM, Haq M, Bolivar I, Henkin J, Goltzman D (1992) Structural requirements for the growth factor activity of the amino-terminal domain of urokinase. J Biol Chem 267:14151–14156

Rabbani SA, Harakidas P, Davidson DJ, Henkin J, Mazar AP (1995) Prevention of prostate-cancer metastasis in vivo by a novel synthetic inhibitor of urokinase-type plasminogen activator (uPA). Int J Cancer 63:840–845

Rajagopal V, Kreitman RJ (2000) Recombinant toxins that bind to the urokinase receptor are cytotoxic without requiring binding to the alpha(2)-macroglobulin receptor. J Biol Chem 275:7566–7573

Ramos-DeSimone N, Hahn-Dantona E, Sipley J, Nagase H, French DL, Quigley JP (1999) Activation of matrix metalloproteinase-9 (MMP-9) via a converging plasmin/stromelysin-1 cascade enhances tumor cell invasion. J Biol Chem 274:13066–13076

Resnati M, Guttinger M, Valcamonica S, Sidenius N, Blasi F, Fazioli F (1996) Proteolytic cleavage of the urokinase receptor substitutes for the agonist-induced chemotactic effect. EMBO J 15:1572–1582

Reuning U, Magdolen V, Wilhelm O, Fischer K, Lutz V, Graeff H, Schmitt M (1998) Multifunctional potential of the plasminogen activation system in tumor invasion and metastasis. Int J Oncol 13:893–906

Roldan AL, Cubellis MV, Masucci MT, Behrendt N, Lund LR, Danø K, Appella E, Blasi F (1990) Cloning and expression of the receptor for human urokinase plasminogen activator, a central molecule in cell surface, plasmin dependent proteolysis. EMBO J 9:467–474

Rosenberg S (2000) Modulators of the urokinase-type plasminogen activation system for cancer. Expert Opin Ther Patents 10:1843–1852

Sato S, Kopitz C, Schmalix W, Muehlenweg B, Kessler H, Schmitt M, Krüger A, Magdolen V (2002) High-affinity urokinase-derived cyclic peptides inhibiting urokinase/urokinase receptor-interaction: effects on tumor growth and spread. FEBS Lett 528:212–216

Schmiedeberg N, Schmitt M, Rölz C, Truffault V, Sukopp M, Bürgle M, Wilhelm OG, Schmalix W, Magdolen V, Kessler H (2002) Synthesis, solution structure, and biological evaluation of urokinase-type plasminogen activator (uPA)-derived receptor binding domain mimetics. J Med Chem 45:4984–4994

Schmitt M, Wilhelm OG, Reuning U, Krüger A, Harbeck N, Lengyel E, Graeff H, Gänsbacher B, Kessler H, Bürgle M, Stürzebecher J, Sperl S, Magdolen V (2000) The urokinase plasminogen activator system as a novel target for tumor therapy. Fibrinol Proteol 14:114–132

Schmitt M, Harbeck N, Thomssen C, Wilhelm O, Magdolen V, Reuning U, Ulm K, Höfler H, Jänicke F, Graeff H (1997) Clinical impact of the plasminogen activation system in tumor invasion and metastasis: prognostic relevance and target for therapy. Thromb Haemost 78:285–296

Schmitt M, Wilhelm O, Jänicke F, Magdolen V, Reuning U, Ohi H, Moniwa N, Kobayashi H, Weidle U, Graeff H (1995) Urokinase-type plasminogen activator (uPA) and its receptor (CD87), a new target in tumor invasion and metastasis. J Obstet Gyn 21:151–165

Simon DI, Wei Y, Zhang L, Rao NK, Xu H, Chen Z, Liu Q, Rosenberg S, Chapman HA (2000) Identification of a urokinase receptor-integrin interaction site. Promiscuous regulator of integrin function. J Biol Chem 275:10228–10234

Sperl S, Jacob U, Arroyo de Prada N, Stürzebecher J, Wilhelm OG, Bode W, Magdolen V, Huber R, Moroder L (2000) (4-aminomethyl)-phenylguanidine derivatives as non-peptidic highly selective inhibitors of human urokinase. X-ray crystal structure of an uPA/inhibitor complex at 1.8 Å resolution. Proc Natl Acad Sci USA 97:5113–5118

Sperl S, Mueller MM, Wilhelm OG, Schmitt M, Magdolen V, Moroder L (2001) The uPA/uPA-receptor system as a target for tumor therapy. Drug News Perspect 14:401–411

Stefansson S, Lawrence DA (1996) The serpin PAI-1 inhibits cell migration by blocking integrin alpha V beta 3 binding to vitronectin. Nature 383:441–443

Stepanova V, Mukhina S, Kohler E, Resink TJ, Erne P, Tkachuk VA (1999) Urokinase plasminogen activator induces human smooth muscle cell migration and proliferation via distinct receptor-dependent and proteolysis-dependent mechanisms. Mol Cell Biochem 195:199–206

Stürzebecher J, Vieweg H, Steinmetzer T, Schweinitz A, Stubbs MT, Renatus M, Wikström P (1999) 3-amidinophenylalanine-based inhibitors of urokinase. Bioorg Med Chem Lett 9:3147–3152

Towle MJ, Lee A, Maduakor EC, Schwartz CE, Bridges AJ, Littlefield BA (1993) Inhibition of urokinase by 4-substituted benzo[b]thiophene-2-carboxamidines: an important new class of selective synthetic urokinase inhibitor. Cancer Res 53:2553–2559

Wei Y, Lukashev M, Simon DI, Bodary SC, Rosenberg S, Doyle MV, Chapman HA (1996) Regulation of integrin function by the urokinase receptor. Science 273:1551–1555

Wei Y, Waltz DA, Rao N, Drummond RJ, Rosenberg S, Chapman HA (1994) Identification of the urokinase receptor as an adhesion receptor for vitronectin. J Biol Chem 269:32380–32388

Wilhelm O, Schmitt M, Höhl S, Senekowitsch R, Graeff H (1995) Antisense inhibition of urokinase reduces spread of human ovarian cancer in mice. Clin Exp Metastasis 13:296–302

Wilhelm OG, Wilhelm S, Escott GM, Lutz V, Magdolen V, Schmitt M, Rifkin DB, Wilson EL, Graeff H, Brunner G (1999) Cellular glycosylphosphatidylinositol-specific phospholipase D regulates urokinase receptor shedding and cell surface expression. J Cell Physiol 180:225–235

Wilhelm O, Schmitt M, Senekowitsch R, Höhl S, Wilhelm S, Will C, Rettenberger P, Reuning U, Weidle U, Magdolen V, Graeff H (1994a) The urokinase/urokinase receptor system – a new target for cancer therapy? In: Schmitt M, Graeff H, Kindermann G (eds) Prospects in diagnosis and treatment of breast cancer. Excerpta Medica 1050. Elsevier, Amsterdam, pp 145–156

Wilhelm O, Weidle UH, Höhl S, Rettenberger P, Schmitt M, Graeff H (1994b) Recombinant soluble urokinase receptor as a scavenger for urokinase–type plasminogen activator (uPA). Inhibition of proliferation and invasion of ovarian cancer cells. FEBS Lett 337:131–134

Wilson KJ, Illig CR, Subasinghe N, Hoffman JB, Rudolph MJ, Soll R, Molloy CJ, Bone R, Green D, Randall T, Zhang M, Lewandowski FA, Zhou Z, Sharp C, Maguire D, Grasberger B, DesJarlais RL, Spurlino J (2001) Synthesis of thiophene-2-carboxamidines containing 2-aminothiazoles and their biological evaluation as urokinase inhibitors. Bioorg Med Chem Lett 11:915–918

Xing RH, Mazar A, Henkin J, Rabbani SA (1997) Prevention of breast cancer growth, invasion, and metastasis by antiestrogen tamoxifen alone or in combination with urokinase inhibitor B-428. Cancer Res 57:3585–3593

Xue W, Kindzelskii AL, Todd RF III, Petty HR (1994) Physical association of complement receptor type 3 and urokinase-type plasminogen activator receptor in neutrophil membranes. J Immunol 152:4630–4640

Zeslawska E, Schweinitz A, Karcher A, Sondermann P, Sperl S, Stürzebecher J, Jacob U (2000) Crystals of the urokinase type plasminogen activator variant bc-uPA in complex with small molecule inhibitors open the way towards structure based drug design. J Mol Biol 301:465–475

Molecular Mechanisms of Carcinogenesis in Gastric Cancer

Heinz Höfler, Karl-Friedrich Becker

K.-F. Becker (✉)
Technische Universitaet Muenchen, Institut fuer Pathologie,
Klinikum rechts der Isar, Trogerstrasse 18, 81675 Munich, Germany

Abstract

The catalog of gene alterations in human cancer grows rapidly. Gastric cancer is no exception and displays gene changes in multiple oncogenes, suppressor genes, and DNA repair genes. Clinically relevant molecules whose expression or structure is altered include the plasminogen activator (uPA) and its inhibitor PAI-1 (plasminogen activator inhibitor type 1), the cell-cycle regulator cyclin E, epidermal growth factor (EGF), the apoptosis inhibitor *bcl-2*, the cell adhesion molecule E-cadherin, and the multifunctional protein beta-catenin. In addition, genetic instability is commonly seen. Gene amplification and protein overexpression of the growth factor receptors *c-erb*B2 and K-*sam* may be prognostic factors for intestinal-type and diffuse-type gastric cancer, respectively. The clinical implications of some of the recent findings for diagnosis and therapy are discussed.

Molecular Basis of Gastric Cancer

One million new patients with gastric cancer are diagnosed each year worldwide. For 1999 the World Health Organization estimated that 801,000 patients died of the disease (http://filestore.who.int/~who/whr/2000/en/pdf/AnnexTable 03.pdf). Death by neoplasms of the stomach, therefore, is the second most frequent cause for cancer-associated deaths after lung cancer (1.193 million). Gastric adenocarcinoma can be divided into two variants. Intestinal-type carcinomas, the predominant type of tumor in high-risk areas, have a glandular pattern and are usually accompanied by papillary formation or solid components. The rather large pleomorphic tumor cells have large hyperchromatic nuclei, are connected one to another, and are well polarized when lining a lumen. Precursor lesions for intestinal-type tumors include chronic gastritis, atrophy, intestinal metaplasia, and dysplasia. By contrast, the so-called diffuse-type tumors include signet-ring cell carcinomas and anaplastic adenocarcinomas, whose small and fairly uniform cells spread individually. If of a more solid cellular appearance, the individual cells are only loosely attached to each other [1]. No clear precursor lesions have been identified for this type of carcinoma, and it is thought to arise de novo from the proliferative zone of the gastric pit. The number of molecular events required to stably transmit the malignant phenotype may vary considerably between different cell populations.

Traditionally, the diagnosis and staging of gastric cancer is based on clinical-pathological criteria, including tumor size, histological type, grade, and nodal or distant metastases. Although still at an early stage, advances in the understanding of molecular pathology of gastric cancer are being made, and researchers are beginning to piece together clues of gastric cancer genetics. Recent molecular analysis indicates that alterations in the structure or function of multiple oncogenes and tumor suppressor genes, including *c-met*, *K-sam*, *erbB-2*, *bcl-2*, *p53*, *deleted in colorectal carcinoma* (*DCC*), *beta-catenin*, and *adenomatous polyposis coli* (*APC*), are involved in the pathogenesis of this disease and that different genetic pathways lead to the two variants of gastric cancer, intestinal and diffuse types. Recent reviews are available which summarize genetic defects associated with gastric carcinoma [2–9]. Deregulation of gastric cell proliferation and differentiation may be provoked by any one of a number of these catalogued gene alterations, some of which are discussed in more detail here.

Cadherin Cell Adhesion Molecules in Gastric Tumorigenesis

Cell adhesion has been implicated in tumorigenesis by virtue of the growth-controlling function of cell-to-cell contact [10]. The signal pathway mediating this process is not yet defined in all details, but both extracellular and intracellular molecules are involved. Intriguingly, both of these components have been shown to be subject to mutation or deregulation in gastric cancer. Among the different classes of molecules involved in cell-to-cell interactions, cadherins form a group of calcium-dependent transmembrane glycoproteins typically mediating homophilic and homotypic cell-to-cell adhesion [11]. The classical cadherins, including E-, N-, and P-cadherin, possess structural and functional domains that are involved in adhesive recognition, calcium binding, membrane anchoring, cytoskeletal interactions, phosphorylation, and proteolysis [12]. Based on partial extracellular sequences, the X-ray structures of various members of the cadherin superfamily have been reported [13,14]. Generally, the molecules have an immunoglobulin-like fold, and the adhesion specificity resides within the N-terminal part. One of the earliest and most extensively analyzed molecules of the cadherin superfamily is E-cadherin, a cell-surface protein preferentially expressed on epithelial cells of a variety of tissues in different species. In tissue culture experiments it has been shown that antibodies or antisense RNA against E-cadherin resulted in increased ability of cells to invade collagen gels [15]. In addition, carcinoma cell lines not expressing E-cadherin were highly invasive, whereas those expressing E-cadherin were much less invasive [16]. The high invasion potential of E-cadherin-negative carcinoma cells could be significantly reduced by transfection with E-cadherin complementary DNA. Thus, E-cadherin is considered to be encoded by an invasion suppressor gene [17].

E-cadherin has been suggested to play a major role in determining which of the two subtypes of gastric cancer develops [5, 6, 18]. Tumors tend to show a more diffuse growth pattern when E-cadherin immunoreactivity is diminished or lost; unaltered E-cadherin staining, on the other hand, may be indicative for the intestinal type [19]. This correlation was not always seen, however, suggesting that lack of mutual cohesion in diffuse-type tumors can occur even if E-cadherin immunoreactivity is present (e.g., [20]).

E-cadherin function can be altered by a variety of mechanisms, including transcriptional downregulation, promoter polymorphisms, and structural gene mutations, depending on the tumor type. To delineate the spectrum of somatic mutations in gastric carcinogenesis with regard to the two main histological types, the integrity of the E-cadherin gene in gastric cancer patients has been analyzed by several groups. Somatic E-cadherin mutations were identified in 50% of the cases with diffuse-type tumors (for a review see [21]), even in early gastric cancer [22, 23]. Interestingly, most mutations detected either directly or indirectly resulted in in-frame deletions of small portions from the E-cadherin molecule. In many patients, splice site mutations eliminating either exon 8 or 9 were found; both exons contain putative calcium-binding domains. In addition, smaller deletions or single amino acid substitutions destroying highly conserved domains expected to be critical for the adhesive function were detected. In contrast, mutations affecting the E-cadherin amino acid sequence were not identified in intestinal-type tumors.

In addition to reporting most of the E-cadherin mutations, our group determined allele-specifically the expression pattern of the E-cadherin gene in a series of gastric cancer patients. Polymorphic nucleotides in the coding sequence [21] enabled us to investigate expression of both E-cadherin alleles at the mRNA level. This approach has the advantage of directly using *expressed* sequence polymorphisms rather than polymorphic markers adjacent to the E-cadherin gene. Of 63 patients analyzed, 38 were informative (heterozygous) at known E-cadherin polymorphisms. Loss of heterozygosity at the mRNA level was seen in 42% of patients with diffuse-type tumors. We defined allelic inactivation in tumor tissues as the disappearance of mRNAs containing codon 582 or codon 692 polymorphisms that are expressed in adjacent non-tumorous tissue from the same patient. Surprisingly, 42% of informative patients with intestinal-type tumors were also found to have lost expression of one E-cadherin allele in the tumor tissues. Thus, in both diffuse-type and intestinal-type gastric cancer patients, somatic expression loss of one E-cadherin allele was frequently seen, but somatic mutations of the remaining allele were exclusively associated with diffusely invasive lesions [24]. These results suggest that E-cadherin mutations together with loss of the wild-type allele play a critical role in the pathogenesis of diffuse-type gastric carcinomas. Somatic inactivating mutations of both E-cadherin alleles are frequent only in diffuse-type gastric cancer and infiltrative lobular breast cancer; in other types of carcinomas, somatic mutations can occur but are the exception. Transcriptional downregulation correlates with the loss of or decreased E-cadherin immunoreactivity in many other tumors [21].

Clinical Implications

Understanding the structure and function of gastric cancer-associated genes is fundamental for establishing methods for tumor diagnosis prior to tumor invasion and dissemination, for quantification of an individual's risk for developing the disease, for discovering novel treatments, and for monitoring the efficacy of a therapeutic or preventive intervention.

Diagnostic Applications

The characteristic type of somatic E-cadherin mutation in diffuse-type gastric cancer (more than 70% of the mutations are complete or partial deletions of exons) might improve the information of conventional diagnostic techniques. Once frank peritoneal metastases have developed, the clinical situation has to be regarded as incurable. In addition, a positive cytology without frank peritoneal metastases has also been found to be an important clinical parameter. Therefore, considerable efforts have gone into improvements in the sensitivity of peritoneal lavage cytology, including the use of immunocytology directed at epithelial markers [25]. An extension of these efforts is the concept that reverse transcription-polymerase chain reaction (RT-PCR) for the detection of wild-type E-cadherin mRNA in lavage fluid might serve as a diagnostic test for peritoneal cell dissemination, even before tumor cells are detectable by conventional cytology [26]. However, the detection of wild-type E-cadherin may not sufficiently be tumor cell-specific. Therefore, a rapid (PCR-based) E-cadherin mutation detection technique has been established that allows positive results within 1 day. It was shown that for diffuse-type gastric carcinomas with confirmed E-cadherin mutations, identification of the abnormal molecule is a potentially valuable method for tumor cell detection in lavage specimens [27].

Therapeutic Applications

A novel therapeutic approach to treating gastric cancer using monoclonal antibody SC-1 was described in 1998 [28]. The human monoclonal antibody was isolated from a patient with signet-ring cell carcinoma and shown to react with a 50-kDa surface molecule expressed by gastric carcinoma cells. It induces apoptosis and inhibits proliferation of gastric carcinoma cells in vitro. It was demonstrated that SC-1 significantly reduced gastric cancer growth in vivo. The antibody shows no toxic cross-reactivity to other organs or tissues, even when applied in high doses. The concept of tumor-specific apoptosis induction by monoclonal antibodies may present a novel type of adjuvant cancer therapy [28].

Mutant E-cadherin is considered to be a very attractive and innovative drug target. The well known normal biological function of E-cadherin is to connect epithelial cells by calcium-dependent homophilic interactions [11]. Most of the mutations detected in the E-cadherin gene do not interrupt the translation of the mRNA (*in-frame* deletions) but result in the synthesis of a slightly shortened protein. Functional analysis of the mutations demonstrated that the alterations not only destroy the cell adhesion function of E-cadherin but also act in a *trans*-dominant-negative manner inhibiting other cell adhesion molecules, e.g. N-cadherin [29]. The mutations are exclusively seen in tumorous tissues, especially diffuse-type gastric cancer, and thus are tumor-specific. The markedly decreased cell adhesion defect is in excellent agreement with the scattered tumor growth. Expression of the mutant and functional defective E-cadherin protein may explain the discrepancy observed with the immunohistochemical analysis (see above). Furthermore, the mutations induce an altered cellular morphology and a dramatic increase in cell motility [29] that could explain the rapid spread within the stomach wall that is often seen for these very aggressive tumors. Therefore, the alterations do not simply abolish E-cadherin's function but do provide tumor cells with a growth advantage that guarantees continued expression of the mutant molecule: loosening from the neighbor cell and active invasion into other tissues. Consequently, tumor cells at distant sites, e.g., lymph node metastasis, strongly express mutant E-cadherin.

Importantly, all mutations affect the extracellular portion of the molecule, with a mutational hot spot located between extracellular domains two and three. This special type of mutation may allow the detection of the altered protein at the cell membrane and the construction of mutation-specific monoclonal antibodies. Indeed, such an E-cadherin mutation-specific monoclonal antibody is available, termed E-cadherin delta 9–1, that reacts with 13% of E-cadherin-positive diffuse-type gastric cancers [30]. More than 31 non-tumorous tissues have been analyzed using this antibody, and in none of them could mutant E-cadherin be detected. A second antibody, E-cadherin delta 8–1, has been developed recently and is currently being analyzed [31]. Since both mutation-specific monoclonal antibodies work very well with archival material, they provide an optimal means for routine diagnosis, simply by staining biopsies. Diagnosing gastric cancer histologically is usually not a problem in routine pathology; however, screening patients for these specific mutations is a prerequisite to identify patients for whom a personalized new therapy may be beneficial. Analysis of mutant E-cadherin in tissue sections from a biopsy and the statement that it is expressed or not expressed at all is much easier than to evaluate if a certain protein target (e.g., Her2/neu) is "overexpressed" or detected at the "normal" level.

After linking to plant or bacterial toxins, small molecular drugs, or radioisotopes, these conjugated antibodies could serve as highly specific means to treat small tumor deposits for adjuvant, neoadjuvant, and additive therapy. The antibodies could also be used in a gene therapy approach for the introduction of a costimulator to activate the individual's own immune system, or could be used to generate bispecific antibodies recruiting immune cells to tumor cells. Preliminary in vitro proof-of-principle results using a chemical conjugate between a modified version of *Pseudomonas* exotoxin and a mutation-specific E-cadherin antibody demonstrated selective cytotoxicity to cells expressing mutant E-cadherin. Those expressing the normal protein were not affected (Mages et al., in preparation).

In order to establish a loco-regional radioimmunotherapy, a mutation-specific E-cadherin monoclonal antibody was conjugated to the high energy transfer alpha-emitter Bi-213 and tested for its binding specificities in subcutaneous and intraperitoneal nude mouse models [32]. After intratumoral application, the Bi-213- labeled antibody was specifically retained by subcutaneous tumor cells expressing mutant E-cadherin as demonstrated by autoradiography. Following intraperitoneal injection, uptake in small peritoneal tumor nodules expressing mutant E-cadherin was 17-fold higher than in those expressing normal E-cadherin [62% injected dose per gram tissue (ID/g) vs. 3.7% ID/g].

These results show that E-cadherin mutation-specific monoclonal antibodies are attractive candidates for radioimmunotherapy of a subgroup of gastric cancer patients.

We presented here a novel concept for personalized diagnosis and therapy of gastric cancer on the basis of tumor-specific E-cadherin gene mutations that may be beneficial for approximately 250,000 gastric cancer patients per year.

References

1. Laurén P (1965) The two histological main types of gastric carcinoma: diffuse and so-called intestinal-type of carcinoma. Acta Pathol Microbiol Scand 64:31–49
2. Thompson GB, Heerden JA, Sarr MG (1993) Adenocarcinoma of the stomach: are we making progress? Lancet 342:713–718
3. Wright PA, Williams GT (1993) Molecular biology and gastric carcinoma. Gut 34:145–147
4. Tahara E (1993) Molecular mechanism of stomach carcinogenesis. J Cancer Res Clin Oncol 119:265–272
5. Tahara E (1995) Genetic alterations in human gastrointestinal cancers. Cancer 75:1410–1417
6. Correa P, Shiao Y-H (1994) Phenotypic and genotypic events in gastric carcinogenesis. Cancer Res [Suppl] 54:1941s-1943s
7. Stemmermann G, Heffelfinger SC, Noffsinger A, Hui YZ, Miller MA, Fenoglio-Preiser CM (1994) The molecular biology of esophageal and gastric cancer and their precursors oncogenes, tumor suppressor genes, and growth factors. Hum Pathol 25:968–981

8. Fuchs CS, Mayer RJ (1995) Gastric carcinoma. N Engl J Med 333:32–41
9. Werner M, Becker KF, Keller G, Hofler H (2001) Gastric adenocarcinoma pathomorphology and molecular pathology. J Cancer Res Clin Oncol 127:207–216
10. Hedrick L, Cho KR, Vogelstein B (1993) Cell adhesion molecules as tumor suppressors. Trends in Cell Biology 3:36–39
11. Takeichi M (1991) Cadherin cell adhesion receptors as a morphogenetic regulator. Science 251:1451–1457
12. Grunwald GB (1993) The structural and functional analysis of cadherin calcium-dependent cell adhesion molecules. Curr Opin Cell Biol 5:797–805
13. Shapiro L, Fannon AM, Kwong PD, Thompson A, Lehmann MS, Grubel G, Legrand JF, Als-Nielsen J, Colman DR, Hendrickson WA (1995) Structural basis of cell-cell adhesion by cadherins. Nature 374:327–337
14. Nagar B, Overduin M, Ikura M, Rini JM (1996) Structural basis of calcium-induced E-cadherin rigidification and dimerization. Nature 380:360–364
15. Behrens J, Mareel MM, Van Roy FM, Birchmeier W (1989) Dissecting tumor cell invasion epithelial cells acquire invasive properties after the loss of uvomorulin-mediated cell-cell adhesion. J Cell Biol 108:2435–2447
16. Frixen UH, Behrens J, Sachs M, Eberle G, Voss B, Warda A, Lochner D, Birchmeier W (1991) E-cadherin-mediated cell-cell adhesion prevents invasiveness of human carcinoma cells. J Cell Biol 113:173–185
17. Vleminckx K, Vakaet JL, Mareel M, Fiers W, Van Roy F (1991) Genetic manipulation of E-cadherin expression by epithelial tumor cells reveals an invasion suppressor role. Cell 66:107–119
18. Hirohashi S (1998) Inactivation of the E-cadherin-mediated cell adhesion system in human cancers. Am J Pathol 153:333–339
19. Mayer B, Johnson JP, Leitl F, Jauch KW, Heiss MM, Schildberg FW, Birchmeier W, Funke I (1993) E-cadherin expression in primary and metastatic gastric cancer down-regulation correlates with cellular dedifferention and glandular disintegration. Cancer Res 53:1690–1695
20. Shimoyama Y, Hirohashi S (1991) Expression of E- and P-cadherin in gastric carcinomas. Cancer Res 51:2185–2192
21. Berx G, Becker KF, Hofler H, van Roy F (1998) Mutations of the human E-cadherin (CDH1) gene. Hum Mutat 12:226–37
22. Becker I, Becker K-F, Röhrl MH, Minkus G, Schütze K, Höfler H (1996) Single-cell mutation analysis of tumors from stained histologic slides. Lab Invest 75:801–807
23. Muta H, Noguchi M, Kanai Y, Ochiai A, Nawata H, Hirohashi S (1996) E-cadherin gene mutations in signet ring cell carcinoma of the stomach. Jpn J Cancer Res 87:843–848
24. Becker K, Höfler H (1995) Frequent somatic allelic inactivation of the E-cadherin gene in gastric carcinomas. J Natl Cancer Inst 87:1082–1084
25. Ramaekers F, Haag D, Jap P, Vooijs PG (1984) Immunochemical demonstration of keratin and vimentin in cytologic aspirates. Acta Cytol 28:385–392
26. Ninomiya I, Yonemura Y, Endo Y (1995) Detection of E-cadherin mRNA from preoperative peritoneal cavity washings as diagnosis of peritoneal metastasis of gastric cancer. In: Nishi M, Sugano H, Takahashi T (eds) Proceedings 1st International Gastric Cancer Congress, Kyoto, Japan. Monduzzi Editore, Bologna, pp 795–799
27. Schuhmacher C, Becker KF, Reich U, Schenk U, Mueller J, Siewert JR, Hofler H (1999) Rapid detection of mutated E-cadherin in peritoneal lavage specimens from patients with diffuse-type gastric carcinoma. Diagn Mol Pathol 8:66–70
28. Vollmers HP, Zimmermann U, Krenn V, Timmermann W, Illert B, Hensel F, Hermann R, Thiede A, Wilhelm M, Ruckle-Lanz H, Reindl L, Muller-Hermelink HK (1998) Adjuvant therapy for gastric adenocarcinoma with the apoptosis-inducing human monoclonal antibody SC-1 first clinical and histopathological results. Oncol Rep 5:549–552
29. Handschuh G, Candidus S, Luber B, Reich U, Schott C, Oswald S, Becke H, Hutzler P, Birchmeier W, Hofler H, Becker KF (1999) Tumour-associated E-cadherin mutations alter cellular morphology, decreasecellular adhesion and increase cellular motility. Oncogene 18:4301–4312

30. Becker, KF, Kremmer, E, Eulitz, M, Becker, I, Handschuh, G, Schuhmacher, C, Müller, W, Gabbert, HE, Ochiai, A, Hirohashi, S, Höfler, H (1999) Analysis of E-cadherin in diffuse-type gastric cancer using a mutation-specific monoclonal antibody. Am J Pathol 155:1803–1809
31. Becker KF, Kremmer E, Eulitz M, Schulz S, Mages J, Handschuh G, Wheelock MJ, Cleton-Jansen AM, Hofler H, Becker I (2002) Functional allelic loss detected at the protein level in archival human tumors using allele-specific E-cadherin monoclonal antibodies. J Pathol 197:567–574
32. Senekowitsch-Schmidtke R, Schuhmacher C, Becker KF, Nikula TK, Seidl C, Becker I, Miederer M, Apostolidis C, Adam C, Huber R, Kremmer E, Fischer K, Schwaiger M (2001) Highly specific tumor binding of a 213Bi-labeled monoclonal antibody against mutant E-cadherin suggests its usefulness for locoregional alpha-radioimmunotherapy of diffuse-type gastric cancer. Cancer Res 61:2804–2808

Clinical Implications of Molecular Diagnosis in Hereditary Nonpolyposis Colorectal Cancer

Gabriela Möslein

G. Möslein (✉)
Department of Surgery, Heinrich-Heine University, Moorenstr. 5,
40225 Düsseldorf, Germany

Abstract

Hereditary nonpolyposis colorectal cancer (HNPCC) is a hereditary cancer predisposition accounting for approximately 1%–5% of all colorectal cancers. Clinical management of HNPCC families is most challenging due to the following factors: (1) reduced penetrance of approximately 80%; (2) predisposition to cancer of the colorectum but also of the endometrium, urinary tract and small bowel; (3) broad inter- and intrafamilial heterogeneity; and (4) highly accelerated adenoma carcinoma sequence in the colorectum. To date, HNPCC may be defined either by the so-called Amsterdam I+II criteria or by detection of a mutation in one of the mismatch repair genes. Once the positive mutation has been identified, predictive testing of at-risk family members is available. Screening recommendations for clinically identified families, mutation carriers, and their unaffected at-risk relatives must be defined for clinical management. The question of prophylactic colectomy in HNPCC is also discussed.

Introduction

Hereditary nonpolyposis colorectal cancer (HNPCC) is a frequent hereditary cancer predisposition accounting for approximately 1%–5% of all colorectal cancers. Members of families with HNPCC also have a high risk for developing tumours at extracolonic sites, especially endometrium, small bowel, stomach, and urinary tract [1, 2]. On a clinical level, identification relies on an accurate family history, since in contrast to familial adenomatous polyposis, there is no specific phenotype observed in the individual patient pinpointing towards the underlying hereditary condition. HNPCC is caused by germline mutations in DNA mismatch-repair (MMR) genes [3–6]. To date, disease-causing mutations have been identified in five different MMR genes (hMSH2, hMLH1, hPMS1, hPMS2, and hMSH6, also known as GTBP).

Clinical Criteria

The Amsterdam criteria defined in 1991 took only colorectal cancers (CRCs) into account and were therefore the early subject of controversial discussion [7]. The extended Amsterdam II criteria form a solid basis for identifying HN-PCC families.

In the Amsterdam II criteria as shown in the list below (Vasen et al. 1999), cancers of the upper urinary tract, the small intestine, and the endometrium are equally taken into account as the colorectal cancers for family risk assessment.

Amsterdam II Criteria

There should be at least three relatives with an HNPCC-associated cancer (CRC, cancer of the endometrium, small bowel, ureter, or renal pelvis); all of the following criteria should be fulfilled:

- One patient should be a first-degree relative of the other two
- At least two successive generations should be affected
- At least one CRC should be diagnosed before age 50
- Familial adenomatous polyposis should be excluded
- Tumours should be verified by pathological examination

Which Screening Protocol Is to Be Recommended for Colonic and Extracolonic Cancers?

Screening is only useful if it leads to improved survival due to early diagnosis of cancer or identification (and if possible removal) of precursor lesions. In this regard, obviously the colorectum objectively offers ideal prerequisites, since the adenoma-carcinoma sequence is the underlying pathogenetic mechanism in the majority of all cases of colorectal cancer in HNPCC families. Järvinen [8] demonstrated the value of screening for CRC at a 3-year interval, which led to a reduction of CRC of 50%. Vasen [9, 10], however, described a substantial amount of "interval" CRC in a group under surveillance. A total of 11 CRCs were observed in the screening group, and of these four were detected after a negative colonoscopy performed 1–4 years previously. He concludes that a screening interval of 1–2 years for colonoscopy seems adequate. The issue of regular colonoscopic screening affects patient compliance considerably, since bowel preparation before the actual procedure and the procedure itself

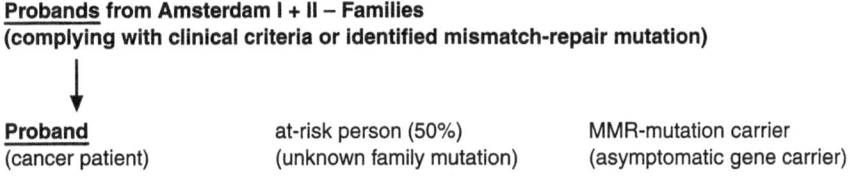

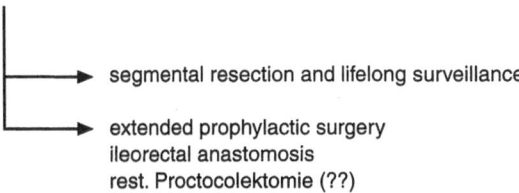

Fig. 1. Probands from Amsterdam I+II families complying with clinical criteria or identified mismatch-repair mutation

are uncomfortable. Innovative screening procedures such as virtual endoscopy and molecular genetic testing (i.e. in stool) may improve the sensitivity and specificity of less-invasive screening measures and improve patient compliance.

Surveillance of CRC in HNPCC families does not solve all screening issues. There is little debate about the timing of the first colonoscopies. However, if a family member was diagnosed with colorectal cancer or adenomas at a younger age, initiation of screening is also recommended at an earlier stage. As a general recommendation, site-specific screening is proposed 5 years before the youngest member of a family was diagnosed with cancer. Since screening protocols have reduced but not eliminated the risk of CRC and reports of advanced CRCs during screening (interval cancers) have repeatedly been reported, the question of prophylactic surgery arises. In order to address this issue, a clear differentiation must be made in regard to the families discussed and the status of family members. The first distinction must be made between families highly suspected to be HNPCC (Amsterdam I and II families) without detection of the underlying genetic cause, and families with an identified mutation in one of the mismatch-repair genes. Members of the family may then be subdivided into the different categories (see Fig. 1).

Probands may in this context primarily be defined as members of a clinically identified HNPCC family (with or without detection of a mutation in one of the mismatch-repair genes) who have been diagnosed with cancer of the colorectum. In this setting, there are two distinct management strategies: the first comprises surgery according to the well-established oncological principles, without extending the procedure to prophylactic removal of the rest of the colo(rectum). Following this strategy implies lifelong surveillance of the remaining colorectum at yearly intervals, due to the substantially high risk for

At risk persons from Amsterdam I + II – Families
(complying with clinical criteria or demonstrating mismatch-repair mutation)

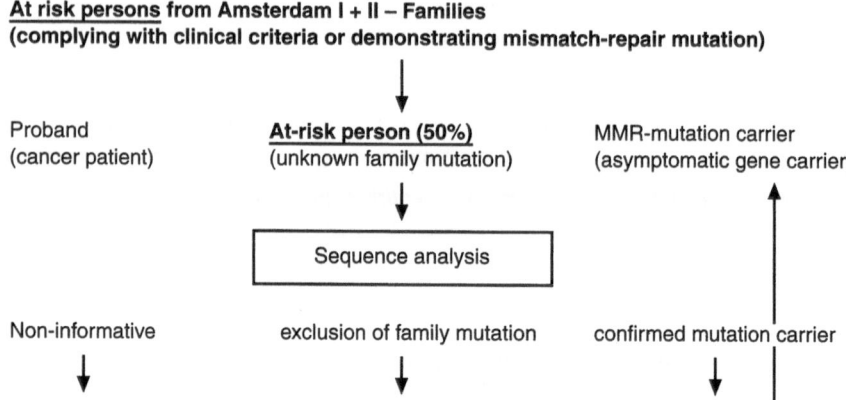

Fig. 2. At-risk persons from Amsterdam I+II families complying with clinical criteria or demonstrating mismatch-repair mutation

metachronous cancer. Alternatively, extension of the procedure may be discussed with the patient. Arguments in favour of more extensive surgery are:

- Uncertainty of a cleared colon (approx. 15%)
- Broad adenomas, de novo cancers
- Accelerated progression from adenoma to carcinoma
- Reduced patient compliance for frequent colonoscopies

At this point, however, it remains to be proven whether more extended surgery improves survival in the setting of HNPCC. The patient's quality of life in either setting must also be assessed. If regular surveillance is warranted, endoscopic colon surveillance may be equally effective, causing less perioperative morbidity (Fig. 2).

Obviously, as shown in Fig. 3, prophylactic surgery can only be discussed for organs that are not essential for survival. It is not an option for the small bowel, urinary tract, hepatobiliary tract, or pancreas, among others, that may to a lesser extent also be affected in HNPCC families.

The last group of persons to be discussed are clinically unaffected members of an HNPCC family who are identified mutation carriers. In this group, the issue of prophylactic surgery may theoretically be relevant. Prophylactic surgery would only be an option for those organs that may be functionally replaced or are not relevant for overall survival. Therefore prophylactic surgery can be discussed for the colorectum, endometrium, ovaries, and stomach. The value of prophylactic surgery must be discussed on a syndrome-specific basis, taking the general penetrance of the gene defect, site-specific risk assessment, and overall perioperative morbidity into account. Based on the literature, in HNPCC the penetrance for colorectal cancer is 68%–75% by age 65 years, for the endometrium 30%–35% by age 70 (for hMSH2 and hMLH1), and for the

Amsterdam I + II – Families
(complying with clinical criteria or demonstrating mismatch-repair mutation)

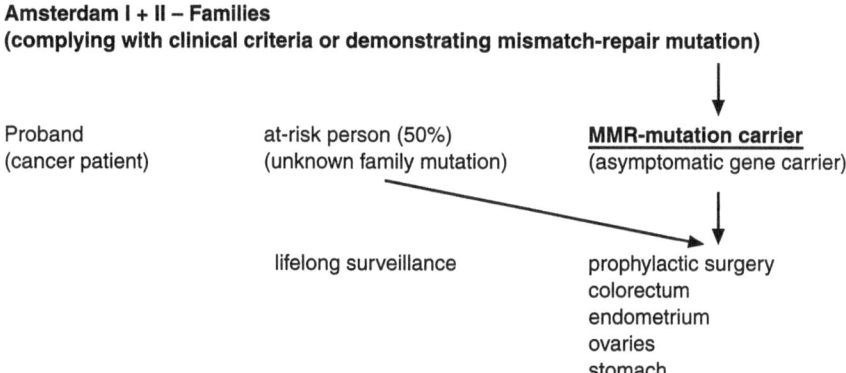

Fig. 3. Amsterdam I+II families complying with clinical criteria or demonstrating mismatch-repair mutation

ovaries less than 10% by age 70. These data suggest that prophylactic removal of the unaffected colorectum is not justified. However, when a patient in an HNPCC family develops adenomas at an early age and even more if this adenoma proves to be microsatellite instable (MSI), prophylactic colectomy is one of the treatment options to be discussed. Vasen et al. [9] calculated the effect on survival of prophylactic colectomy in 30-year-old gene carriers, using registry cases in The Netherlands and Finland. He revealed an increase in life expectancy in the two countries of 12 and 24 months, respectively. However, this datum derives from a setting that would not correspond to contemporary adapted screening strategies and therefore remains to be verified. Data regarding the risk for stomach cancer in mutation carriers are not available. Prophylactic hysterectomy and oophorectomy are commonly advised for women who have completed their reproductive activity, although there are no prospective studies available to support this recommendation.

Although identification of the mismatch-repair genes has brought the major benefit of predictive testing in families with an identified mutation, the major problems of clinical management for mutation carriers remain unsolved. The surveillance program is extensive and uncomfortable for patients. The clinical heterogeneity of the disease remains the major problem for clinical management. Identification of disease modifiers will hopefully improve individual risk assessment of mutation carriers in the near future. An intended study in Germany looking at oncological resection versus extended prophylactic resection at occurrence of colorectal cancer in HNPCC probands will hopefully make a major contribution to delineating the most beneficial concept for these patients. Quality of life assessment is an integral part of the randomised study which will begin shortly.

References

1. Lynch HT, Watson P, Lanspa SJ, Lynch JF, et al (1993) Genetics, natural history, tumor spectrum, and pathology in hereditary nonpolyposis colorectal cancer: an updated review. Gastroenterology 104:1535–49
2. Vasen HFA, Offerhaus GJA, Den Hartog Jager FCA, Menko FH, et al (1990) The tumour spectrum in hereditary nonpolyposis colorectal cancer: a study of 24 kindreds in the Netherlands. Int J Cancer 46:31–34
3. Fishel R, Lescoe MK, Rao MR, et al (1993) The human mutator gene homolog MSH2 and its association with hereditary nonpolyposis colorectal cancer. Cell 75:1027–1038
4. Bronner CE, Baker SM, Morrison PT, et al (1994) Mutation in the DNA mismatch repair gene homologue hMLH1 is associated with hereditary nonpolyposis colon cancer. Nature 368:258–261
5. Leach FS, Nicolaides NC, Papadopoulos N, et al (1993) Mutations of a mutS homolog in hereditary nonpolyposis colorectal cancer. Cell 75:1215–1225
6. Papadopoulos N, Nicolaides NC, Liu B, et al (1995) Mutations of GTBP in genetically unstable cells. Science 268:1915–1917
7. Vasen HFA, Mecklin JP, Khan PM, Lynch HT (1991) The International Collaborative Group on Hereditary Non-Polyposis Colorectal Cancer (ICG-HNPCC) Des. Colon Rectum 34:424–425
8. Järvinen HJ, Mecklin JP, Sistonen P (1995) Screening reduces colorectal cancer rates in families with hereditary nonpolyposis colorectal cancer. Gastroenterology 108:1405–141
9. Vasen HFA, Taal BG, Nagengast G, et al (1995) Hereditary nonpolyposis colorectal cancer: results of long-term surveillance in 50 families. Eur J Cancer 31A:1145–1148
10. Vasen HF, Wijnen JT, Menko FH, et al (1996) Cancer risk in families with hereditary nonpolyposis colorectal cancer diagnosed by mutation analysis. Gastroenterology 110:1020–1027

Minimal Residual Disease in Gastric Cancer

Hendrik Seeliger, Hanno Spatz, Karl-Walter Jauch

H. Seeliger (✉)
Klinik und Poliklinik für Chirurgie, Klinikum der Universität Regensburg,
93042 Regensburg, Germany

Abstract

In curatively resected gastric cancer, the incidence of distant relapse is as high as 30%. Although the most important factor contributing to the local control of the tumor is the microscopic tumor-free margin of the surgical resection, the occurrence of distant metastases is in many cases due to preoperative or perioperative tumor cell dissemination. In addition to the established TNM staging system, disseminated tumor cells may serve as independent prognostic factors influencing patient outcome after curative surgery. Basically, in gastric cancer three compartments have been identified in which single tumor cells may be shed: lymph nodes, peritoneal cavity, and bone marrow. Assessment of resected regional lymph nodes with monoclonal antibodies directed against cytokeratin antigens leads to an upstaging in comparison with conventional histology. Nodal micrometastases detected by immunohistochemistry result in an upstaging of up to 36% of patients. However, their prognostic significance remains controversial. Local dissemination of tumor cells in the peritoneal cavity determines the outcome in advanced gastric cancer and diffuse-type carcinoma. Patients with negative peritoneal washings seem to have a more favorable prognosis. Moreover, with the use of these diagnostic tools, patient subpopulations may be identified which profit from intraperitoneal therapy regimens. Diffuse hematogenous tumor cell dissemination into the bone marrow has been shown to be a prognostic factor in several studies. In our own population of 180 gastric cancer patients, bone marrow cells were screened immunohistochemically with a monoclonal antibody directed against cytokeratin 18 (CK18). In 95 patients (53%), CK2-posititve cells were detected. In a multivariate analysis, the independence of the presence of three or more disseminated tumor cells per 10^6 mononuclear cells was proven to be a prognostic factor in patients with intestinal-type tumors, pT1/2 status, and pN0 status. In conclusion, the TNM status only partially reflects the actual extent of systemic disease in patients with resected gastric cancer. The assessment of minimal residual disease is valuable in estimating the prognosis in many patients. In the future, staging systems will have to not only include TNM data but also provide specific information on biological properties of residual cancer cells in order to establish more exact prognostic estimates and provide patients with an individually tailored multimodal treatment.

Introduction

The prognosis of locally advanced gastric cancer in Western populations is poor despite radical surgical procedures and extensive lymphadenectomy. In curatively resected tumors, the incidence of distant relapse is as high as 30%. Although an important factor contributing to the local control of the tumor is the extent of the surgical resection [1], the occurrence of distant metastases is in many cases due to preoperative or perioperative tumor cell dissemination. These individual cells can be detected by immunocytochemical and molecular methods. The term "disseminated tumor cells" is used as a synonym with "minimal residual disease" herein, in concordance with most of the literature [2]. These terms should not be confused with "micrometastasis", which implies that these cells have a metastatic potential.

In addition to the established TNM staging system, disseminated tumor cells may serve as an independent factor influencing patient outcome after curative surgery. To date, neoadjuvant or adjuvant chemotherapy regimens have shown no survival benefit [3]. The concept of minimal residual disease may be a tool to identify patient subgroups who benefit from an adjuvant chemotherapy regimen. In gastric cancer, three compartments have been identified in which tumor cells are shed: the locoregional lymph nodes, the peritoneal cavity, and the bone marrow.

Lymph Node Minimal Residual Disease

Several studies have shown the prognostic benefit of D2 lymph node dissection in patients with stage II and IIIa gastric cancer. Even patients with no lymph node involvement in routine conventional histology have a significantly better survival rate when having undergone extensive lymphadenectomy [4]. These findings led to the concept of lymph node micrometastases that cannot be detected in routine H&E histology but are demonstrated with immunohistochemical methods. Using antibodies directed against tumor-associated antigens as cytokeratin polypeptides present in epithelial cells or carcinoembryonic antigen (CEA) or combinations of both, even single tumor cells or their small aggregates can be detected sensitively. In gastric cancer, several reports have shown that micrometastases are present in up to 11% of examined lymph nodes. Incorporating these data in the conventional TNM status thus results in an upstaging in 23.5% to 36% of patients node-negative by conventional histology. Linking these findings to survival data, the results are not

Table 1. Prognostic significance of lymph node micrometastases in patients with curatively resected gastric cancer detected by immunohistochemistry

Reference	n	pT Status	pN Status	Lymph nodes with micro-metastases	Patients with micro-metastases	Correlation with prognosis
Maehara 1996	34	pT1 early cancer	pN0	15/420 (3.6%)	8 (23.5%)	Yes
Ishida 1997	109	pT1-pT4	pN0-pN2	201/2446 (8%)	44 (40%)	Yes
Cai 2000	69	pT1	pN0	36/1722 (2.1%)	17 (25%)	Yes
Harrison 2000	25	pT1-pT4	pN0	24/226 (11%)	9 (36%)	Yes
Fukagawa 2001	107	pT2	pN0	87/4484 (1.9%)	38 (35.5%)	No

uniform. Several studies with limited patient numbers were able to demonstrate better overall survival data in patients with no lymph node micrometastases in univariate analysis [5–7]. In accordance, in a series of 109 patients with resected UICC stage I–IV gastric cancer, Ishida et al. reported significantly better disease-specific survival in a subgroup of patients with stage II disease without micrometastases. Analysis of the other subgroups failed to have a significant influence on survival [8]. Furthermore, no report could confirm lymph node micrometastases as an independent prognostic factor in multivariate analysis (Table 1). A recently published study of 107 Japanese patients with pT2pN0 gastric cancer who had undergone gastrectomy with D2 lymph node dissection failed to demonstrate any influence of micrometastases on tumor recurrence, overall survival, and disease-specific survival [9].

To address the issue of whether lymph node micrometastases represent an independent prognostic factor or just identify a biologically distinct group of invasive tumors being at high risk of peritoneal recurrence, the incidence of lymph node micrometastases has been correlated with biological properties of the tumor. In a study of 68 patients with pT1 tumors, the macroscopic type, vascular invasion, and microinvasion in the primary lesion deeper than the submucosal layer were shown to be independent prognostic factors in multivariate analysis, whereas lymph node involvement was not. A correlation between microinvasion and lymph node micrometastases was not found. In univariate survival analysis, both microinvasion to the muscularis propria and lymph node micrometastases correlated with significantly worse prognosis [7].

The concept of sentinel lymph node biopsy is well documented in breast cancer and malignant melanoma. Lymphatic afferents from a primary tumor drain into a first node termed the "sentinel" lymph node before spreading into the local lymphatics. Shortly, this lymph node is identified by vital dyes or radiolabeled colloid and then examined meticulously using serial sections and immunohistochemistry [10]. This concept was applied to gastric carcinoma for the first time in a recent study. This procedure may aid in detecting minimal residual disease in lymph nodes. Whether this may have an impact on clinical decision making in gastric cancer remains to be determined by further studies [11].

Peritoneal Minimal Residual Disease

The prognosis of patients with advanced diffuse-type gastric cancer correlates with peritoneal dissemination resulting in peritoneal carcinosis. The prognostic value of single tumor cells shed in the peritoneal cavity has been assessed in several studies using immunocytochemical or molecular methods [12–15]. In detecting single cancer cells, conventional cytology of peritoneal washouts has been replaced by more sensitive immunocytochemistry and molecular methods. Different panels of monoclonal antibodies have been used to stain cytospin samples of peritoneal cells. These antibodies are directed against epithelial glycoprotein surface markers to allow differentiation between tumor cells and contaminating peritoneal cells. Furthermore, antibodies against tumor epitopes such as CEA and CA 19–9 or mucin are used. In a study comparing different antibodies on the specimens, the antibodies directed against CEA and CA19–9 showed to have the highest sensitivity alone. The tumor cell detection rate was significantly increased by combining several antibodies [13].

The incidence rate of tumor cells in intraoperative peritoneal washout samples of patients with UICC stage I–IV gastric cancer is between 18% and 64% [13, 15] using immunocytology, versus 7.1%–32.9% in conventional cytology [16]. In a univariate analysis of 30 patients with curatively resected gastric cancer, positive immunocytology was significantly related to an unfavorable prognosis [16]. In this report, mean survival time was significantly increased in patients with negative cytology. Furthermore, positive cytology and immunocytology have been shown to correlate with pT and pN status (Table 2).

In another analysis of 84 patients with stage I–IV gastric cancer, a correlation of positive immunocytology with overall 4-year survival rate was elabo-

Table 2. Prognostic significance of disseminated peritoneal tumor cells. In all studies, patients with UICC stage I–IV gastric carcinoma are analyzed

Reference	n	Method	Positive patients	Statistical endpoint	Prognostic significance
Schott 1998	84	ICC	54 (64%)	4-Year survival	Yes
Vogel 2000	47	ICC	23 (49%)	Local recurrence Overall survival	Yes
Nakanishi 1999	199	RT-PCR (CEA)	60 (30%)	Peritoneal recurrence	Yes
Yonemura 2001	152	RT-PCR (MMP-7)	28 (18%)	Peritoneal recurrence	Yes

ICC, immunocytochemistry; RT-PCR, reverse transcriptase polymerase chain reaction; CEA, carcinoembryonic antigen; MMP-7, matrix-metalloproteinase-7.

rated. These data were confirmed in a subgroup analysis of patients with early (UICC stage I–II) and advanced (stages III and IV) tumors [13]. Interestingly, evaluation of tumor cells in bone marrow samples of this patient population did not show a significant prognostic influence. As an explanation, the authors discuss the hypothesis that a contact of single tumor cells with the peritoneum supports the ability to develop a full metastatic phenotype, whereas the bone marrow environment keeps them in a dormant state.

Molecular methods have recently been developed using the reverse transcriptase polymerase chain reaction (RT-PCR) technique. Nakanishi used RT-PCR analysis on peritoneal wash samples with a primer specific for CEA in 199 patients. With a detection rate of 30%, RT-PCR has been shown to be more sensitive than conventional cytology. Curatively resected patients with negative PCR had a more favorable prognosis regarding overall survival. Furthermore, a rapid method using the light cycler was developed which may have implications on patient selection for intraperitoneal chemotherapy [14]. An RT-PCR assay detecting matrix metalloproteinase-7 (MMP-7) mRNA, a specific marker of gastric carcinoma cells, in peritoneal cells, has been established by Yonemura [14]. MMP-7 and positive cytology combined in peritoneal washout were demonstrated to be an independent prognostic marker in multivariate analysis with respect to peritoneal recurrence [15].

However, despite the increased sensitivity of the immunocytological and molecular methods and the resulting prognostic implications, the issue of whether peritoneal dissemination is an independent prognostic factor or just a manifestation of advanced disease remains unanswered. Further studies must concentrate on large patient populations and multivariate analyses, and elucidate the biological properties and the metastatic potential of single peritoneal tumor cells.

Bone Marrow Minimal Residual Disease

The concept of bone marrow minimal residual disease is well characterized in esophageal, gastric, pancreatic, and colorectal cancer. Physiologically, no cells of epithelial origin are found in the bone marrow. Due to the intensive contact of blood cells with the interstitial sinusoids in the bone marrow, tumor cells are extravasated into this compartment after surviving the high cell turnover during the passage through the circulation.

The harvest of bone marrow cells is a safe, easy, reproducible, and well-tolerated procedure that can be used intraoperatively as well as in local anesthesia on an outpatient basis for follow-up aspirations. A disadvantage of bone marrow needle aspiration in comparison with bone marrow harvested by rib resection is a significantly lower yield of disseminated tumor cells [17]. Using conventional cytopathological stains, cells of epithelial origin can be detected in bone marrow aspirates; however, sensitivity and specificity are low. Hence, immunocytochemical and molecular methods have been established to identify disseminated tumor cells in the bone marrow. In most cases, monoclonal

Table 3. Incidence and prognostic significance of bone marrow disseminated tumor cells

Reference	Antigens detected	Cell number	Detection rate	Prognostic significance
Juhl 1995	KL-1, CA 19–9, 17–1A, C1P83, CEA, C-54–0, Ra96	250,000	9/36 (25%)	Not significant
Heiss 1995	CK-18, uPA-R	1,000,000	47/78 (60%)	Disease-free survival
Jauch 1996	CK-18	1,000,000	95/180 (53%)	Disease-free survival Overall survival
Funke 1996	CK-18 E-cadherin	1,000,000	45/102 (44%)	n.d.
Regensburg	CK-18	2,000,000	54/104 (52%)	Not significant

antibodies against cytokeratin components of the tumor cells are used, e.g., CK2, which is directed against the intracellular cytokeratin component 18 [18, 19]. Other researchers have used different antibodies against membrane-bound mucins, tumor-associated glycoproteins, or adhesion molecules [20, 21]. With these techniques, one tumor cell can be detected among 10^5–10^6 mononuclear bone marrow cells [22].

In addition to immunocytochemical methods, some recent studies have used immunomagnetic techniques to detect disseminated epithelial cells with high sensitivity.

An even higher sensitivity can be achieved using PCR to detect mutations on the DNA level (e.g., K-ras or p53 mutations [23]) or the expression of marker genes on the mRNA level by RT-PCR. The sensitivity of these molecular methods has been determined with a yield of one tumor cell among 10^7 mononuclear cells.

The malignancy of epithelial cells in the bone marrow has been studied extensively using immunocytochemical double staining for cytokeratin components and tumor-associated antigens as well as molecular methods such as RT-PCR and fluorescent in situ hybridization (FISH). With these techniques, tumor-associated characteristics of the cells have been demonstrated, e.g., the expression of Lewis-Y blood group precursor antigens and p53, the overexpression of the erb-B2 oncogene, numerical chromosome aberrations, and the expression of genes of the MAGE family [22].

Another important approach has been the immunocytological assessment of the expression of members of the urokinase-type plasminogen activator (uPA) system in disseminated bone marrow cells. In contrast to most tumor-associated antigens, the uPA system represents a measure of the biological aggressiveness of the tumor cells by characterizing their proteolytic potential [18].

In gastric cancer, the detection rate of disseminated tumor cells in the bone marrow of patients with a curatively resected tumor varies between 25% and 60% [18, 19]. In univariate analyses considering the prognosis in correlation with bone marrow dissemination, results are heterogeneous (Table 3). In a study of 36 patients, the presence of bone marrow epithelial cells failed to show significant prognostic relevance [21]. Our own data, reported in 1996, showed a prevalence of disseminated tumor cells in the bone marrow of 53% of 180 patients with UICC stage I–IV gastric cancer. In 109 of these patients, a curative resection was performed. In that study, disseminated cells were assessed semiquantitatively and correlated with disease-free survival, overall survival, and established clinicopathological parameters such as pT status and Borrmann's classification. A multivariate subgroup analysis of the curatively resected patients showed disseminated tumor cells in the bone marrow to be a significant independent prognostic factors in patients with intestinal-type tumors, in earlier disease stages (pT1 and pT2), and in nodal-negative disease [19].

The prognostic relevance of the uPA system in patients with gastric cancer was demonstrated by Heiss et al. In 203 patients, the expression of uPA, its receptor (uPA-R), its activators and inhibitors, substrates, and other parameters of the uPA-R cycle on bone marrow disseminated cells was analyzed. In that study, a multivariate risk factor analysis showed an independent prognostic influence on disease-free survival of plasminogen activator inhibitor type 1 (PAI-1) and the uPA activator cathepsin D expression. Interestingly, a subgroup of nodal negative pT1/pT2 patients with bone marrow tumor cells and high PAI-1 expression was identified, which had a worse prognosis than nodal-positive pT1/pT2 patients [18].

The same group assessed the question of whether there is an influence of the kinetics of repeat biopsies on prognosis. In 78 curatively resected patients, a favorable prognosis was shown in the group with negative follow-up biopsies regardless of a positive intraoperative biopsy [18, 24, 25].

Although there is evidence that bone marrow disseminated tumor cells seem to correlate with the patient outcome after curative resection and may even be an independent prognostic factor, the biological relevance of the disseminated cells and cell clusters has not been clearly characterized. As the incidence of clinically relevant bone metastases in gastric cancer is low, these cells seem not to be a precursor lesion of manifest metastases. The tumor cells in the bone marrow seem to remain in a dormant state of mitotic inactivity, resulting in low expression of proliferation markers such as Ki-67 and p120 [22]. Interestingly, in early gastric cancer, a correlation was found between disseminated tumor cells in the bone marrow and microvessel density in the primary tumor as a determinant for the angiogenic and metastatic potential of the tumor [26]. However, the network of local environmental factors, adhesion molecules, growth factors and their receptors, angiogenetic properties of the primary tumor, and the regulation of the host immune response to the tumor cells resulting in the growth of metastasis, has yet to be characterized in detail.

Outlook and Conclusion

The TNM status in gastric cancer only partially reflects the actual extent of systemic disease in patients with resected gastric cancer. The assessment of minimal residual disease is valuable in estimating the prognosis in many patients. Whether there are subgroups who benefit from additional therapeutic regimens remains to be elucidated. Immunocytochemistry and molecular methods have been shown to be powerful tools to detect occult micrometastases. Further efforts must focus on standardization and quantification of these methods. To elaborate the biological behavior and the aggressiveness of disseminated cells, new molecular markers must be established on the single-cell level. To support the prognostic data on minimal residual disease which have been reported to date, multivariate analyses of large patient groups are essential. In the future, staging systems will have to not only include TNM data but also provide information concerning minimal residual disease with specific information on the biological behavior of disseminated cells, to establish more exact prognostic estimates and individually tailored multimodal treatment.

References

1. Doglietto GB, Pacelli F, Caprino P, Sgadari A, Crucitti F (2000) Surgery: independent prognostic factor in curable and far advanced gastric cancer. World J Surg 24 4:459–463
2. Müller P, Schlimok G (2000) Bone marrow "micrometastases" of epithelial tumors: detection and clinical relevance. J Cancer Res Clin Oncol 126:607–618
3. Schmid A, Kremer B (2000) Chirurgische Prinzipien beim Magencarcinom. Chirurg 71 8:974–986
4. Siewert JR, Kestlmeier R, Busch R, et al (1996) Benefits of D2 lymph node dissection for patients with gastric cancer and pN0 and pN1 lymph node metastases. Br J Surg 83:1144–1147
5. Harrison LE, Choe JK, Goldstein M, Meridian A, Kim SH, Clarke K (2000) Prognostic significance of immunohistochemical micrometastases in node negative gastric cancer patients. J Surg Oncol 73:153–157
6. Maehara Y, Oshiro T, Endo K, et al (1996) Clinical significance of occult micrometastasis lymph nodes from patients with early gastric cancer who died of recurrence. Surgery 119:397–402
7. Cai J, Ikeguchi M, Maeta M, Kaibara N (2000) Micrometastasis in lymph nodes and microinvasion of the muscularis propria in primary lesions of submucosal gastric cancer. Surgery 127:32–39
8. Ishida K, Katsuyama T, Sugiyama A, Kawasaki S (1997) Immunohistochemical evaluation of lymph node micrometastases from gastric carcinomas. Cancer 79:1069–1076
9. Fukagawa T, Sasako M, Mann GB, et al (2001) Immunohistochemically detected micrometastases of the lymph nodes in patients with gastric carcinoma. Cancer 92:753–760
10. Kell MR, Winter DC, O'Sullivan GC, Shanahan F, Redmond HP (2000) Biological behaviour and clinical implications of micrometastases. Br J Surg 87:1629–1639
11. Vogel P, Rüschoff J, Kümmel S, et al (1999) Immunocytology improves prognostic impact of peritoneal tumour cell detection compared to conventional cytology in gastric cancer. Eur J Surg Oncol 25:515–519

12. Schott A, Vogel I, Krueger U, et al (1998) Isolated tumor cells are frequently detectable in the peritoneal cavity of gastric and colorectal cancer patients and serve as a new prognostic marker. Ann Surg 227:372–379

13. Nakanishi H, Kodera Y, Yamamura Y, et al (1999) Molecular diagnostic detection of free cancer cells in the peritoneal cavity of patients with gastrointestinal and gynecologic malignancies. Cancer Chemother Pharmacol 43 [Suppl]:S32–S36

14. Yonemura Y, Fujimura T, Ninomiya I, et al (2001) Prediction of peritoneal micrometastasis by peritoneal lavaged cytology and reverse transcriptase-polymerase chain reaction for matrix metalloproteinase-7 mRNA. Clin Cancer Res 7:1647–1653

15. Vogel P, Rüschoff J, Kümmel S, et al (2000) Prognostic value of microscopic peritoneal dissemination: comparison between colon and gastric cancer. Dis Colon Rectum 43:92–100

16. Bonavina L, Soligo D, Quirici N, et al (2001) Bone marrow-disseminated tumor cells in patients with carcinoma of the esophagus or cardia. Surgery 129:15–22

17. Heiss MM, Allgayer H, Gruetzner KU, Babic R, Jauch KW, Schildberg FW (1997) Clinical value of extended biologic staging by bone marrow micrometastases and tumor-associated proteases in gastric cancer. Ann Surg 226:736–744

18. Jauch KW, Heiss MM, Gruetzner U, et al (1996) Prognostic significance of bone marrow micrometastases in patients with gastric cancer. J Clin Oncol 14:1810–1817

19. Funke I, Fries S, Rolle M, et al (1996) Comparative analyses of bone marrow micrometastases in breast and gastric cancer. Int J Cancer 65:755–761

20. Juhl H, Kalthoff H, Krüger U, Henne-Bruns D, Kremer B (1995) Immunzytologischer Nachweis mikrometastatischer Zellen bei Patienten mit gastrointestinalen Tumoren. Zentralbl Chir 120:116–122

21. Spatz H, Kerner T, Vogel P, Fürst A, Dietmaier W, Jauch KW (2000) Tumorzelldissemination und Metastasierung beim gastrointestinalen Karzinom: Mechanismen, Nachweis und Bedeutung. Viszeralchirurgie 35:375–384

22. Kerner T, Hauzenberger T, Jauch KW (1998) Nachweis und Bedeutung der Tumorzelldissemination beim Magenkarzinom. Onkologe 4:294–300

23. Heiss MM, Allgayer H, Gruetzner KU, et al (1995) Individual development and uPA-receptor expression of disseminated tumour cells in bone marrow: a reference to early systemic disease in solid cancer. Nat Med 1:1035–1039

24. Allgayer H, Heiss MM, Riesenberg R, et al (1997) Urokinase plasminogen activator receptor (uPA-R): one potential characteristic of metastatic phenotypes in minimal residual tumor disease. Cancer Res 57:1394–1399

25. Maehara Y, Hasuda S, Abe T, et al (1998) Tumor angiogenesis and micrometastasis in bone marrow of patients with early gastric cancer. Clin Cancer Res 4:2129–2134

Minimal Residual Disease in Breast Cancer and Gynecological Malignancies: Phenotype and Clinical Relevance

Frigga Roggel, Stefan Hocke, Kristina Lindemann, Sonja Sinz, Anita Welk, Martin Bosl, Martina Pabst, N. Nusser, Stephan Braun, Manfred Schmitt, Nadia Harbeck

F.R. and S.H. contributed equally to this work.

N. Harbeck (✉)
Klinische Forschergruppe der Frauenklinik,
Technische Universität München,
Ismaninger Straße 22, 81675 Munich, Germany

Abstract

In breast cancer, about 35% of patients without any clinical signs of overt distant metastases already have disseminated tumor cells in bone marrow aspirates at the time of primary therapy. A significant prognostic impact of these disseminated tumor cells has been shown by many international studies: patients with tumor cells in their bone marrow have a significantly worse prognosis than those without them. Even in malignancies where the skeletal system is not a preferred location for distant metastasis, such as ovarian cancer, early presence of minimal residual disease (MRD) is correlated with poor patient outcome. Thus, besides analysis of the primary tumor, detection of MRD can be used for assessment of patient prognosis and for prediction or monitoring of response to systemic therapy. Disseminated tumor cells are also the targets for novel tumor biological therapy approaches such as specific antibody-based therapies against target cell-surface antigens such as HER2, Ep-CAM (17–1A), and uPA-R. In breast cancer, a first antibody-based tumor therapy against HER2 (Herceptin) has already been approved for clinical use in recurrent disease. However, patient selection for such tumor biological therapies becomes rather difficult due to phenotype changes, which may manifest themselves as differences between primary lesion and disseminated tumor cells. Therefore, not only identification of disseminated tumor cells but even more so their characterization at the protein and gene levels have become increasingly important. In conclusion, characterization of tumor biological properties of disseminated tumor cells allows identification of patients with breast cancer or gynecological malignancies at risk for relapse who are likely to benefit from systemic treatment and/or novel tumor biological therapy approaches.

Abbreviations. BM, bone marrow; CK cytokeratin; DFS, disease-free survival; DDFS, distant disease-free survival; ICC, immunocytochemistry; IF, immunofluorescence; HD-CTX, high-dose chemotherapy; IHC, immunohistochemistry; LN, lymph nodes; MRD, minimal residual disease; n.r., not reported; n.s. not significant; PB, peripheral blood; (RT)-PCR, (reverse-transcriptase) polymerase chain reaction; OS, overall survival.

History and Detection Techniques

Early systemic dissemination of cancer cells in patients who are apparently metastasis-free as assessed by appropriate clinical, laboratory, and X-ray examinations constitutes the cause of later symptomatic systemic spread. Thus, a thorough understanding of the clinical relevance and biological properties of these cells is a prerequisite for their successful therapeutic elimination.

First research on disseminated tumor cells was performed on bone marrow samples in breast cancer – a malignancy which preferentially spreads to bone. Using conventional histology, Ridell and Landys (1979) detected tumor cell infiltration in only 4% of bone marrow biopsies in primary breast cancer. Researchers from the London Ludwig Institute were able to raise this percentage to more than 20% using first a polyclonal antiserum and later a monoclonal antibody against epithelial membrane antigen (EMA), a cell surface mucin (Dearnaley et al. 1981; Redding et al. 1983).

Reports of unspecific staining of hematopoietic cells such as plasma cells by anti-EMA or other anti-mucin antibodies (Heyderman and McCartney 1985; Brugger et al. 1999) motivated the search for more tumor cell-specific antibodies. Schlimok and coworkers (1987) were the first to use an anti-cytokeratin antibody (CK2 against cytokeratin 18) for detection of epithelial tumor cells in bone marrow, a mesenchymal organ. More recently, a pan-cytokeratin antibody, mAB A45-B/B3 directed against cytokeratins 8/18/19, showed a very low false positive rate (Braun et al. 2000b), and thus seems to be preferable.

Two aspiration sites and subsequent examination of 2×10^6 bone marrow cells are minimal requirements for a standardized methodology. Enrichment of mononuclear cells is performed using density gradient centrifugation. Immunomagnetic enrichment seems to enable higher detection rates and recovery of more tumor cell aggregates (Otte et al. 2000). The detection limit of the immunocytochemical methods is about 1 in 10^5–10^6 cells – independent of the primary antibody used (Osborne et al. 1991; Braun and Pantel 1998). Due to endogenous bone marrow peroxidase, most groups use an alkaline phosphatase-based visualization system.

Currently, detection of disseminated tumor cells in bone marrow or other organ systems cannot be used as a routine diagnostic test for patient management. International efforts regarding standardization and quality control need to be reinforced. In conjunction with a standardized immunocytochemical method, standardized and reproducible morphological and cytological criteria need to be applied (Borgen et al. 1999). Close interdisciplinary collaboration among basic researchers, pathologists, cytologists, and clinicians is mandatory with regard to the increasing clinical relevance of the test results. Automated evaluation systems that allow rapid and reproducible processing of large sample numbers are a promising step towards quality assurance (e.g., ACIS, ChromaVision Medical Systems Inc., San Juan Capistrano, Calif., USA; MDS, Applied Imaging Ltd., Newcastle, UK). In view of the low frequency of disseminated tumor cells, new detection techniques that offer higher sensitivity and/or easier processing of larger sample volumes offer a considerable advantage. Unfortunately, flow cytometry has not been an improvement due to the low number of tumor cells per sample (Molino et al. 1991). PCR techniques are still very promising – yet, the lack of suitable marker antigens limits their clinical usefulness so far (Braun and Pantel 1998).

Minimal Residual Disease in Breast Cancer

In breast cancer, most groups have looked at the dissemination of tumor cells into the bone marrow. More recently, detection of single tumor cells in lymph nodes has gained clinical interest due to evaluation of sentinel lymph nodes (Kowolik et al. 2000). However, the clinical relevance of single tumor cells in axillary lymph nodes is still under investigation (Wong et al. 2001). Only a weak correlation exists between the presence of disseminated tumor cells in

Table 1. Prognostic impact of immunocytochemically detected disseminated tumor cells in bone marrow aspirates of patients with primary breast cancer

First author (year)	Antigen	Detection rate	Number of patients	Follow-up Median (months)	Prognostic relevance All patients	Node-negative
Salvadori (1990)[a]	MBrl	17%	121	48	No	n.r.
Cote (1991)	C26, T16, AE-1	37%	49	30	Yes[b]	n.r.
Harbeck (1994)	EMA, CAM 5.2	38%	100	34	Yes[b]	Yes[c]
Diel (1996)	2E11 (anti-TAG12)	43%	727	36	Yes[b]	Yes
Landys (1998)[a]	AE1-AE3, KL1, CAM 5.2	13%	128	240	Yes[b]	n.r.
Mansi (1999)	EMA	25%	350	150	Yes[c]	Yes
Molino (1999)	MBr1, MOV8/16, MluC1	31%	125	48	No	n.r.
Braun (2000b)	CK 8/18/19	36%	552	38	Yes[b]	Yes[b]
Gerber (2001)[d]	CK 8/18/19	31%	484	54	Yes[b]	Yes[b]
Gebauer (2001)	CK, EMA	42%	393	75	Yes[b]	n.r.
Funke (2001)	CK18	27%	1045	52	Yes[b]	n.r.

[a] Used bone marrow biopsies.
[b] Prognostic significance confirmed by multivariate analysis.
[c] Prognostic significance only in univariate analysis.
[d] Analyzed occult tumor cells in bone marrow and/or axillary lymph nodes.

bone marrow and axillary lymph nodes (Braun et al. 2001a; Gerber et al. 2001), thus suggesting independent occurrence of early hematogenous and lymphatic spread.

So far, data of bone marrow aspirations from more than 4,000 patients with primary breast cancer have been published, comprising median follow-up periods of up to 12 years (see Table 1; reviewed extensively in Braun et al. 2002). Most authors report that presence of disseminated tumor cells in bone marrow aspirates is a significant prognostic factor for patient prognosis. Yet, considerable variability of detection methods, particularly with regard to the primary antibodies used, as well as the lack of thorough subgroup analyses renders direct comparison of the published evidence rather difficult. None of the research groups reported any serious complications due to the aspiration procedure. The detection rate increases with the number of aspiration sites (Coombes et al. 1983). Timing of the bone marrow aspiration before or after primary surgery did not significantly impact on detection rates thus rendering surgical manipulation as the sole cause of the presence of disseminated tumor cells rather unlikely (Salvadori et al. 1990; Diel et al. 1992; Pantel et al. 1994).

Minimal Residual Disease in Gynecological Malignancies

In gynecological malignancies, such as ovarian, cervical or endometrial cancer, detection of minimal residual disease has been performed in a variety of clinical specimens: Bone marrow, blood, or abdominal lymph nodes (see Tables 2 and 3). Even in *ovarian cancer*, in which – unlike breast cancer – the skeletal system is not a preferred location for distant metastasis, disseminated tumor cells in the bone marrow can be found in about 30% of patients without any signs of clinically overt metastasis (see Table 2). Just like in breast cancer, early dissemination in ovarian cancer seems to be correlated with poor patient outcome (Braun et al. 2001b).

In *cervical or endometrial cancer*, only few studies are available (see Table 3). The availability of a specific, well defined cytokeratin marker (CK 20) in endometrial cancer is a methodological advantage, in particular for RT-

Table 2. Disseminated tumor cells in patients with ovarian cancer

Tissue	Method	Marker	Detection rate	Prognostic impact	First author (year)
BM	ICC	CK 8/18/19	32/108 (30%)	DDFS[a]	Braun (2001b)
BM	ICC (IF)	CK 8/18/19	18/60 (30%)	n.r.	Roggel (2001)
BM	ICC	CK, CA 125	9/49 (18%)	n.s.	Gabriel (2000)
BM, PB	ICC	MOC-31	14/70 (20%)	n.r.	Marth (1999)
BM	ICC	TFS-4, OV-632, TFS-2, SB-3[b]	10/23 (43%)	n.r.	Ross (1995)
BM	ICC	CK	12/53 (23%)	n.s.	Cain (1990)

[a] Prognostic value as an independent parameter confirmed by multivariate analysis.
[b] Antibody cocktail against ovarian or glandular epithelia.

Table 3. Disseminated tumor cells in patients with gynecological malignancies

Tumor type	Tissue	Method	Marker	Detection rate	Prognostic impact	First author (year)
Cervix	Liposuction specimen	IHC	CK	3/30 (10%)	n.r.	Horn (2001)
	BM	ICC	CK	29/93 (31%)	DFS, OS[a]	Hepp (2000)
	LN	IHC	CK	10/11 (91%)	n.r.	Czegledy (1995)
Endo-	PB	RT-PCR	CK-20	24/53 (45%)	n.r.	Klein (2000)
metrium	LN	RT-PCR	CK-20	6/18 (33%)	n.r.	Fishman (2000)

[a] Prognostic impact on OS confirmed by multivariate analysis.

PCR analysis. Nevertheless, at present, the clinical utility of detection of MRD in these malignancies is rather low, partly due to lack of therapeutic options. Yet, it is interesting to note that also in cervical cancer, about 30% of patients have disseminated tumor cells in their bone marrow (Hepp et al. 2000). Thus, future targeted therapeutics are promising options also for patients with gynecological malignancies.

Phenotyping of Disseminated Tumor Cells

Beyond being yet another *prognostic* factor, disseminated tumor cells in bone marrow do have a considerable clinical relevance. Even after completion of primary, i.e. loco-regional and systemic therapy, disseminated tumor cells can be found in bone marrow aspirates of breast cancer patients (Mansi et al. 1989; Molino et al. 1999; Janni et al. 2001). Initial observations about a significant prognostic impact of such persistent tumor cells (Janni et al. 2001) support the idea that not all disseminated cells possess "malignant" potential.

Expression of numerous antigens has been studied on disseminated tumor cells in the bone marrow (see Table 4). Some of these antigens are already clinically relevant due to available targeted therapeutics, such as uPA-R [synthetic uPA inhibitor, WX-UK1, in phase I clinical trials (WILEX AG, press release 21.9.2001)], 17–1A [clinical therapy trial using mAB edrecolomab (Riethmüller et al. 1998)] or HER2 [mAB trastuzumab FDA-approved for metastatic breast cancer (Slamon et al. 2001)].

Heiss et al. (1995) were the first to show that not just the mere presence of disseminated tumor cells in bone marrow but rather their phenotype is correlated to poor patient outcome in gastric cancer: Patients whose tumor cells expressed the urokinase receptor (CD 87, uPA-R) had a significantly worse DFS than patients with uPA-R negative tumor cells. Using a double fluorescent staining method and a different anti CD 87 antibody, uPA-R expression is found on almost all cytokeratin-positive cells in bone marrow aspirates of breast cancer or ovarian cancer patients, yet at varying intensities (Roggel et al. 2001; Sinz et al. 2001). Braun et al. (2001c) were able to demonstrate that

Table 4. Phenotyping of disseminated tumor cells

Tumor type	Tissue	Method	Marker	Phenotype	Patients with phenotype-positive/marker-positive cells (%)	First author (year)
Breast	BM	ICC	CK18	erbB2	31/52 (60%)	Braun (2001b)
Breast	BM	ICC	CK 8/18/19	erbB2	13/15 (87%)	Braun (1999b)
Breast	BM	ICC	CK18	erbB2	48/71 (68%)	Pantel (1993)
Colorectal/ stomach	BM	ICC	CK18	erbB2	14/50 (28%)	Pantel (1993)
Ovary	BM	ICC (IF)	CK8/18/19	uPA-R	18/18 (100%)	Roggel (2001)
Breast	BM	ICC	CK 8/18/19	uPA-R	10/15 (67%)	Togel (2001)
Breast	PB	ICC	CK 8/18/19	uPA-R	7/10 (70%)	Togel (2001)
Stomach	BM	ICC	CK18	uPA-R	29/61 (48%)	Allgayer (1997)
Stomach	BM	ICC	CK18	uPA-R	20/44 (45%)	Heiss (1995)
Breast	BM	ICC	CK18	MHC-I	22/30 (73%)	Zia (2001)
Breast	BM	ICC	CK18	MHC-I	9/26 (35%)	Pantel (1991)
Colon/ stomach	BM	ICC	CK18	MHC-I	20/28 (71%)	Pantel (1991)
Breast	BM	ICC	CK18	Transferrin	17/59 (29%)	Schlimok (1990)
Colorectal	BM	ICC	CK18	Transferrin	7/17(41%)	Schlimok (1990)
Breast	BM	ICC	CK18	3Ki-67	1/12 (8.3%)	Pantel (1993)
Colorectal	BM	ICC	CK18	Ki-67	0/21 (0%)	Pantel (1993)
Breast	BM	ICC	CK18	pl20	1/11 (9.7%)	Pantel (1993)
Colorectal/ stomach	BM	ICC	CK18	pl20	9/25 (36%)	Pantel (1993)
Breast	BM	tCC	CKS/18/19	17-1A	14/18 (78%)	Braun (1999b)
Breast	BM	ICC	CK 8/18/19	MUC-1	11/14 (79%)	Braun (1999b)
Breast	BM	ICC	CK 8/18/19	Lewis Y	11/14 (79%)	Braun (1999b)

HER2 positive tumor cells in bone marrow aspirates of primary breast cancer patients were correlated significantly with poor prognosis.

Thus, the phenotype of early disseminated tumor cells seems to be crucial for their ability to proliferate and subsequently form manifest metastases. Moreover, the phenotype of disseminated cells may differ substantially from that of the primary tumor: In breast cancer, only about 25% of primary lesions overexpress HER2 (Ross and Fletcher 1998), whereas about 60% of disseminated cells in the bone marrow show HER2 overexpression (Pantel et al. 1993). Considering such phenotypic changes and the fact that tumor biological therapies will probably be most effective targeting MRD rather than large tumors, it may clinically be more relevant to evaluate the disseminated cells themselves instead of the primary lesion with regard to potential therapeutic targets. Novel immunofluorescent staining techniques may be helpful by enabling not only qualitative but also quantitative assessment of tumor cell characteristics (Noack et al. 2000).

Table 5. Monitoring of systemic therapy using disseminated tumor cells

Tumor type	Tissue	Method	Marker	Pheno-type	Therapy	First author (year)
Breast	BM, PB	ICC, RT-PCR	CK 8/18/19	None	HD-CTX	Krüger (2001)
Breast	BM	ICC	CK 8/18/19	None	CTX	Braun (2000a)
Breast	BM	ICC	CK 8/18/19	17-1A	Edrecolomab	Braun (1999a)
Breast	BM, PB	ICC	CK8/18/19, HEA 125, BM7, BM8	None	HD-CTX	Hohaus (1996)
Breast	BM	ICC	CK 8/18/19	None	CTX, Edre-colomab	Hempel (1997)
Breast/ Colorectal	BM	ICC	CK18	17-1A	Edrecolomab	Schlimok (1987)

Monitoring of Systemic Therapy

Studies looking at the fate of disseminated tumor cells after systemic therapy (see Table 5), demonstrated lack of efficient elimination of such cells by conventional chemotherapy. Pantel et al. (1993) showed that only a minority of cytokeratin-positive cells in the bone marrow actually proliferate (see Table 4). Thus, such non-proliferating dormant cells may not be susceptible for conventional systemic therapy, particularly chemotherapy. In a pilot study in high-risk breast cancer patients, Braun et al. (2000a) demonstrated that the overall prevalence of tumor cell positive bone marrow aspirates remained essentially unchanged before and after chemotherapy. Yet, presence of tumor cells after therapy was associated with an extremely poor prognosis suggesting early treatment failure. Similarly, Roggel et al. (2001) showed in a small, still ongoing study in ovarian cancer patients that the presence of cytokeratin-positive cells in bone marrow aspirates taken before and after preoperative chemotherapy was not substantially altered by administration of systemic chemotherapy. Moreover, small studies in breast cancer patients undergoing high-dose chemotherapy with autologous stem cell transplantation reported presence of cytokeratin-positive cells in a substantial percentage (30–83%) of the bone marrow or peripheral blood specimens obtained after completion of treatment while most of the patients were considered still being in complete clinical remission (Hempel et al. 1997; Hohaus et al. 1996; Krüger et al. 2001).

In view of the above pilot studies, monitoring of success of conventional systemic therapy is feasible using mainly bone marrow aspirates (but also peripheral blood preparations) for detection of minimal residual disease. This approach offers the considerable advantage of "on-line" monitoring with the option of early therapeutic interference. At present, therapeutic intervention is performed when disease progression becomes clinically evident. In contrast to MRD, disease progression usually manifests itself clinically at a later stage and thus with a substantially larger tumor burden. So far, therapeutic efficacy of *adjuvant* treatment can only assessed in large-scale clinical trials after a sufficient observation period of at least 5 years. Consequently, clinical progress with regard to this form of therapy is rather slow. The important advantage of a surrogate marker assay that permits immediate assessment of therapy-induced cytotoxic effects on MRD is therefore evident. "On-line" monitoring of MRD would allow therapeutic consequences at a potentially still curable state instead at the much later time of first clinically evident distant relapse, with no option for cure – at least in breast cancer.

>With the availability of novel tumor biological therapies, disseminated tumor cells are an obvious target for such approaches (see Table 5), especially since dormant tumor cells may be resistant to conventional therapeutics. One promising approach is the use of bisphosphonates for prevention of bone metastases. A pilot study already showed therapeutic efficacy of adjuvant bisphosphonates in breast cancer patients with disseminated tumor cells in their bone marrow aspirates and thus at high-risk for subsequent bone metastasis (Diel et al. 1998). Another promising therapy approach is the use of monoclonal antibodies directed against cell surface antigens. In a pilot study, Braun et al (1999a) were able to demonstrate reduction of disseminated tumor cells in bone marrow aspirates after infusion of edrecolomab (anti-17–1A monoclonal antibody).

Considering the recent advances in characterizing disseminated tumor cells and the promising clinical pilot studies described above, detection, phenotyping, and monitoring of MRD has certainly the potential to support individualized and tailored therapy strategies.

Clinical Relevance

In conclusion, detection of disseminated tumor cells, i.e. minimal residual disease, has numerous clinical applications:

- *Prognostic* impact
- *Predictive* impact: therapy response, monitoring of success of systemic therapy
- Information on individual tumor biology (phenotyping)
- Target for tumor biological therapy

So far, with regard to breast cancer and gynecological malignancies, detection of minimal residual disease, shows the greatest clinical potential in breast cancer patients, particularly using bone marrow aspirates. Presence of these cells in bone marrow aspirates of primary breast cancer patients allows identification of high-risk patients, thus enabling risk-adapted therapy concepts. Unfortunately, not all criteria for transfer of new markers into clinical practice have yet been fulfilled (McGuire 1991; McGuire and Clark 1992; Hayes et al. 1996).

Phenotyping and further characterization of disseminated tumor cells has become increasingly important due to the availability of novel targeted therapy approaches. However, standardized, robust detection and characterization methods are a prerequisite for routine clinical application. Thus, in the interest of cancer patients, detection of disseminated tumor cells should at the present time only be performed in experienced centers within well-defined clinical studies.

Acknowledgements. This work was supported by grants to N.H. from the State of Bavaria (KKF Project #8756159) and to S.B. and N.H. from the German Research Foundation (Deutsche Forschungsgemeinschaft DFG BR 2149/1–1).

References

Allgayer H, Heiss MM, Riesenberg R, Babic R, Jauch KW, Schildberg FW (1997) Immuno-cytochemical phenotyping of disseminated tumor cells in bone marrow by uPA receptor and CK18: investigation of. sensitivity and specificity of an immunogold/alkaline phosphatase double staining protocol. J Histochem Cytochem 45:203–212

Borgen E, Naume B, Nesland JM, Kvalheim G, Beiske K, Fodstad O, Diel I, Solomayer EF, Theocharous P, Coombes RC, Smith BM, Wunder E, Marolleau JP, Garcia J, Pantel K (1999) Standardization of the immunocytochemical detection of cancer cells in BM and blood: I. establishment of objective criteria for the evaluation of immunostained cells. Cytotherapy 1:377–388

Braun S, Pantel K (1998) Prognostic significance of micrometastatic bone marrow involvement. Breast Cancer Res Treat 52:201–216

Braun S, Hepp F, Kentenich CR, Janni W, Pantel K, Riethmuller G, Willgeroth F, Sommer HL (1999a) Monoclonal antibody therapy with edrecolomab in breast cancer patients: monitoring of elimination of disseminated cytokeratin-positive tumor cells in bone marrow. Clin Cancer Res 5:3999–4004

Braun S, Hepp F, Sommer HL, Pantel K (1999b) Tumor-antigen heterogeneity of disseminated breast cancer cells: implications for immunotherapy of minimal residual disease. Int J Cancer 84:1–5

Braun S, Kentenich C, Janni W, Hepp F, de Waal J, Willgeroth F, Sommer H, Pantel K (2000a) Lack of effect of adjuvant chemotherapy on the elimination of single dormant tumor cells in bone marrow of high-risk breast cancer patients. J Clin Oncol 18:80–86

Braun S, Pantel K, Muller P, Janni W, Hepp F, Kentenich CR, Gastroph S, Wischnik A, Dimpfl T, Kindermann G, Riethmuller G, Schlimok G (2000b) Cytokeratin-positive cells in the bone marrow and survival of patients with stage I, II, or III breast cancer. N Engl J Med 342:525–533

Braun S, Cevatli BS, Assemi C, Janni W, Kentenich CR, Schindlbeck C, Rjosk D, Hepp F (2001a) Comparative analysis of micrometastasis to the bone marrow and lymph nodes of node-negative breast cancer patients receiving no adjuvant therapy. J Clin Oncol 19:1468–1475

Braun S, Schindlbeck C, Hepp F, Janni W, Kentenich C, Riethmüller G, Pantel K (2001b) Occult tumor cells in bone marrow of patients with locoregionally restricted ovarian cancer predict early distant metastatic relapse. J Clin Oncol 19:368–375

Braun S, Schlimok G, Heumos I, Schaller G, Riethdorf L, Riethmüller G, Pantel K (2001c) ErbB2 overexpression on occult metastatic cells in bone marrow predicts poor clinical outcome of stage I-III breast cancer patients. Cancer Res 61:1890–1895

Braun S, Nusser N, Harbeck N, Pantel K (2002) Occult metastatic cancer cells in the bone marrow: a clinical marker for tumor staging and decision making in primary breast cancer. Clin Cancer Res (in press)

Brugger W, Bühring HJ, Grünebach F, Vogel W, Kaul S, Müller R, Brümmendorf TH, Ziegler BL, Rappold I, Brossart P, Scheding S, Kanz L (1999) Expression of MUC-1 epitopes on normal bone marrow: implications for the detection. J Clin Oncol 17: 1535–1544

Cain JM, Ellis GK, Collins C, Greer BE, Tamimi HK, Figge DC, Gown AM, Livingston RB (1990) Bone marrow involvement in epithelial ovarian cancer by immunocytochemical assessment. Gynecol Oncol 38:442–445

Coombes RC, Dearnaley DP, Redding WH, Ormerod MG, Skilton RA, Sloane JP, Imrie S, Edwards AW, Monaghan P, Neville AM (1983) Micrometastases in breast cancer. In: Peeters H (ed) Protides of the biological fluids. Pergamon, Oxford, pp 317–323

Cote RJ, Rosen PP, Lesser ML, Old LJ, Osborne MP (1991) Prediction of early relapse in patients with operable breast cancer by detection of occult bone marrow micrometastases. J Clin Oncol 9:1749–1756

Czegledy J, Iosif C, Hansson BG, Evander M, Gergely L, Wadell G (1995) Can a test for E6/E7 transcripts of human papillomavirus type 16 serve as a diagnostic tool for the detection of micrometastasis in cervical cancer? Int J Cancer 64:211–215

Dearnaley DP, Sloane JP, Ormerod MG, Steele K, Coombes RC, Clink HM, Powles TJ, Ford HT, Gazet JC, Neville AM (1981) Increased detection of mammary carcinoma cells in marrow smears using antisera to epithelial membrane antigen. Br J Cancer 44:85–90

Diel IJ, Kaufmann M, Costa SD, Holle R, von Minckwitz G, Solomayer EF, Kaul S, Bastert G (1996) Micrometastatic breast cancer cells in bone marrow at primary surgery: prognostic value in comparison with nodal status. J Natl Cancer Inst 88:1652–1658

Diel IJ, Kaufmann M, Goerner R, Costa SD, Kaul S, Bastert G (1992) Detection of tumor cells in bone marrow of patients with primary breast cancer: a prognostic factor for distant metastasis. J Clin Oncol 10:1534–1539

Diel IJ, Solomayer EF, Costa SD, Gollan C, Goerner R, Wallwiener D, Kaufmann M, Bastert G (1998) Reduction in new metastases in breast cancer with adjuvant clodronate treatment. N Engl J Med 339:357–363

Fishman A, Klein A, Zemer R, Zimlichman S, Bernheim J, Cohen I, Altaras MM (2000) Detection of micrometastasis by cytokeratin-20 (reverse transcription polymerase chain reaction) in lymph nodes of patients with endometrial cancer. Gynecol Oncol 77:399–404

Funke I, Schraut W, Jauch KW, Untch M, Schildberg FW (2001) Prospective study on minimal residual disease in breast cancer. Proceedings of 1st International Congress on Molecular staging of cancer. Munich, p 25

Gabriel M, Obrebowska A, Spaczynski M (2000) Nachweis von Epithelzellen im Knochenmark von Patientinnen mit Ovarialkarzinomen unter Anwendung von immunhistochemischen Methoden. Gynakol Geburtshilfliche Rundsch 40:140–144

Gebauer G, Fehm T, Merkle E, Beck EP, Lang N, Jager W (2001) Epithelial cells in bone marrow of breast cancer patients at time of primary surgery: clinical outcome during long-term follow-up. J Clin Oncol 19:3669–3674

Gerber B, Krause A, Muller H, Richter D, Reimer T, Makovitzky J, Herrnring C, Jeschke U, Kundt G, Friese K (2001) Simultaneous immunohistochemical detection of tumor cells in lymph nodes and bone marrow aspirates in breast cancer and its correlation with other prognostic factors. J Clin Oncol 19:960–971

Harbeck N, Untch M, Pache L, Eiermann W (1994) Tumour cell detection in the bone marrow of breast cancer patients at primary therapy: results of a 3-year median follow-up. Br J Cancer 69:566–571

Hayes DF, Bast RC, Desch CE, Fritsche HJr, Kemeny NE, Jessup JM, Locker GY, Macdonald JS, Mennel RG, Norton L, Ravdin P, Taube S, Winn RJ (1996) Tumor marker utility grading system: a framework to evaluate clinical utility of tumor markers. J Natl Cancer Inst 88:1456–1466

Heiss MM, Allgayer H, Gruetzner KU, Funke I, Babic R, Jauch KW, Schildberg FW (1995) Individual development and uPA-receptor expression of disseminated tumour cells in bone marrow: a reference to early systemic disease in solid cancer. Nat Med 1:1035–1039

Hempel D, Müller P, Oruzio D, Ehnle S, Schlimok G (1997) Adoptive immunotherapy with the monoclonal antibody (moab) 17/1A to reduce minimal residual disease in breast cancer patients after high dose chemotherapy (HDC) (abstract). Blood 90[Suppl 1]:379b

Hepp F, Kentenich C, Janni W, Kindermann G, Braun S (2000) Prognostische Bedeutung Cytokeratin (CK)-positiver Knochenmark-Mikrometastasen (KMM) bei Patientinnen mit Zervixkarzinom (CC) im Stadium FIGO I-II. Geburtsh Frauenheilk 60:S37

Heyderman E, Strudley I, Powell G, Richardson TC, Cordell JL, Mason DY (1985) A new monoclonal antibody to epithelial membrane antigen (EMA)-E29. A comparison of its immunocytochemical reactivity with polyclonal anti-EMA antibodies and with another monoclonal antibody, HMFG-2. Br J Cancer 52:355–361

Hohaus S, Funk L, Brehm M, Abdallah A, Murea S, Kaul S, Haas R (1996) Persistence of isolated tumor cells in patients with breast cancer after sequential high-dose therapy with peripheral blood stem cell transplantation (PBSC) (abstract). Blood 88[Suppl 10]:128a

Horn LC, Fischer U, Hockel M (2001) Occult tumor cells in surgical specimens from cases of early cervical cancer treated by liposuction-assisted nerve-sparing radical hysterectomy. Int J Gynecol Cancer 11:159–163

Janni W, Hepp F, Rjosk D, Kentenich C, Strobl B, Schindlbeck C, Hantschmann P, Sommer H, Pantel K, Braun S (2001) The fate and prognostic value of occult metastatic cells in the bone marrow of patients with breast carcinoma between primary treatment and recurrence. Cancer 92:46–53

Klein A, Fishman A, Zemer R, Zimlichman S, Altaras MM (2000) Detection of tumor circulating cells by cytokeratin 20 in the blood of patients with endometrial carcinoma. Gynecol Oncol 78:352–355

Kowolik JH, Kuhn W, Nahrig J, Werner M, Obst T, Avril N, Schmitt M, Graeff H (2000) Detection of micrometastases in sentinel lymph nodes of the breast applying monoclonal antibodies AE1/AE3 to pancytokeratins. Oncol Rep 7:745–749

Krüger WH, Kroger N, Tögel F, Renges H, Badbaran A, Hornung R, Jung R, Gutensohn K, Gieseking F, Janicke F, Zander AR (2001) Disseminated breast cancer cells prior to and after high-dose therapy. J Hematother Stem Cell Res 10:681–689

Landys K, Persson S, Kovarik J, Hultborn R, Holmberg E (1998) Prognostic value of bone marrow biopsy in operable breast cancer patients at the time of initial diagnosis: results of a 20-year median follow-up. Breast Cancer Res Treat 49:27–33

Mansi JL, Berger U, McDonnell T, Pople A, Rayter Z, Gazet JC, Coombes RC (1989) The fate of bone marrow micrometastases in patients with primary breast cancer. J Clin Oncol 7:445–449

Mansi JL, Gogas H, Bliss JM, Gazet JC, Berger U, Coombes RC (1999) Outcome of primary-breast-cancer patients with micrometastases: a long-term follow-up study. Lancet 354:197–202

Marth C, Hoifodt H, Walberg L, Kaern J, Andresen M, Hovland B, Mathiesen O, Tropé C (1999) Carcinoma cells in bone marrow and peripheral blood of ovarian cancer patients (abstract). 2nd International Symposium on Minimal Residual Cancer, Berlin, Germany

McGuire W (1991) Breast cancer prognostic factors: Evaluation guidelines. J Natl Cancer Inst 83:154–155

McGuire WL, Clark GM (1992) Prognostic factors and treatment decisions in axillary-node-negative breast cancer. N Engl J Med 326:1756–1761

Molino A, Colombatti M, Bonetti F, Zardini M, Pasini F, Perini A, Pelosi G, Tridente G, Veneri D, Cetto GL (1991) A comparative analysis of three different techniques for the detection of breast cancer cells in bone marrow. Cancer 67:1033–1036

Molino A, Pelosi G, Micciolo R, Turazza M, Nortilli R, Pavanel F, Cetto GL (1999) Bone marrow micrometastases in breast cancer patients. Breast Cancer Res Treat 58:123–130

Noack F, Schmitt M, Bauer J, Helmecke D, Kruger W, Thorban S, Sandherr M, Kuhn W, Graeff H, Harbeck N (2000) A new approach to phenotyping disseminated tumor cells: methodological advances and clinical implications. Int J Biol Markers 15:100–104

Osborne MP, Wong GY, Asina S, Old LJ, Cote RJ, Rosen PP (1991) Sensitivity of immunocytochemical detection of breast cancer cells in human bone marrow. Cancer Res 51:2706–2709

Otte M, Deppert K, Ebel S, Hosch S, Jänicke F, Izbicki JR, Pantel K (2000) Immunomagnetic enrichment of disseminated tumor cells from bone marrow of carcinoma patients (abstract 2475). Proc AACR687

Pantel K, Felber E, Schlimok G (1994) Detection and characterization of residual disease in breast cancer. J Hematother 3:315–322

Pantel K, Schlimok G, Braun S, Kutter D, Lindemann F, Schaller G, Funke I, Izbicki JR, Riethmüller G (1993) Differential expression of proliferation-associated molecules in individual micrometastatic carcinoma cells. J Natl Cancer Inst 85:1419–1424

Pantel K, Schlimok G, Kutter D, Schaller G, Genz T, Wiebecke B, Backmann R, Funke I, Riethmuller G (1991) Frequent down-regulation of major histocompatibility class I antigen expression on individual micrometastatic carcinoma cells. Cancer Res 51:4712–4715

Rappold I, Brossart P, Scheding S, Kanz L (1999) Expression of MUC-1 epitopes on normal bone marrow: implications for the detection of occult bone marrow micrometastases. J Clin Oncol 17:1535–1544

Redding WH, Coombes RC, Monaghan P, Clink HM, Imrie SF, Dearnaley DP, Ormerod MG, Sloane JP, Gazet JC, Powles TJ (1983) Detection of micrometastases in patients with primary breast cancer. Lancet 2:1271–1274

Ridell B, Landys K (1979) Incidence and histopathology of metastases of mammary carcinoma in biopsies from the posterior iliac crest. Cancer 44:1782–1788

Riethmüller G, Holz E, Schlimok G, Schmiegel W, Raab R, Höffken K, Gruber R, Funke I, Pichlmaier H, Hirche H, Buggisch P, Witte J, Pichlmayr R (1998) Monoclonal antibody therapy for resected Dukes' C colorectal cancer: seven-year outcome of a multicenter randomized trial. J Clin Oncol 16:1788–1794

Roggel F, Späthe K, Sinz S, Braun S, Hocke S, Rutke S, Bosl M, Schmalfeldt B, Sandherr M, Werner M, Kuhn W, Schmitt M, Harbeck N (2001) Characterization of disseminated tumor cells in bone marrow of patients with ovarian carcinoma (abstract 62). 3rd International Symposium on Minimal Residual Cancer, Hamburg, Germany

Ross AA, Miller GW, Moss TJ, Kahn DG, Warner NE, Sweet DL, Louie KG, Schneidermann E, Pecora AL, Meagher RC (1995) Immunocytochemical detection of tumor cells in bone marrow and peripheral blood stem cell collections from patients with ovarian cancer. Bone Marrow Transplant 15:929–933

Ross JS, Fletcher JA (1998) The HER-2/neu oncogene in breast cancer: prognostic factor, predictive factor, and target for therapy. Oncologist 3:237–252

Salvadori B, Squicciarini P, Rovini D, Orefice S, Andreola S, Rilke F, Barletta L, Menard S, Colnaghi MI (1990) Use of monoclonal antibody MBr1 to detect micrometastases in bone marrow specimens of breast cancer patients. Eur J Cancer 26:865–867

Schlimok G, Funke I, Holzmann B, Gottlinger G, Schmidt G, Hauser H, Swierkot S, Warnecke HH, Schneider B, Koprowski H (1987) Micrometastatic cancer cells in bone marrow: in vitro detection with anti-cytokeratin and in vivo labeling with anti-17–1A monoclonal antibodies. Proc Natl Acad Sci U S A 84:8672–8676

Schlimok G, Riethmuller G (1990) Detection, characterization and tumorigenicity of disseminated tumor cells in human bone marrow. Semin Cancer Biol 1:207–215

Sinz S, Rutke S, Späthe K, Hocke S, Roggel F, Sandherr M, Werner M, Braun S, Kuhn W, Schmitt M, Harbeck N (2001) Phenotyping of disseminated tumor cells in bone marrow aspirates of breast cancer patients (abstract 63). 3rd International Symposium on Minimal Residual Cancer, Hamburg, Germany

Slamon DJ, Leyland-Jones B, Shak S, Fuchs H, Paton V, Bajamonde A, Fleming T, Eiermann W, Wolter J, Pegram M, Baselga J, Norton L (2001) Use of chemotherapy plus a monoclonal antibody against HER2 for metastatic breast cancer that overexpresses HER2. N Engl J Med 344:783–792

Tögel F, Datta C, Badbaran A, Kröger N, Renges H, Gieseking F, Jänicke F, Zander AR, Krüger W (2001) Urokinase-like plasminogen activator receptor expression on disseminated breast cancer cells. J Hematother Stem Cell Res 10:141–145

Wilex AG MG (2001) Wilex starts phase I trial with anti-metastatic urokinase inhibitor drug. Press release 21–09–2001 http://www.wilex.de

Wong SL, Chao C, Edwards MJ, Simpson D, McMasters KM (2001) The use of cytokeratin staining in sentinel lymph node biopsy for breast cancer. Am J Surg 182:330–334

Advanced Statistical Methods for the Definition of New Staging Models

Ronald Kates, Manfred Schmitt, Nadia Harbeck

N. Harbeck (✉)
Klinische Forschergruppe der Frauenklinik,
Technische Universität München, Ismaningerstr. 22,
81675 Munich, Germany

Abstract

Adequate staging procedures are the prerequisite for individualized therapy concepts in cancer, particularly in the *adjuvant* setting. Molecular staging markers tend to characterize *specific*, fundamental disease processes to a greater extent than conventional staging markers. At the biological level, the course of the disease will almost certainly involve interactions between multiple underlying processes. Since new therapeutic strategies tend to target specific processes as well, their impact will also involve interactions. Hence, assessment of the prognostic impact of new markers and their utilization for prediction of response to therapy will require increasingly sophisticated statistical tools that are capable of detecting and modeling complicated interactions. Because they are designed to model *arbitrary* interactions, neural networks offer a promising approach to improved staging. However, the typical clinical data environment poses severe challenges to high-performance survival modeling using neural nets, particularly the key problem of maintaining good generalization. Nonetheless, it turns out that by using newly developed methods to minimize unnecessary complexity in the neural network representation of disease course, it is possible to obtain models with high predictive performance. This performance has been validated on both simulated and real patient data sets. There are important applications for design of studies involving targeted therapy concepts and for identification of the improvement in decision support resulting from new staging markers. In this article, advantages of advanced statistical methods such as neural networks for definition of new staging models will be illustrated using breast cancer as an example.

Introduction

Clinical Needs in Cancer

Breast cancer is an example of a potentially curable carcinoma with high incidence in the Western world. However, once the patient has developed overt distant metastases, breast cancer is no longer curable by presently available therapies. Hence, the major challenge for the clinician is to assess accurately each patient's risk situation right at the beginning and to individualize loco-regional and systemic treatment modalities accordingly (McGuire and Clark 1992; Clark 1994; Hayes et al. 1998). Accurate risk group selection has often been discussed in the context of adjuvant systemic therapy with the goal of avoiding over-treatment for *low-risk* patients already cured by loco-regional treatment. Unfortunately, established prognostic factors and guidelines are not yet sufficient for accurate identification of this low-risk group (Gasparini et al. 1993; Thomssen et al. 2000). Accurate risk group selection has also been discussed in the context of improving care of *high-risk* patients: One option for these patients could be the use of more aggressive therapies whose side effects are severe enough to preclude using them without a clear indication (Harbeck et al. 2002).

In a clinical context, *prognostic* characterization of patients may often be viewed as a kind of scoring problem, in which one or more scores are to be assigned to each patient on the basis of factors (individual data patterns) available at some initial time. These scores can be used for decision support, e.g., for stratification of patients with respect to their risk of relapse or their probability of response to available treatments. The use of self-learning or adaptive systems such as neural nets for risk assessment is a natural approach, since such systems have been used quite successfully for scoring in nonmedical contexts such as data mining. However, in such applications, large data bases with 20,000 or more entries are typical, making it easier to find even a weak "signal" above the "noise" of random statistical variations. In clinical studies, data are often expensive to collect, and collectives with more than a few hundred patients are rare. In small samples, it is common to use traditional statistical models. However, with the advent of molecular staging, proper modeling of nonlinearities will be crucial; intelligent systems such as neural nets offer an important potential advantage over traditional statistical models in their ability to represent and also identify a broad spectrum of non-linear effects such as arbitrary factor interactions.

Advanced Statistical Models

Advanced statistical models have applications in several areas of medicine, including:

1. Screening
2. Diagnosis
3. Staging for an existing disease ultimately applicable for:
   a. Risk assessment
   b. Prediction of therapy response
   c. Decision support

These areas exhibit similarities in their underlying mathematical structure, but there are also important differences in the specific probability models and in the medical (e.g., therapeutic) consequences of applying a model. Here, we are particularly interested in the third problem (staging for an existing disease) and its ultimate application for decision support in choosing optimal individualized therapy.

Intelligent (learning) systems may be thought of as a form of advanced statistical modeling. In nonlinear problems with interactions, there are several methodological options, for example:

1. Adding nonlinear terms to ordinary (e.g., Cox) regression models, etc.
2. Recursive partitioning (CART)
3. Fuzzy logic
4. Neural networks

All of these techniques have their merits in particular applications (Kates et al. 2000) and are worthy of investigation. The techniques described here involve the training of trained neural networks based on censored survival data to represent the risk structure for disease progression.

Markers, Interactions, and Neural Nets

Conventional staging systems in cancer have difficulty distinguishing tumors that appear similar but will ultimately differ in clinically important respects, e.g., relapse-free survival, relapse site, or treatment response (Hayes et al. 1998). Molecular staging markers, based for example on data obtained by immunohistochemistry, ELISA, PCR, in situ hybridization, microarrays, or proteomics, have the potential to characterize *specific*, fundamental disease processes to a greater extent than conventional staging markers (McGuire and Clark 1992; Harbeck et al. 1999). Hence, these markers could contribute to a significant improvement in staging and ultimately lead to enormous clinical benefits, particularly if they contribute to improved quality in prediction of response to candidate therapy regimens.

In cancer, the clinical course of the disease will often involve interactions between multiple underlying biological processes. Moreover, as new, targeted treatment modalities in cancer become available, both the range of therapeutic options and the scope of the clinical decision context will increase. This enhanced clinical decision context will pose a major challenge for the physician in assessing each patient's unique risk/response characteristics and individualizing treatment modalities accordingly, particularly in the adjuvant setting. Hence, clinical application of new markers including assessment of prognostic impact and prediction of response to therapy will require increasingly sophisticated statistical tools that are capable of detecting and modeling complex interactions, including the interaction of treatment options with biological processes.

Because they are designed to model arbitrary interactions, neural networks offer a potentially promising approach to improved staging, but the typical clinical data environment poses severe challenges to high-performance survival modeling using neural nets, particularly the key problem of maintaining good generalization. Nonetheless, it turns out that by using newly developed methods to minimize unnecessary complexity (i.e., the number of independent "connectors") in the neural network representation of disease course, it is possible to obtain models with high predictive performance.

The Problem of "Competing Risks"

In most forms of cancer, disease progression takes different forms that may reflect inherent differences in the underlying disease phenotype and pathology. Hence, there is often more to be learned from clinical follow-up data than simply what factors are prognostic for relapse-free survival. Studying the dependence of the *kind* of relapse on factors determined at the time of primary therapy could also give valuable early clues to the biological disease processes in question and ultimately to the appropriate targeted therapy. This is of course most relevant for the adjuvant setting when a curative therapeutic approach is feasible if the patient receives optimal therapy. Present and future treatment options will inevitably impact some biological processes of disease progression more strongly than others and thus may reduce one type of relapse mode more than another. For example, this behavior complicates analysis of breast cancer patient data: in analyzing first relapse in treated patients, it is important to distinguish the *apparent* rise in a competing mode of relapse (a purely statistical effect) from a *real* rise in a competing mode due to an unforeseen side effect. Furthermore, treatment decisions reflected in available patient data are also related to risk factors. Hence, an appropriate computational framework is required in order to analyze these complex interactions and interrelationships and to support decision making at both the strategic and the clinical level.

Modeling of censored survival data with differentially coded endpoints for first relapse usually raises the question of competing risks: For example, suppose we wish to design a study in breast cancer targeting patients with a high risk for bone metastases by a new adjuvant therapy regimen including, say, bisphosphonates. Even if there were a positive therapy response delaying bone metastasis in some patients, a subgroup of these patients who (in the absence of the new treatment) would have suffered first relapse in *bone* might still be at risk for, say, *other distant metastases*. Hence, if one models separate relapse categories by standard methods such as Kaplan-Meier survival curves or Cox regression (censoring after any first relapse), there could even be an apparent *rise* in the other distant metastasis forms in treated patients compared to controls (or historic data), which in this case would not constitute an adverse effect of treatment, but rather a consequence of competing risks. Hence, standard methods could suggest an incorrect and damaging interpretation. One approach to understanding this issue might be to study *all* relapses, not just first relapse. For example, for a patient in the control group of our hypothetical breast cancer study observed to suffer first relapse in bone and subsequent relapse in a distant organ, one might suppose that the second relapse would have been observed as a first relapse if the patient had been treated with bisphosphonates and had responded to treatment. However, it is a very risky scientific hypothesis to suppose that the second relapse is an independent event, i.e., not causally related to the first relapse. To the extent that later relapses could be causally related to first relapses, this approach also does not provide a conclusive comparison of controls with treated patients.

We address this problem below by describing a modeling technique using neural networks that reconstructs the underlying probability structure of relapse site from follow-up data on first relapse in a situation with competing risks.

Competing Risk Neural Networks

Based on these considerations, a computational environment for neural network analysis of competing risks has been developed as described in the following section. The method has been extensively tested on both simulated and real patient data (Kates et al. 2001). The environment offers several special features not present in commercially available software:

1. A competing-risk neural statistical model (patent pending)
2. New complexity reduction techniques resulting in improved generalization capability despite limited training data
3. Unbiased statistical treatment of censored data
4. Statistical uncertainty estimates for the parameters ("weights") of the neural network.

Need for Differential Therapy Benefit Prediction in Cancer

Our empirical knowledge of the differential impact of therapies on different disease processes and outcomes is of course limited by the availability of data, most of which involves conventional adjuvant therapy regimens (e.g., endocrine therapy or chemotherapy). Nonetheless, even the data that is available

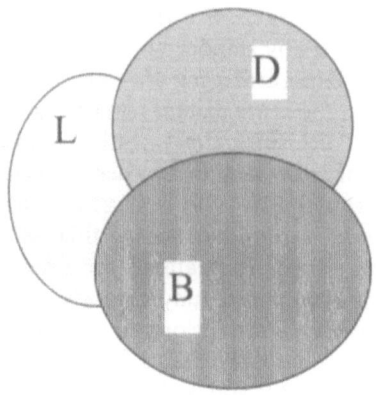

Fig. 1. Relapse categories as a Venn diagram

has not yet been utilized to its full potential because of the presence of competing risks:

There is a considerable body of statistical literature on competing risks (Tolley et al. 1978; Beck 1979; Kalbfleisch and Prentice 1980; Wohlfart et al. 1999), but for application to breast cancer it is possible to highlight the issues using a hypothetical example. There is evidence that, all other things being equal, elevated estrogen receptor (ER) values tend to increase the probability of first metastasis in bone compared to other distant metastasis as first metastasis. Some of this tendency may be related to treatment, and some may be related to the intrinsic nature of the disease. In either case, it is very difficult to distinguish to what extent the increase in first bone metastasis with elevated ER may be attributed to the decrease in other distant metastasis, and to what degree ER is truly a risk factor for relapse in bone in and of itself. A linear Cox proportional hazards model for bone metastasis does not distinguish these two explanations. Hence, one cannot use it to answer the question "what would be the risk of distant metastasis in bone due to elevated ER, all other things being equal, if we could reduce or eliminate all other distant metastasis?".

This question may appear hypothetical, but in fact it is a simplified version of a question that is sure to arise increasingly in the future, as new therapies are developed that preferentially reduce one mode of relapse compared to another, especially if response is dependent on risk factors. We will now briefly sketch the mathematical structure of a solution to this problem utilizing the learning capability of neural networks[1]:

Consider follow-up data containing a classification of first relapse in breast cancer in categories:

"B" for "bone", "D" for "distant not bone", and L for local/regional relapse (not distant) as illustrated in Fig. 1. For the purposes of this discussion, assume that patients are observed at month "t" and are either censored or can

---

[1] The discussion is of highly technical nature and can be safely omitted by the reader interested only in the basic ideas.

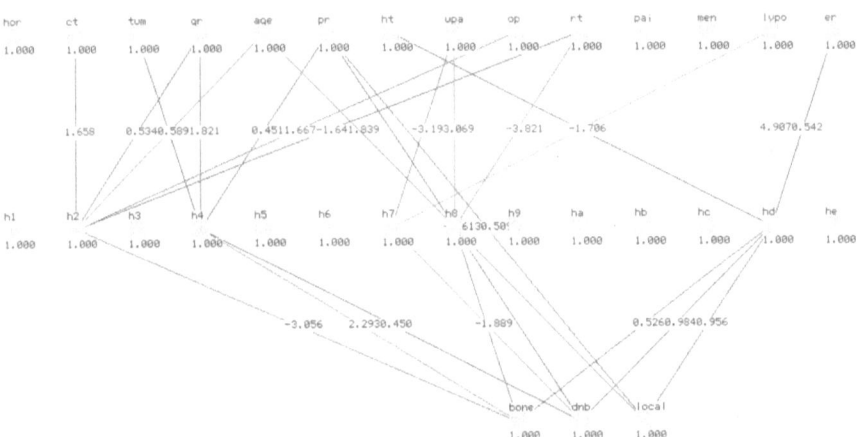

Fig. 2. Illustration of competing-risk neural network

be classified into exactly one of the categories B, D, or L according to the following logic:

1. *Bone metastasis* (yes/no)?
a. If yes, then: $\epsilon_{j1}=1$ $\epsilon_{j2}=0$ $\epsilon_{j3}=0$ $\psi_{j1}=0$ $\psi_{j2}=0$ $\psi_{j3}=0$
b. If no, then: *other distant metastasis* (yes/no)?
- If yes, then: $\epsilon_{j1}=0$ $\epsilon_{j2}=1$ $\epsilon_{j3}=0$ $\psi_{j1}=1$ $\psi_{j2}=0$ $\psi_{j3}=0$
- If no, then: *local/regional* (yes/no)?
- If yes, then: $\epsilon_{j1}=0$ $\epsilon_{j2}=0$ $\epsilon_{j3}=1$ $\psi_{j1}=1$ $\psi_{j2}=1$ $\psi_{j3}=0$
- If no, then: $\epsilon_{j1}=0$ $\epsilon_{j2}=0$ $\epsilon_{j3}=0$ $\psi_{j1}=1$ $\psi_{j2}=1$ $\psi_{j3}=1$

These variables are thus uniquely defined for each patient with follow-up data.

Suppose now that in addition to the follow-up data, risk factors and treatment variables denoted by x_j are recorded for the jth patient. It is then possible to train a neural network to learn the underlying relationship between risk factors/treatment variables and endpoints. The basic method has been described previously (Harbeck et al. 2000; Kates et al. 2000) and is sketched in Fig. 2.

Suppose for the moment that we already have a trained neural network: The trained neural network produces a *risk profile* for each patient, which we denote $NN_{kl}(x_j)$. The risk profile can be thought of simply as a list of scores that code information such as the risk of each mode of relapse and also whether a risk has particular time variation (e.g., a trend to early onset). Once the net is trained, the risk profile can in principle be generated from known factors x_j for any patient by an intelligent, but not terribly complicated, computer program. Using the trained neural network, it is also possible to construct a function well known in statistical survival modeling as the "hazard function," according to the formulae

$$\lambda_k(t|\mathbf{x}) = \lambda_{k0}(t)h_k(t|\mathbf{x}), \text{ where } h_k(t|\mathbf{x}) = \exp\left[\sum_{l=1}^{L} B_l(t)NN_{kl}(\mathbf{x})\right]$$

Here, the functions $B_l(t)$ represent so-called fractional polynomials and are used to characterize a possible time-varying effect. From these, it is possible to compute the expected survival rate S and the failure rate F with respect to each mode of failure k.

We now return to the question of how to train a competing-risk neural network using this data. One defines a statistical "likelihood function," which characterizes the probability that the data would have been seen as recorded, given the parameters and topology of the neural network. In the above formulation, the likelihood function may be written as:

$$L(\mu; \{\mathbf{x}, t\}) = \prod_{j=1}^{n} \prod_{k=1}^{K} \left[f_{NN(k,\mathbf{x})}(t_j)\right]^{\varepsilon_{jk}} \left[S_{NN(k,\mathbf{x})}(t_j)\right]^{\psi_{jk}}$$

In training a neural network, just as in statistical estimation, we turn the question around and ask how the parameters and topology of the net can be adjusted to maximize the probability of the data as seen. Actually, the key to successful application of neural nets in most medical applications is to seek a solution that is not an absolute maximum, but rather one whose network complexity (number of parameters) is low without paying too high a price in terms of L.

Data Fusion and Decision Support

Thus far, this paper has primarily addressed the questions of individualized risk assessment and prediction of therapy response by advanced statistical modeling. This information is an important *prerequisite* for determining optimal individualized therapy regimens in cancer, but the benefit to the patient also depends on the quality of the decision procedures *utilizing* this information.

The entire procedure leading to a particular therapy regimen – beginning with measurement of staging markers, application of an advanced statistical model for risk and treatment response assessment, and finally the decision itself – may be viewed as a problem in "data fusion."

Data fusion is an interdisciplinary concept describing a procedure for combining possibly heterogeneous data sources within a complex information environment. A typical data fusion paradigm involves several levels of integration. The goal of data fusion in general is to derive the highest possible quality of information for the application in question. The same data and information basis may "support" several different applications. The specific requirements of different applications are addressed at the top level of a data fusion process;

in particular, it often happens that different applications pose different requirements on what constitutes "quality."

It is typical to distinguish levels of fusion according to the degree of integration performed on the information at lower levels. Each level reduces the volume of data and extracts information for the next level. In a medical context, a typical example of *low-level* data fusion is the assignment of histological grade to a tumor (Elston and Ellis 1991) or the characterization of uPA levels in tumor tissue by ELISA measurement (Harbeck et al. 1999). Needless to say, even the lowest level of data fusion already involves quite a bit of work on calibration and may also require sophisticated statistical techniques such as outlier detection. Univariate analysis of a factor's impact on prognosis is a typical application of low-level data fusion. In cancer, it may happen that the impact of one factor is so strong that it already gives a clear picture of the disease. In this case, there is little integration required, and decisions may be based on this one factor.

However, often one factor is not adequate for risk classification. In this case a *second level of data fusion* is carried out which strives to combine several factors to improve risk classification. In analysis of clinical survival data, the familiar multivariate Cox analysis, CART, and scoring by neural networks (as described here) are examples of *level-two data fusion*. Here, the goal is to construct a "model" that embodies a knowledge base about the relationship between factors and disease course. A particularly useful case occurs when treatments can be explicitly included in the "model." Often, however, the effects of treatments are known only in an aggregate sense, and the model merely indicates who is most at risk in the absence of treatment. In any case, the result of this "level-two data fusion" is not yet a decision, but a knowledge base to support a decision.

Finally, a typical example of *high-level* data fusion in the clinical context is the therapy decision process. This process should *ideally* utilize everything that can be determined from risk assessment, including if possible differential risk assessment depending on relapse site, differential response to therapy, and enhanced probabilities of early relapse. *In practice*, the statistically validated knowledge base usually supplies only partial information, and certain tacit assumptions are made. For example, in the absence of an explicit multivariate statistical model of differential response to therapy based on factors, it is natural to suppose that patients with "poor prognosis" are those who are most likely to benefit from more aggressive therapy options. Biological understanding of therapy mechanisms is also utilized, of course. Such reasoning is implicit in treatment guidelines such as the St. Gallen guidelines in breast cancer (Goldhirsch et al. 2001). The goal here is to assess benefits and risks. Since the relative value of different benefits and risks can depend on individual patient preferences, a properly designed data fusion process for decision support should be capable of including these as well.

Determining the optimal degree of data integration/reduction to be performed at each level of data fusion is a universal and very difficult problem that will probably become the key issue in application of molecular staging to clinical decision support. Although the details go far beyond the scope of this paper and deserve considerable research in their own right, it is useful to highlight some of the issues involved.

As a general principle of data fusion, hard classifications at level one, such as introduction of dichotomized (binary) univariate factors, are to be avoided, because they often degrade overall multivariate classification performance. For example, using "nodal status" in breast cancer (ignoring the information provided by the number of affected nodes) is an example of one extreme, namely too much data reduction at an early stage. Many conventional statistical treatments of medical databases ignore this principle for simple reasons of convenience.

New molecular techniques such as microarrays or proteomics provide an enormous volume of information about each individual patient. At the other extreme, it would be conceivable to supply this entire raw information to a neural network as described above and train the network for survival. However, the learning process utilized in these networks, known as *supervised learning*, concentrates on obtaining a model for the outcomes (nodes o1, o2,...) as conditional probabilities given the inputs. Recognizing the independent prognostic impact of large numbers of factors generally requires prohibitively high statistical power.

In contrast, clustering algorithms and neural nets with *unsupervised* learning (typical for so-called self-organizing maps) are designed to learn the probability distribution among factors including complex interactions. Hence, such algorithms are designed to map the high-dimensional space of raw factors down to a low-dimensional space of "integrated" factors based on classification. Such a mapping or fusion of raw factors is already performed in standard software and would appear to be required. Nonetheless, theoretically one can discuss what degree of refinement should be produced by these methods.

The information obtained at each level of data fusion has some level of uncertainty. For this reason, the knowledge basis for a decision support system using data fusion should include at each level an estimate of uncertainty in the information being provided to the next level. For example, in context of treatment strategy, the concepts of *therapeutic efficiency* and *therapeutic security* are often discussed:

1. High therapeutic efficiency: exclude patients from therapy unless the risk is sufficiently high to justify adjuvant therapy
2. High therapeutic security: administer adjuvant therapy unless the risk can be proved to be very low

The first of these concepts is related to the *specificity* of prognosis, whereas the second is related to the *sensitivity*. Ideally, both of these goals should be achieved. In practice, one deals with the uncertainty as illustrated in breast cancer. In breast cancer, axillary lymph node status is considered the strongest established prognostic marker; about 70% of node-negative patients will be cured by surgery alone. Nevertheless, up to 30% of the patients may relapse within 10 years after surgery and eventually die of metastasis (McGuire and Clark 1992). In other words, achieving both high therapeutic efficiency and security is impossible based only on nodal status, because too many "low-risk" patients would still relapse if the node-negative group were not treated. Hence, the side effects and other risks of therapy still represent the lesser of two evils even for this group.

Conclusions and Implications for Cancer Management

In cancer, the designation "high-risk" is often used as a surrogate with the implication "likely to benefit from therapy." In view of the broadening spectrum of new treatment options, including tumor-biological therapy approaches such as Herceptin (Slamon et al. 2001), accurate *prediction of response to therapy* will be the prerequisite for clinical indications. Moreover, as mentioned previously, as our understanding of disease processes and therapy impacts is refined, a *differential prediction* of response for competing risks based on individual patient characteristics will be required to target the treatment regimen to the patient with the goal of *optimal individualized cancer therapy*. Thus, advanced statistical methods able to exploit the increasingly detailed information provided by molecular, i.e., tumor biology-oriented staging markers, will become essential in the future.

Moreover, the clinical decision environment is complex and includes both subjective and objective influences on physician and patient. Often, subjective or intangible considerations having little to do with statistics are the most important ones from the patient's point of view. As treatment options become more complex and potentially expensive, important strategic and management issues and conflicts of interest are possible.

Hence, there is a need for advanced evaluation tools for risk profiling and support of clinical decision making in a complex environment, especially for patients and their physicians. Ultimately, such a decision support tool will require a self-learning computational framework based for example on competing-risk neural networks to predict differential therapy effects on different modes of relapse – providing not necessarily a single risk score, but optimally a *differential risk profile*. On the basis of this risk profile, decision support utilizing properly designed data fusion techniques could then provide the following advantages:

1. *Differential risk profile*: Improve individual therapy decisions and quality of care by providing physicians and patients with a differential risk profile for each available treatment option.
2. *Prediction of treatment benefits*: Predict what benefits may be expected from proposed or hypothetical treatment regimens targeting particular relapse modes.

3. *Improved study design and analysis*: Distinguish apparent and real rises in competing modes of relapse in a study. Improve study design by proper consideration of these requirements.
4 *Generalization*: Improve generalization performance of the estimates obtained.
5. *Support benefit-oriented guidelines*: Use differential risk profiling to establish improved guidelines and target therapies to those patients who are most likely to derive a benefit from them. This will not only minimize unnecessary side effects and costs, but most importantly optimize patient treatment and hence the overall quality of care.

Outlook

Molecular staging markers in cancer tend to characterize *specific*, fundamental disease processes to a greater extent than conventional staging markers. At the biological level, the course of the disease will almost certainly involve complex interactions between multiple underlying processes. Hence, tools capable of extracting the maximum information in the presence of interactions will be required.

There are severe complications to training neural nets in a typical clinical data environment, including the problem of confidence assessment. Hence, "off-the-shelf solutions" are unlikely to work. Nonetheless, neural networks are an appropriate tool for this kind of analysis and could form an important part of the statistical backbone of a decision support environment. Their true value compared to conventional methods may well become apparent in the form of improved performance of decision support systems, as the information characterizing disease processes becomes more complete.

Acknowledgements. This work was supported in part by a grant to N.H. and M.S. from the Wilhelm Sander Stiftung (Project #1996.066.2).

References

Beck GJ (1979) Stochastic survival models with competing risks and covariates. Biometrics 35:427–438
Clark GM (1994) Do we really need prognostic factors in breast cancer? Breast Cancer Res Treat 30:117–126
Elston CW, Ellis IO (1991) Pathological prognostic factors in breast cancer. I. The value of histological grade in breast cancer: experience from a large study with long-term follow-up. Histopathology 19:403–410
Gasparini G, Pozza F, Harris AL (1993) Evaluating the potential usefulness of new prognostic and predictive indicators in node-negative breast cancer patients. J Natl Cancer Inst 85:1206–1219
Goldhirsch A, Glick JH, Gelber RD, Coates AS, Senn HJ (2001) Meeting Highlights: International Consensus Panel on the Treatment of Primary Breast Cancer. J Clin Oncol 19:3817–3827

Hayes DF, Trock B, Harris AL (1998) Assessing the clinical impact of prognostic factors: when is "statistically significant" clinically useful? Breast Cancer Res Treat 52:305–319

Harbeck N, Dettmar P, Thomssen C, Berger U, Ulm K, Kates R, Jänicke F, Höfler H, Graeff H, Schmitt M (1999) Risk-group discrimination in node-negative breast cancer using invasion and proliferation markers: six-year median follow-up. Br J Cancer 80:419–426

Harbeck N, Kates R, Ulm K, Graeff H, Schmitt M (2000) Neural network analysis of follow-up data in primary breast cancer. Int J Biol Markers 15:116–122

Harbeck N, Kates R, Schmitt M (2002) Clinical relevance of invasion factors uPA and PAI-1 for individualized therapy decisions in primary breast cancer is greatest when used in combination. J Clin Oncology 20 (in press)

Kalbfleisch JD, Prentice RL (1980) The statistical analysis of failure time data. New York: John Wiley and Sons

Kates R, Harbeck N, Ulm K, Jänicke F, Graeff H, Schmitt M (2000). Decision support in breast cancer: Recent advances in prognostic and predictive techniques. In: Jain A, Jain A, Jain S, Jain L (eds) Artificial intelligence techniques in breast cancer diagnosis and prognosis. World Scientific Publishing, Singapore, pp 55–95

Kates RE, Foekens JA, Look MP, Ulm K, Schmitt M, Harbeck N (2001) Generalization of competing-risk neural networks in breast cancer. Breast Cancer Res Treat 69:267

Mc Guire WL, Clark GM (1992) Prognostic factors and treatment decisions in axillary node-negative breast cancer New Engl J Med 326:1756–1761

Slamon DJ, Leyland-Jones B, Shak S, Fuchs H, Paton V, Bajamonde A, Fleming T, Eiermann W, Wolter J, Pegram M, Baselga J, Norton L (2001) Use of chemotherapy plus a monoclonal antibody against HER2 for metastatic breast cancer that overexpresses HER2. New Engl J Med 344:783–792

Thomssen C, Jänicke F, Kaufmann M, Scharl A, Hayes DF (2000) Current controversies in cancer. Do we need better prognostic factors in node-negative breast cancer? Eur J Cancer 36:293–306

Tolley, HD Manton, KG Poss SS (1978) A linear models application of competing risks to multiple causes of death. Biometrics 34 581–591

Wohlfahrt J, Andersen PK, Melbye M (1999) Multivariate competing risks. Statistics in medicine 18:1023–1030

Clinical Implications of the EGF Receptor/Ligand System for Tumor Progression and Survival in Gastrointestinal Carcinomas: Evidence for New Therapeutic Options

Reinhard Kopp, Elisabeth Rothbauer, Maximilian Ruge, Hans Arnholdt, Joachim Spranger, M. Muders, Doris G. Pfeiffer, Friedrich Wilhelm Schildberg, Andreas Pfeiffer

R. Kopp (✉)
Department of Surgery, Klinikum Grosshadern, University of Munich, Marchioninistrasse 15, 81377 Munich, Germany

Abstract

The epidermal growth factor (EGF) receptor and its various ligands (EGF, TGF-α, amphiregulin, heparin-binding (HB)-EGF, heregulin, betacellulin) seem to be involved in the growth regulation of intestinal mucosa and might be related to the development and progression of gastrointestinal tumors. However, few quantitative data investigating the impact of tumor-EGF receptor levels in gastrointestinal carcinomas on tumor stage and prognosis are available. Therefore, EGF receptors were quantitatively determined in colorectal carcinomas in comparison to adjacent normal mucosa by ^{125}I[EGF]-binding studies. EGFR capacity was increased in advanced invasive colorectal carcinomas (T1/2 vs. T3/4 tumors, $p<0.001$) and advanced UICC stages (UICC I vs. UICC II/III, $p<0.001$). These findings were confirmed with quantitative ^{125}[I]EGF autoradiography performed on frozen tissue slides and analyzed by laser densitometry ($p=0.020$). EGF receptor analysis with immunohistochemistry with EGFR antibodies directed against the extracellular domain of the receptor was not correlated with tumor invasion or prognosis. mRNA-expression of EGFR ligands was investigated using semiquantitative RT-PCR amplification using specific primers. RT-PCR transcripts of EGFR ligands (EGF, TGF-α, HB-EGF, and amphiregulin) were detected in both carcinomas and normal mucosa, indicating that autocrine growth stimulation of colorectal carcinomas is mediated by coexpression of EGF receptor ligands and upregulation of EGF receptors. Survival of colorectal cancer patients with increased tumor EGF receptor levels was significantly reduced in comparison to patients with low/unchanged tumor EGF receptor levels (mean survival±SD, 36.2±4.0 vs. 46.8±4.3 months; $p=0.017$). Further studies investigating EGF receptor levels in gastric cancer patients have shown that increased tumor EGF receptor levels were associated with poor prognosis in gastric cancer patients with tumors localized distal from the cardia. Several specific EGF receptor tyrosine kinase inhibitors have recently entered clinical phase I–III studies, with promising

antitumor effects in several tumors, including gastrointestinal cancer. Therefore, patients with invasive gastric or colorectal carcinomas might benefit from therapies specifically blocking EGFR-mediated signal transduction.
Abbreviations. EGFR, epidermal growth factor receptor; TGF-α, transforming growth factor-alpha; HB-EGF, heparin-binding epidermal growth factor; IHC, immunohistochemistry.

Introduction

The epidermal growth factor/ligand system was early proposed as an important pathway for tumor development and progression by autocrine stimulation of cell proliferation (Sporn and Roberts 1985). The epidermal growth factor (EGF) receptor is a plasma glycoprotein (MW 170,000 kDa) composed of an extracellular ligand-binding domain, a transmembrane region, and an intracellular protein tyrosine kinase domain (Cohen et al. 1980; Ulrich and Schlessinger 1990). Several ligands including epidermal growth factor (EGF), transforming growth factor-α (TGF-α), heparin-binding epidermal growth factor (HB-EGF), amphiregulin, heregulin, and betacellulin (Tahara 1995) were found to bind to EGF receptors or other members of the EGFR family (ErbB1–4) with differential affinities, activating a cascade of signal transduction pathways involved in the regulation of proliferation in epithelial cells (Fig. 1). Following ligand binding, receptor dimerization occurs, leading to stimulation of intrinsic tyrosine kinase activity and tyrosine autophosphorylation. Receptor inactivation is mediated by receptor internalization and ligand-receptor dissociation (Carpenter and Cohen 1979; Schreiber et al. 1983). Additionally, activation of EGF receptors is modulated by intracellular kinases mediating negative feedback control via receptor phosphorylation at specific regulatory domains (Downward et al. 1985). The structure of the EGF receptor is homologous with the product of the avian erythroblastosis virus oncogene v-erb (Downward et al. 1984). By overexpression of EGF receptors or secretion of increased levels of EGF receptor ligands, epithelial cells of the gastrointestinal tract might acquire growth advantages relative to surrounding tissue due to autocrine stimulation of proliferation (Malden et al. 1989; Tanaka et al. 1991; Tahara 1995). In addition, involvement of EGF receptors and their ligands has been implicated in differentiation of fetal gastrointestinal mucosa (Trembley et al. 1997), mucosa regeneration, and healing of gastric ulcers (Tarnawski and Jones 1998). Several colon cancer cell lines were found to possess EGF receptors and secrete EGFR ligands, supporting the concept of autocrine stimulation of tumor growth (Coffey et al. 1986; Anzano et al. 1989; Johnson et al. 1992).

First preliminary data on EGF receptor levels in gastric and colon cancer specimen were reported by Yasui et al. (1988). To date, only a few studies with small numbers of patients have investigated the impact of tumor EGF receptor levels on tumor progression and survival using ^{125}I[EGF] radioreceptor analysis in colorectal cancer patients, with controversial results (Yasui et al. 1988;

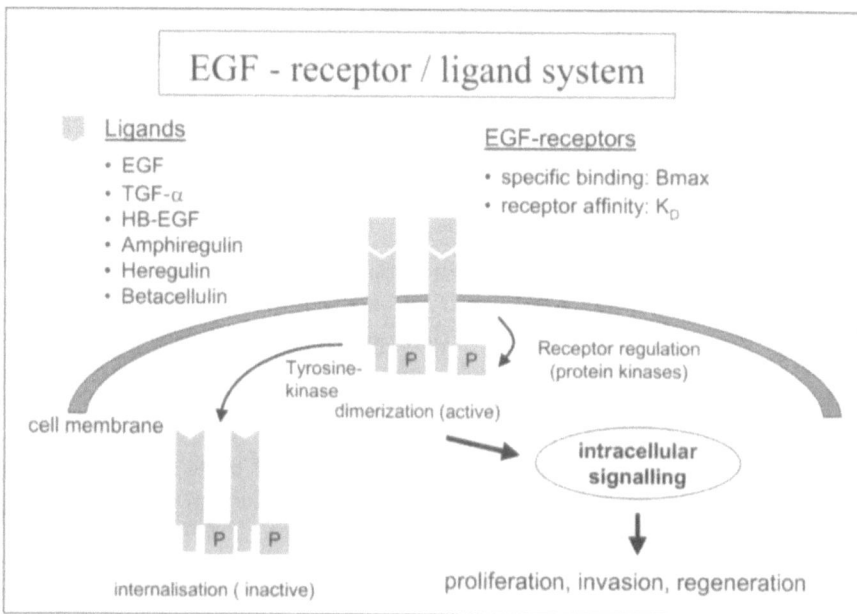

Fig. 1. EGF receptor/ligand system

Rothbauer et al. 1989; Steele et al. 1990; Koenders et al. 1992; Borlinghaus et al. 1993). Preliminary data were reported from our group (Rothbauer et al. 1989) investigating early tumor stages of colorectal carcinomas showing unchanged or decreased EGF receptors and increased levels of EGFR ligands. We have therefore increased the number of colorectal carcinomas investigated and compared ^{125}I[EGF] radioligand binding studies with ^{125}I[EGF]autoradiography and the detection of EGF receptors by immunohistochemistry. To investigate the expression of the various EGFR ligands, we additionally performed semiquantitative RT-PCR analysis using ligand-specific primers.

Analysis of EGF receptor levels might be of clinical and therapeutic relevance, since recent studies using EGF receptor-specific tyrosine kinase inhibitors have shown remarkable inhibitory effects on tumor proliferation and invasion in some models of gastrointestinal cancer and in phase I–III clinical trials (Baselga 2000; Ciardiello and Tortora 2001).

Patients and Methods

In samples from 38 colorectal carcinomas and adjacent normal-appearing mucosa from the same patients, the EGF receptor/ligand system was characterized. Seven tumors were localized in the right colon, seven in the left colon, and 24 tumors were localized in the rectum. Patients were curatively treated by colonic or rectal resection with appropriate lymph node removal according to the principles of oncologic surgery. All patients were followed up for up to 60 months after the operation. Follow-up investigations included clinical examination, blood tests including tumor markers (CEA and CA 19–9), chest X-ray, upper abdomen sonography, colonoscopy with endoscopic examination of the anastomosis, additional rectoscopy in patients with rectal cancer or low anastomosis, and yearly abdominal CT scan.

Membrane Preparations and ^{125}I[EGF] Receptor Analysis

^{125}I EGF radioreceptor binding assays were performed as described by Pfeiffer et al. (1990). Briefly, tissue samples were washed in cold saline and stored at – 60°C. Corresponding pieces of tissue used for subsequent analysis were investigated by the pathologist without knowledge of assay results. Samples of tumors or mucosa were thawed on ice in 10 vol (wt/vol) of 0.32 M sucrose in 5 mM HEPES (pH 7.4), cut into small pieces, and homogenized with a polytron homogenizer (Bachhofer, Reutlingen, Germany). The supernatant was then recentrifuged at 17,500×g for 30 min, and the pellet was resuspended in assay buffer, as described (Kopp et al. 2002). Radiolabeled EGF (0.1–0.6 nM) was incubated with membrane preparations in the presence of various concentrations of unlabeled EGF (0.1–200 nM) in a final volume of 200 µl at 4°C overnight, when stable binding under equilibrium conditions was achieved. The incubations were terminated by addition of 500 µl ice-cold buffer followed by two centrifugation and washing steps of the pellet at 10,000×g for 5 min at 4°C. Remaining radioactivity associated with the membranes was determined in a y-counter.

Murine EGF (Paesel, Frankfurt, Germany) was iodinated as reported (Carpenter and Cohen 1976), and specific activity (80–150 µCi/mg) was determined by self-displacement using the 'Allfit' program as described by De Lean et al. (1978). Protein contents in the membrane preparations were determined using a modification of the Bradford assay (1976) with reagents obtained from BioRad (Munich, Germany) with bovine y-globulin as standard. Results from radioreceptor assays were then analyzed by nonlinear least-square regression curve fitting using the computer program 'LIGAND' (Munson and Rodbard 1980). Displacement curves using various concentrations of unlabeled EGF (0.1–200 nM) in the presence of ^{125}I-labeled EGF indicated a single binding site with similar affinities in mucosa (dissociation constant K_D 0.9 nM) and carcinoma (K_D 0.7 nM) preparations, respectively. Therefore, for determination of receptor capacities using the 'Ligand' program, similar affinities were assumed for mucosa and carcinoma samples.

[125]I[EGF] Autoradiography

[125]I[EGF] autoradiography was performed as described by Pfeiffer at al. (1995) for the analysis of muscarinic receptors in gastric mucosa samples. Reliability of the method used was analyzed in [125]I[EGF] binding studies using porcine gastric mucosa. Displacement analysis of bound [125]I[EGF] with unlabeled EGF was investigated by radioligand binding in homogenates and on frozen tissue slices of porcine gastric mucosa embedded in Tissue Tek (Miles, Elkhart, Ind., USA). Binding capacity was determined by directly counting specifically and non-specifically labeled pellets of tissue homogenates or tissue slices in a y-counter. Displacement curves were analyzed by Scatchard analysis with the *Ligand* curve fitting program. Data from the displacement curves of these experiments showed similar binding kinetics for homogenate or tissue slice assays (K_D, 0.6–0.9 nM; receptor capacity, 9.1–11.5 fmol/mg protein). Samples of mucosa or tumor were cut into 10 µm slices; four slices were placed on glass slides and incubated with labeled ligand (1 nM [125]I[EGF]; specific activity, 150–200 µCi/µg) for 1 h at 37°C, when equilibrium conditions were achieved, followed by three washes in 250 ml in ice-cold Tris buffer (pH 7.5) for 15, 30, and 60 s. Another slide with four slices from the same tumor area was incubated with [125]I[EGF] in the presence of unlabeled ligand (200 nM EGF), representing nonspecific binding. Bovine serum albumin 1%, PMSF 0.5 mM, and aprotinin 400 IE/ml were added to reduce nonspecific binding, which ranged from 8% to 10%. Slides were then air dried and either wiped with glass fiber filters (GFC, Whatman) for liquid scintillation spectrophotometry or exposed to autoradiography film for 10 days at room temperature. In parallel to tumor slices, internal control tissues with known EGFR capacities were coincubated during the same experiment: porcine gastric mucosa (10.3±0.1 fmol/mg protein) and human placenta (124.5±0.6 fmol/mg protein). To quantify the data obtained by autoradiography, standardized scales with known amounts of ^{125}I radioactivity (^{125}I microscales, Amersham) were coexposed with each film to obtain reference curves. Autoradiography of tissue samples and ^{125}I microscales were then analyzed by laser-densitometry using a Panasonic WV-LD 130 L video camera, connected to a computerized imaging program. Standardized scales with known radioactivity caused a linear increase of blackening of the autoradiography film up to 40 nCi/mg tissue. The gray levels of defined areas in the tumor sample or normal mucosa were calculated (total binding), and nonspecific binding determined in parallel sections was subtracted. Protein content as determined by the Bradford assay varied from15.9 to 16.6 µg per tissue slice.

EGFR Ligand Determination by Semiquantitative RT-PCR

Total RNA was extracted with the acid guanidinium thiocyanate phenol method and resuspended in HPLC-grade water. RNA concentration was determined by spectrophotometry at 260 nm. The RNA template was then incubated with RNAse free DNAse 1U (Promega, Heidelberg, Germany). DNAse was then heat-inactivated at 95°C for 2 min. RNA (3 µg) was then reverse-transcribed into cDNA using 20 U MuLV reverse transcriptase (Boehringer, Mannheim, Germany). cDNA was then amplified by PCR using specific primers for the following EGFR ligands with the length of the expected PCR product given: EGF (248 bp), TGF-α (264 bp), amphiregulin (360 bp), and HB-EGF (290 bp), as described by Schiemann et al. (2001). As an internal standard for RNA quantity, pyruvate dehydrogenase (PDH) was additionally amplified. Semi-quantitative estimation of RNA expression was performed by laser densito-metric analysis of PCR products with various PCR cycles (cycles 18, 21, 24, 27, and 30) when linear increases of the optical density of the PCR products was observed (Pfeiffer et al. 1997).

EGF Receptor Immunohistochemistry

EGF receptor immunohistochemistry was performed as described by Arn-holdt et al. (1991). Monoclonal anti-EGF receptor antibody (clone EGFr1) was purchased from Amersham Buchler (Braunschweig, Germany). Rabbit anti-mouse immunoglobulin antibody, anti-biotin monoclonal antibody (clone BK-1/39), and avidin-biotin complex were obtained from Dakopatts (Copen-hagen, Denmark). Immunohistochemistry was performed on 5 µm slices em-bedded in paraffin with prior heat activation using a microwave. Specific EGF receptor staining on the membranes of tumor cells was semiquantitatively evaluated based on the staining intensity and the number of positive tumor cells. Only tumor samples with more than 10% membrane-bound staining of the tumor cells were evaluated as EGF receptor-positive. Based on the staining intensity and the percentage of stained tumor cells, an immunohistochemistry score (IHC score, 0–3) was calculated. IHC score 0, negative staining; IHC score 1, weak staining intensity with less than 50% positive tumor cells; IHC score 2, moderate staining and/or 10%–50% positive tumor cells; IHC score 3, strong staining intensity and/or more than 50% positive tumor cells.

Statistical Analysis

Data were analyzed with SPSS statistical software (version 10.0 for Windows, SPSS, Chicago). Chi-square tests were used to compare proportions, and Mann-Whitney tests were used for quantitative values. Univariate analysis of survival was carried out by the Kaplan-Meier method, and the evaluation of differences between groups was performed with the log-rank test. A two-sided p value of less than 0.05 was considered to indicate statistical significance. Mean values±SD are shown, if not indicated otherwise.

Results

[125]I[EGF] receptor binding was detected in all colorectal carcinomas investigated, ranging from 1.2 to 23.0 fmol/mg protein. EGFR capacity was increased in advanced and invasive colorectal carcinomas, according to T classification (T1/2 tumors 5.9±4.1 vs. T3/4 tumors 15.6±6.8 fmol/mg protein; $p<0.001$; Fig. 2) or UICC stages (UICC I 3.7±2.5 vs. UICC II 10.2±8.1; UICC III, 13.3±5.8 fmol/mg protein; $p=0.013$, Table 1). These results were confirmed by quantitative [125]I[EGF] autoradiography of frozen tissue slices analyzed by direct counting of bound radioactivity of labeled ligand (specific and nonspecific binding) and laser densitometric imaging analysis of defined and histopathologically controlled areas of mucosa or tumor samples. A significant increase of EGF receptor capacity was found in advanced UICC II/III colorectal carci-

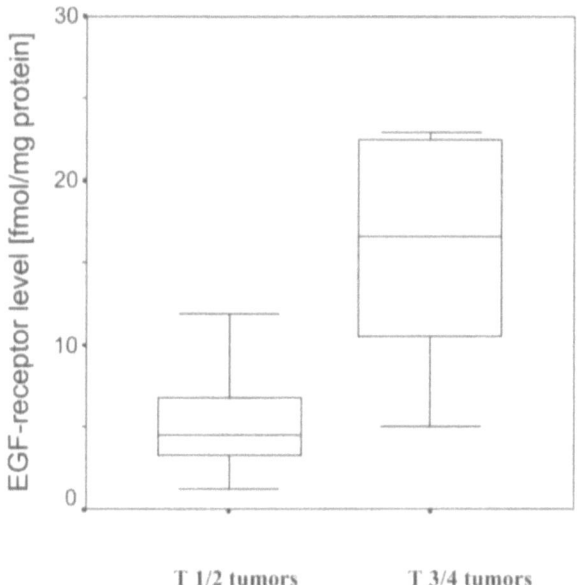

Fig. 2. EGF receptor levels in colorectal carcinomas in T1/2 and T3/4 tumors. EGF receptor levels were determined by [125]I[EGF]binding as described in the text. Blox-bot shows median values with lower/upper quartiles and maximum/minimum levels

Table 1. EGF-receptor levels in colorectal carcinomas according to different UICC stages (mean values±SD as determined by [125]I[EGF] radioligand binding)

	(n)	specific [125]I[EGF]binding	p
UICC I	9	3.7±2.5	
UICC II	11	10.2±8.1	
UICC III	18	13.3±5.8	0.013

Table 2. Comparison of EGF radioreceptor analysis and EGF receptor autoradiography in UICC II/III colorectal carcinomas

	EGF radioreceptor assay (RRA) (n=20)	p	EGF receptor autoradiography (n=9)	p
Adjacent mucosa	7.5±4.5 fmol/mg protein		8.7±4.5 fmol/mg protein	
Colorectal carcinoma	12.4±7.4 fmol/mg protein	0.016	15.1±6.1 fmol/mg protein	0.020

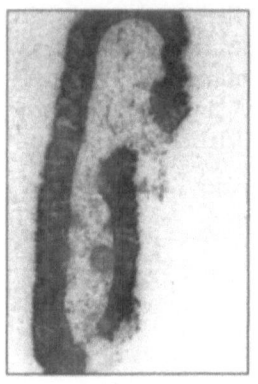 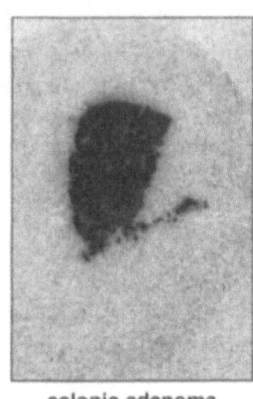 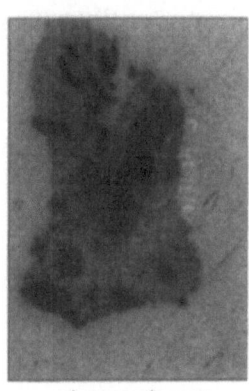

| normal mucosa | colonic adenoma | colon carcinoma |

Fig. 3. ^{125}I[EGF] autoradiography of normal colonic mucosa, colonic adenoma, and colon carcinoma. Total binding of ^{125}I[EGF] to slices of indicated tissues is shown. For quantitative determination of EGF receptor levels, nonspecific binding in the presence of unlabeled EGF was subtracted

Table 3. Comparison of EGF radioreceptor analysis and EGF receptor immunohistochemical detection (IHC-score) in UICC I/II and UICC III colorectal carcinomas. Mean values±SD are shown

	EGF radioreceptor analysis (n=26)	p	EGF receptor immunohisto-chemistry (n=20)	p
UICC I/II	6.4±5.7 fmol/mg protein		1.75±0.51 (IHC-score)	
UICC III	15.2±5.3 fmol/mg protein	0.001	1.83±0.57 (IHC-score)	n.s.

nomas in comparison to normal adjacent mucosa as determined by radioreceptor assays (12.4+7.4 vs. 7.5+4.5 fmol/mg protein, n=20, p=0.016) or by EGF receptor autoradiography (15.1+6.1 vs. 8.7+4.5 fmol/mg protein, n=9, p=0.02; Table 2, Fig. 3).

Analysis of EGF receptors by immunohistochemistry showed EGF receptor staining in 16 of 20 tumors investigated with different staining intensities. Staining intensity and the number of stained tumor cells were evaluated using an immunohistochemistry (IHC) score, as described above. IHC score was not correlated to T or N classification, UICC stage, or EGF receptor level, in contrast to ^{125}I[EGF] radioreceptor analysis (Table 3).

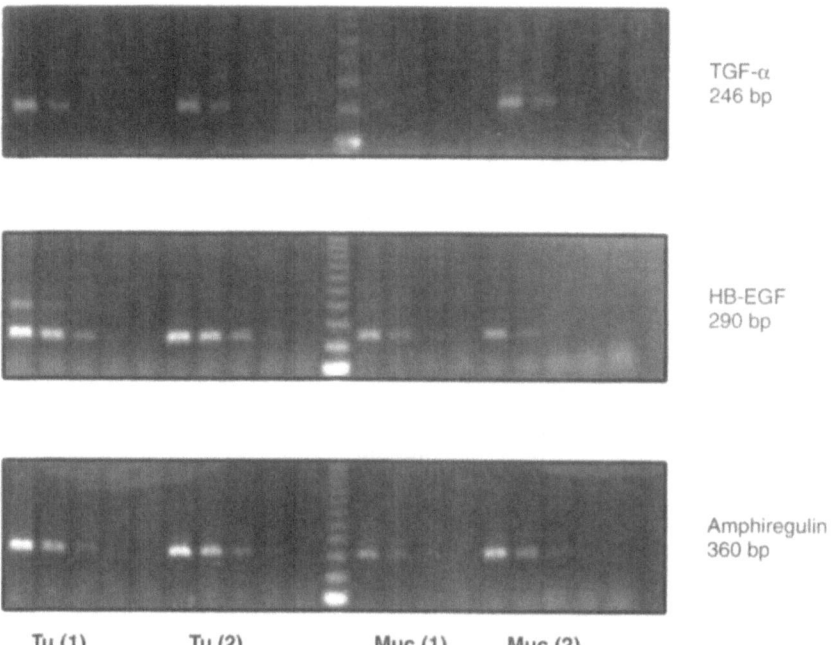

TGF-α
246 bp

HB-EGF
290 bp

Amphiregulin
360 bp

Tu (1)   Tu (2)   Muc (1)   Muc (2)

Fig. 4. Analysis of mRNA expression of EGF receptor ligands determined in colonic adenomas and carcinomas. Shown are RT-PCR transcripts of indicated EGFR ligands amplified during various lengths of PCR cycles (30, 27, 24, 21, and 18 cycles) for semiquantitative analysis. Semiquantitative analysis was performed relative to amplified transcripts of phosphate dehydrogenase (*PDH*, not shown). Corresponding samples of tumor (*Tu*) or normal adjacent mucosa (*Muc*) were analyzed

Analysis of RT-PCR transcripts of EGFR ligands showed similar expression of EGF, TGF-α, HB-EGF, and amphiregulin in carcinomas and normal mucosa (Fig. 4), suggesting that autocrine growth stimulation in advanced colorectal carcinomas is mediated by coexpression of EGFR ligands and increased EGF receptor binding capacity. Further semiquantitative analysis of EGFR ligand mRNA expression by RT-PCR taken from probes with different PCR cycles under conditions of linear increases of amplification transcripts (cycles 18–30) did not indicate detectable differences regarding the mRNA expression of the ligands investigated.

Survival analysis of colorectal cancer patients in relation to elevated or low/unchanged receptor levels in comparison to adjacent normal mucosa indicated significantly reduced mean survival times ($\pm$SD) for patients with elevated EGF receptor levels (36.2$\pm$4.0 months; 95% CI, 28.3–44.0 months; n=22 in comparison to patients with low/unchanged tumor EGF receptor levels (46.8+4.3 months; 95% CI, 33.3–55.4 months; n=16; p=0.017; Fig. 5).

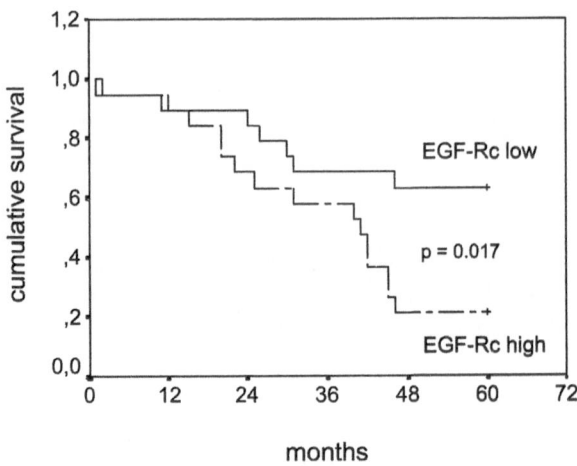

Fig. 5. Clinical impact of EGF receptor levels on survival of colorectal cancer patients. EGF receptor levels, as determined by ^{125}I[EGF]receptor binding, were classified as increased ($n=22$) or low/unchanged ($n=16$) in comparison to samples from normal-appearing mucosa of the same patient

Discussion

Regulation of proliferation and invasion of several malignancies was implicated with the EGFR ligand pathway. Increased EGF receptor expression has been associated with invasiveness of human bladder tumors and poor prognosis in patients with breast and esophageal cancer (Neal et al. 1985; Sainsbury et al. 1985; Itakura et al. 1994). The data reported in this study show increased EGF receptor levels in advanced and invasive colorectal carcinomas according to T classification and UICC stages. Increased EGF receptor levels in colorectal carcinomas were additionally associated with reduced survival times in these patients.

In contrast to our previous study, when mainly T1/T2 carcinomas were investigated (Rothbauer et al. 1989), we have now analyzed a larger number of tumors including more advanced colorectal carcinomas. The observed difference with low or unchanged EGF receptors in early T1/T2 tumors and increased EGF receptors in advanced T3/T4 tumors might explain the controversial results reported in the literature. The decrease in EGF receptor levels in patients with early tumor stages can be explained by EGF receptor downregulation in the presence of autocrine secreted EGFR ligands. In light of the finding that heparin-binding (HB)-EGF was first identified in macrophage-like U-937 cells (Higashiyama et al. 1991), additional paracrine effects due to secretion of growth factors by cells present in the tumor microenvironment might promote early alterations during colorectal carcinogenesis and tumor development. Based on the observation that tumors secrete EGFR ligands promoting autocrine tumor growth with subsequent at least partial receptor downregulation in carcinomas, the observed increase of tumor EGF receptors levels in advanced carcinomas might underestimate the absolute implication of this pathway regulating tumor proliferation and progression in colorectal cancer.

Because EGF radioreceptor assays were performed in tissue homogenates of tumor sample and might therefore contain small amounts of connective tissue or normal adjacent mucosa with possible effects on the results obtained, we additionally performed ^{125}I[EGF] autoradiography on slices of histopathologically proven tumor samples. As shown in this study, the results from ^{125}I[EGF] autoradiography analysis performed in UICC II/III tumors confirmed the finding that EGF receptors are increased in advanced and invasive colorectal carcinomas.

In this study, expression of EGFR ligands was determined by RT-PCR analysis using extracted tumor mRNA. Using this approach, all EGF receptor ligands could be detected at the mRNA level including EGF, TGF-α, amphiregulin, and HB-EGF. However, these results cannot exclude the possibility of relevant differences in the protein expression of the mentioned ligands, due to differences in the posttranscriptional processing. Further studies from our group in colon cancer cell lines have shown that TGF-α was detectable at both the cellular mRNA and protein levels in the conditioned medium with growth-promoting quantities, whereas EGF was found only by RT-PCR analysis and was not detectable at relevant protein levels. We did not determine the expression of heregulin and betacellulin, also members of the EGFR ligand family with binding affinities for the EGF receptor and the ErbB3 receptor (Venkateswarlu et al. 2002). Therefore, based on our study it is not possible to speculate on the precise role of each EGF receptor ligand during the process of malignant transformation and tumor progression of gastrointestinal carcinomas. However, the described increased capacity of EGF receptors determined in our study in advanced colorectal carcinomas and the expression of several specific EGFR ligands promoting autocrine tumor growth suggests that the EGFR ligand pathway will play a major role in the regulation of colorectal tumor progression.

In our study, analysis of EGF receptors by immunohistochemistry did not show differences in EGF immunostaining in different UICC stages of colorectal carcinomas in comparison to ^{125}I[EGF] radioreceptor assays. Similar findings were also reported by other authors (Koretz et al. 1990; Maurer et al. 1998) investigating colorectal carcinomas by immunohistochemistry, indicating that immunohistochemistry seems to be less sensitive due to nonspecific binding of the antibodies used or probably due to staining of downregulated binding-inactive EGF receptors.

The mechanisms leading to EGF receptor upregulation are unclear in colorectal carcinomas. Amplification of the EGF receptor gene (Ullrich et al. 1984), detectable with high incidence in squamous cell carcinomas (Yamamoto et al. 1986), is not frequently found in sporadic gastrointestinal carcinomas (Lemoine et al. 1991). EGF receptor levels and receptor affinity are further regulated by intracellular kinases, leading to receptor phosphorylation at specific sites and subsequent receptor inactivation (Downward et al. 1985). Enhanced tumor formation in athymic mice was observed for cell lines with mutant non-downregulating EGF receptors (Masui et al. 1991). However, tumor-specific mutations modifying EGF receptor capacities have not been reported to date for colorectal carcinomas.

Countaway et al. (1989) showed that incubation with phorbol esters known to activate protein kinase C (PKC) induce EGF receptor phosphorylation at specific sites with subsequently reduced EGF receptor binding. Studies by our group and others have shown that PKC activity is decreased in colorectal adenoma and carcinomas as determined by substrate phosphorylation assays (Kopp et al. 1991; Kusonoki et al. 1992; Verstovsek et al. 1998). Therefore, altered PKC activity in colorectal neoplasias with subsequent reduced regulatory activity on EGF receptor phosphorylation might contribute to the observed upregulation of EGF receptors in colorectal cancer. However, reports indicate that phorbol ester-activated PKC stimulates tyrosine phosphorylation and activation of ErbB2 and ErbB3 (Emkey and Kahn 1997) and is able to induce EGFR transactivation (Chen et al. 2001). Therefore, it remains unclear which of the several known PKC subtypes is probably involved in negative feedback regulation or transactivation of the EGF receptor family.

Binding of ligands to EGF receptors leads to homo- or heterodimerization with other receptors of the EGF receptor family (EGFR 1–4). ErbB2 and erbB3 are transmembrane molecules with close structural homology with the EGF receptor and have been implicated in cell transformation and tumor pathogenesis (Maurer et al. 1998; Gill et al. 2002; Venkateswarlu et al. 2002). Therefore, inhibition of EGF receptor signaling will also inhibit other oncogene signals reported to be upregulated in colorectal cancer. A combined treatment with different inhibitors directed against both EGFR (ErbB1) and ErbB2 (HER2/neu) might be most effective.

Stimulation of the EGF receptor pathway by ligand binding leads to activation of an intracellular signaling cascade involving Grb2/Sos, ras, raf, src, and mitogen-activated protein kinases (MAPK) (Satoh et al. 1990; App et al. 1991). Since ras mutations or overexpression of src is frequently found in sporadic colorectal carcinomas with clinical relevance for tumor progression and survival, therapeutic strategies to inhibit EGF receptor-mediated signaling might be of clinical relevance. Specific inhibition of EGF receptor tyrosine kinase was shown to inhibit tumor growth in a xenograft model by inhibition of VEGF-mediated angiogenesis (Ciardiello et al. 2001). Furthermore, EGFR activation was shown to increase proteolytic activity by enhanced urokinase-type plasminogen activator (uPA) expression (Jensen and Rodeck 1993). Therefore, due to interactions with other tumor biologic pathways, EGF receptor activation in tumor cells will influence proliferation, tumor invasion, tumor angiogenesis, and regulation of apoptosis. Effects on the regulation of apoptosis by EGF receptor signaling might be of importance for neoadjuvant/adjuvant or palliative multimodal therapy protocols. Inhibition of EGF receptors by specific tyrosine kinase inhibitors was shown to increase the therapeutic effects of several antineoplastic substances, including cisplatin and irinotecan, in patients with metastatic disease (Ciardiello and Tortora 2001), and seems to im-

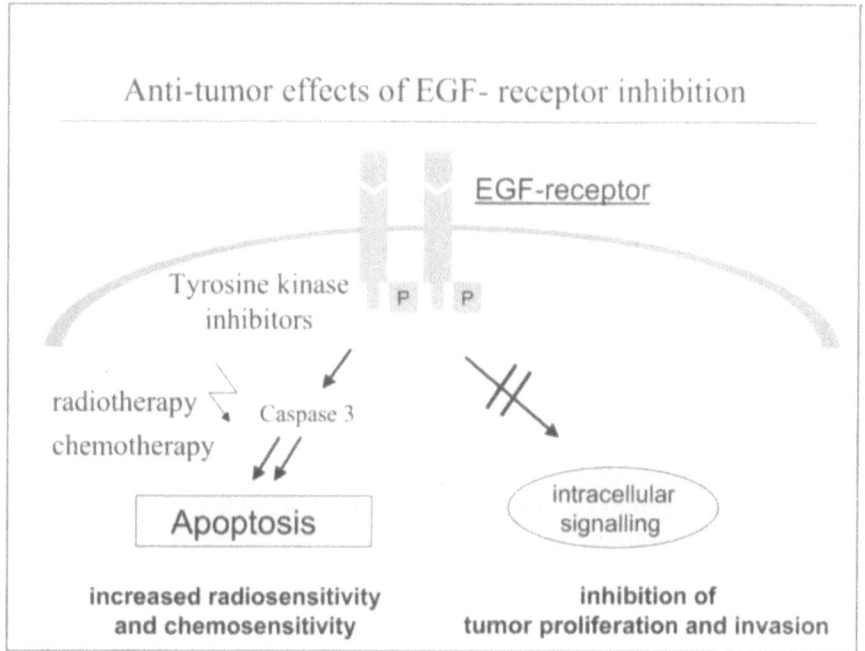

Fig. 6. Antitumor effects of EGF receptor inhibition

prove the effectiveness of radiotherapy in head and neck squamous cell carcinomas (Huang et al. 1999; Huang and Harari 2000; Fig. 6].

We recently showed that EGF receptor levels are also increased in gastric carcinomas localized distal from the cardia (Kopp et al. 2002), with reduced survival in patients with elevated tumor EGF receptors, relative to samples from corresponding adjacent mucosa. Similar data were reported by other groups (Sugiyama et al. 1989; Tokunaga et al. 1995; Slesak et al. 1998) investigating EGF receptors by immunohistochemistry. In these studies, elevated EGF receptor levels were found more frequently in invasive carcinomas, tumors with lymph node infiltration, and in patients with UICC III/IV tumor stages. In the study performed by Yonemura et al. (1992), gastric carcinomas with coexpression of immunoreactive EGF receptors and TGF-α had the poorest prognosis.

Several substances were investigated for their properties to inhibit EGF receptor activation and signaling. Suramin, a known antiprotozoal drug, was investigated several years ago. Although suramin potently inhibited EGF receptor binding in several tumor cell lines, this effect was not specific for EGF receptors, and inhibition of other growth factors and intracellular kinases was observed (Coffey et al. 1987; Kopp et al. 1991). Due to the reported effects on different growth-regulating pathways and difficulties of drug monitoring, sev-

Table 4. Tyrosine kinase inhibition of EGF receptor. Clinical trials investigating the antitumor effects of different EGF receptor tyrosine kinase inhibitors against various human tumors (according to Ciardiello et al. 2001)

Substance	Antitumor activity	Clinical trial	Disease
IMC-225 (mAb)	250 mg/m^2	Phase III	Head/neck, CRC
ZD 1839	80 nM	Phase III	NSCLC
OSI-774	100 nM	Phase II	Head/neck, NSCLC
CI-1033	40 nM	Phase I	Solid tumors

CRC, colorectal cancer; NSCLC, non-small cell lung cancer.

eral clinical trials in tumor patients have not yet shown clear therapeutic benefit (Gradishar et al. 2000; Grossmann et al. 2001).

However, the recent development of specific inhibitors of the EGF receptor pathway has probably provided new therapeutic options for cancer patients. Incubation of gastric or colon carcinoma cells with monoclonal antibodies against the EGF receptor or specific inhibitors of EGF receptor tyrosine kinase was shown to block autocrine growth stimulation via the EGFR ligand system by inhibition of proliferation and induction of apoptosis (Baselga and Mendelsohn 1994; Karnes et al. 1998; Partik et al. 1999; Woodburn 1999; Baselga 2000). Gonzalez et al. (1998) performed a pilot clinical trial investigating an active immunotherapy with modified human EGF to induce antibodies against autologous EGF. Another approach using adenoviral transfer of a dominant negative EGFR mutant has shown significantly increased radiosensitivity in a xenograft model of human mammary carcinoma cells (Lammering et al. 2001). Furthermore, preliminary data from clinical trials investigating the antitumor response and toxicity of EGF receptor-specific tyrosine kinase inhibitors indicate promising results and few side effects in several tumor patients (Ciardiello and Tortora 2001; Table 4).

In summary, the data presented and the results of recently published studies indicate an association of increased tumor EGF receptor levels with more advanced tumor stages and poor prognosis in colorectal and gastric cancer patients. These patients will probably benefit from new therapeutic strategies specifically targeting EGF receptor-mediated induction of tumor cell proliferation and progression.

References

App H, Hazan R, Zilberstein A, Ullrich A, Schlessinger J, Rapp U (1991) Epidermal growth factor (EGF) stimulates association and kinase activity of raf-1 with the EGF receptor. Mol Cell Biol 11:913–919

Anzano MA, Riemann D, Prichett W, Bowen-Pope DF, Greig R (1989) Growth factor production by human colon carcinoma cells. Cancer Res 49:2898–2904

Arnholdt H, Diebold J, Kuhlmann B, Loehrs U (1991) Receptor-mediated processing of epidermal growth factor in the trophoblast of the human placenta. Virchows Archiv B Cell Pathol 61:75–80

Baselga J, Mendelsohn J (1994) Receptor blockade with monoclonal antibodies as anti-cancer therapy. Pharmacol Ther 64:127–154

Baselga J (2000) New therapeutic agents targeting the epidermal growth factor receptor. J Clin Oncol 18:[Suppl]54s–59s

Borlinghaus P, Wieser S, Lamerz R (1993) Epidermal growth factor, transforming growth factor-a, and epidermal growth factor receptor content in normal and carcinomatous gastric and colonic tissue. Clin Invest 71:903–907

Bradford MM (1976) A rapid and sensitive method for the quantification of microgram quantities of protein utilizing the principle of protein-dye-binding. Analyt Biochem 72:248–254

Carpenter G, Cohen S (1976) [125]J-labeled human epidermal growth factor. J Cell Biol 71:159–171

Carpenter G, Cohen S (1979) Epidermal growth factor. Ann Rev Biochem 48:193–216

Chen N, Ma WY, She QB, Wu E, Liu G, Bode AM, Dong Z (2001) Transactivation of the epidermal growth factor receptor is involved in 12-O-tetradecanoylphorbol-13-acetate-induced signal transduction. J Biol Chem 14:46722–46728

Ciardiello F, Tortora G (2001) A novel approach in thee treatment of cancer: targeting the epidermal growth factor receptor. Clin Cancer Res 7:2958–2970

Ciardiello F, Caputo R, Bianco R, Damiano V, Fontanini G, Cuccato S, De Placido S, Bianco AR, Tortora G (2001) Inhibition of growth factor production and angiogenesis in human cancer cells by ZD1839 (Iressa), a selective epidermal growth factor receptor tyrosine kinase inhibitor. Clin Cancer Res 7:1459–1465

Coffey RJ, Shipley GD, Moses HL (1986) Production of transforming growth factors by human colon cancer lines. Cancer Res 46:1164–1169

Coffey JR, Leof EB, Shipley GD, Moses HL (1987) Suramin inhibition of growth factor receptor binding and mitogenicity in AKR-2B cells. J Cell Physiol 132:143–148

Cohen S, Carpenter G, King L (1980) Epidermal growth factor-receptor-protein kinase interactions. J Biol Chem 258:4834–4842

Countaway J, Northwood IC, Davis RJ (1989) Mechanism of phosphorylation of the epidermal growth factor receptor at threonine 669. J Biol Chem 264:10828–10835

De Lean A, Munson PJ, Rodbard D (1978) Simultaneous analysis of families of sigmoidal curves: application to bioassay, and physiological dose-response curves. Am J Physiol 235:E97–E102

Downward J, Yarden Y, Mayes E, Scarce G, Totty N, Stockwell P, Ullrich A, Schlessinger J, Waterfield MD (1984) Close similarity of epidermal growth factor receptor and v-erb-B oncogene protein sequences. Nature 307:521–527

Downward J, Parker P, Waterfield MD (1985) Autophosphorylation sites in the epidermal growth factor receptor. Nature 311:483–485

Emkey R, Kahn CR (1997) Cross-talk between phorbol ester-mediated signaling and tyrosine kinase proto-oncogenes. I. Activation of protein kinase C stimulates tyrosine phosphorylation and activation of ErbB2 and ErbB3. J Biol Chem 272:31172–31181

Gill N, Malik A, Potti A, Talukdar R, Saberi A, Mehdi SA (2002) HER-2/neu overexpression in colonic malignancies. Gastroenterol 122:248–249

Gonzalez G, Crombet T, Catala M, Mirabal V, Hernandez JC, Gonzalez Y, Marinello P, Guillen G, Lage A (1998) A novel cancer vaccine composed of human-recombinant epidermal growth factor linked to a carrier protein: report of a pilot clinical trial. Ann Oncol 9:431–435

Gradishar WJ, Soff G, Liu J, Cisneros A, French S, Rademaker A, Benson AB, Bouck N (2000) A pilot trial of suramin in metastatic breast cancer to assess antiangiogenic activity in individual patients. Oncology 58:324–333

Grossmann SA, Phuphanich S, Lesser G, Rozental J, Grochow LB, Fisher J, Piandatosi (2001) Toxicity, efficacy and pharmacology of suramin in adults with recurrent high-grade gliomas. J Clin Oncol 19:3260–3266

Higashiyama S, Abraham JA, Miller J, Fiddes JC, Klagsbrun M (1991) A heparin-binding growth factor secreted by macrophage-like cells that is related to EGF. Science 252:936–939

Huang SM, Bock JM, Harari PM (1999) Epidermal growth factor receptor blockade with C225 modulates proliferation, apoptosis, and radiosensitivity in squamous cell carcinomas of the had and neck. Cancer Res 15:1935–1940

Huang SM, Harari P (2000) Modulation of radiation response after epidermal growth factor receptor blockade in squamous cell carcinomas: inhibition of damage repair, cell cycle kinetics, and tumor angiogenesis. Clin Cancer Res 6:2166–2174

Itakura Y, Sasano H, Shiga C, Furukawa Y, Shiga K, Mri S, Nagura H (1994) Epidermal growth factor receptor overexpression in esophageal carcinoma. Cancer 74:795–804

Jensen PJ, Rodeck (1993) Autocrine/paracrine regulation of keratinocyte urokinase plasminogen activator through the TGF-alpha/EGF receptor. J Cell Physiol 155:333–339

Johnson GR, Saeki T, Gordon AW, Shoyab M, Salomon DS, Stromberg K (1992) Autocrine action of amphiregulin in a colon carcinoma cell line and immunocytochemical localization of amphiregulin in human colon. J Cell Biol 118:741–751

Karnes WE, Weller SG, Adjei PN, Kottke TJ, Glenn KS, Gores GJ, Kaufmann SH (1998) Inhibition of epidermal growth factor receptor kinase induces protease-dependent apoptosis in human colon cancer cells. Gastroenterol 114:930–939

Kopp R, Pfeiffer A (1990) Suramin alters phosphoinositide synthesis and inhibits growth factor receptor binding in HT-29 cells. Cancer Res 50:6490–96

Kopp R, Noelke B, Sauter G, Schildberg FW, Paumgartner G, Pfeiffer A (1991) Altered protein kinase C activity in biopsies of human colonic adenomas and carcinomas. Cancer Res 51:205–10

Kopp R, Ruge M, Rothbauer E, Krämling HJ, Cramer C, Schildberg FW, Pfeiffer A (2002) Impact of epidermal growth factor (EGF) radioreceptor analysis on long term survival of gastric cancer patients. Anticancer Res 22:1161–1167

Koenders PG, Peters WHM, Wobbes T, Beex LVAM, Nagengast FM, Benrad TJ (1992) Epidermal growth factor receptor levels are lower in carcinomatous than normal colorectal tissue. Br J Cancer 65:189–192

Koretz K, Schlag P, Möller P (1990) Expression of epidermal growth factor in normal colorectal mucosa, adenoma and carcinoma. Virchows Archiv A Pathol Anat 416:343–349

Kusonoki M, Sakanoue Y, Hatada T, Yanagi H, Yamamura T, Utsunomiya J (1992) Protein kinase C activity in human colonic adenoma and colorectal carcinoma. Cancer 69:24–30

Lammering G, Hewit TH, Hawkins WT, Contessa JN, Reardon DB, Lin P-S, Valerie K, Dent P, Mikkelsen RB, Schmidt-Ulrich RK (2001) Epidermal growth factor as a genetic therapy target for carcinoma cell radiosensitization. J Natl Cancer Inst 93:921–929

Lemoine NR, Jain S, Silvestre F, Lopes C, Hughes CM, McLelland E, Gullick WJ, Filipe MI (1991) Amplification and overexpression of the EGF receptor and c-erbB-2 proto-oncogenes in human stomach cancer. Br J Cancer 64:79–83

Malden LT, Novak U, Burgiss AW (1989) Expression of transforming growth factor alpha messenger RNA in the normal and neoplastic gastro-intestinal tract. Int J Cancer 43:380–384

Masui H, Wells A, Lazar CS, Rosenfeld MG, Gill GN (1991) Enhanced tumorigenesis of NR6 cells which express non-down regulating epidermal growth factor receptors. Cancer Res 51:6170–6175

Maurer CA, Friess H, Kretschman B, Zimmermann A, Staufer A, Baer U, Korc M, Buechler MW (1998) Increased expression of erbB3 in colorectal cancer is associated with concomitant increase in the level of erbB2. Hum Pathol 29:771–777

Munson PJ, Rodbard D. LIGAND (1980) A versatile computerized approach for characterization of ligand-binding systems. Analyt Biochem 107:159–171

Neal DE, Marsh C, Bennett MK, Abel PD, Hall RR, Sainsbury JRC, Harris AL (1985) Epidermal growth factor receptors in human bladder cancer: comparison of invasive and superficial tumors. Lancet 1:366–368

Partik G, Hochegger K, Schörkhuber M, Marian B (1999) Inhibition of epidermal growth factor receptor dependent signalling by tyrphostins A25 and AG1478 blocks growth and induces apoptosis in colorectal tumor cells in vitro. J Cancer Res Clin Oncol 125:379–388

Pfeiffer A, Rothbauer E, Wiebecke B, Pratschke E, Kraemling HJ, Mann K (1990) Increased epidermal growth factor receptors in gastric carcinomas. Gastroenterol 98:961–967

Pfeiffer A, Kroemer W, Friemann J, Ruge M, Herawi M, Schaetzl M, Schwegler U, May B, Schatz H (1995) Muscarinic receptors in gastric mucosa are increased in peptic ulcer disease. Gut 36:813–818

Pfeiffer D, Spranger J, Al-Deiri M, Kimmig R, Fisseler-Eckhoff A, Scheidel P, Schatz H, Jensen A, Pfeiffer A (1997) mRNA expression of ligands of the epidermal-growth-factor-receptor in the uterus. Int J Cancer 72:581–586

Rothbauer E, Mann K, Wiebecke B, Borlinghaus P, Lamerz R, Pratschke E, Kraemling HJ, Pfeiffer A (1989) Epidermal growth factor receptors and epidermal growth factor-like activity in colorectal mucosa, adenomas and carcinomas. Klin Wochenschr 67:518–523

Sainsbury JRC, Farndon JR, Sherbet GV, Harris AL (1985) Epidermal growth-factor receptors and oestrogen receptors in human breast cancer. Lancet 1:364–366

Satoh T, Endo M, Nakafuku M, Akiyama T, Yamamoto T, Kaziro Y (1990) Accumulation of p21 ras GTP in response to stimulation with epidermal growth factor and oncogene products with tyrosine kinase activity. Proc Natl Acad Sci USA 87:7926–7929

Schiemann U, Konturek JW, Osterhoff M, Assert R, Rembiasz K, Pfeiffer D, Schatz H, Domschke W, Pfeiffer A (2001) Decreased expression of epidermal growth factor receptor and mRNA of its ligands in helicobacter pylori-infected gastric mucosa. Scand J Gastroenterol 36:23–31

Schreiber AB, Libermann TA, Lax I, Yarden Y, Schlinger J (1983) Biological role of epidermal growth factor-receptor clustering. J Biol Chem 258:846–853

Slesak B, Harlozinska A, Porebska I, Bojarowski T, Lapinska J, Rzeszutko M, Wojnar A (1998) Expression of epidermal growth factor receptor family proteins (EGFR, c-erbB-2 and c-erbB-3) in gastric cancer and chronic gastritis. Anticancer Res 18:2727–2732

Sporn MB, Roberts AB (1985) Autocrine growth factors and cancer. Nature 313:745–747

Steele RJC, Kelly BE, Eremin O (1990) Epidermal growth factor receptor expression in colorectal cancer. Br J Cancer 77:1352–1354

Sugiyama K, Yonemura Y, Miyazaki I (1989) Immunohistochemical study of epidermal growth factor and epidermal growth factor receptor in gastric carcinoma. Cancer 63:1557–1561

Tahara E (1995) Genetic alterations in human gastrointestinal cancers. Cancer 75:1410–1417.

Tanaka S, Imanishi K, Yoshihara M, Haruma K, Sumii K, Kajiyama G, Akamatsu S (1991) Immunoreactive transforming growth factor alpha is commonly present in colorectal neoplasia. Am J Pathol 139:123–129

Tarnawski AS, Jones MK (1998) The role of epidermal growth factor (EGF) and its receptor in mucosal protection, adaptation to injury, and ulcer healing: involvement of EGF-R signal transduction pathways. J Clin Gastroenterol 27:Suppl 1:S12–20

Tokunaga A, Onda M, Okuda T, Teramoto T, Fujita I, Mizutani T, Kiyama T, Yoshiuki T, Nishi K, Matsukura N (1995) Clinical significance of epidermal growth factor (EGF), EGF receptor, and c-erbB-2 in human gastric cancer. Cancer 15:1418–1425

Tremblay E, Monfils S, Menard D (1997) Epidermal growth factor influences cell proliferation, glycoproteins, and lipase activity in human fetal stomach. Gastroenterol 112:1188–1196

Ullrich A, Coussens L, Hayflick JS, Dull TJ, Gray A, Tam AW, Lee J, Yarden Y, Libermann TA, Schlessinger J Downward J, Mayer ELV, Whittle N, Waterfield MD, Seeburg PH (1984) Human epidermal growth factor receptor cDNA sequence and aberrant expression of the amplified gene in A431 epidermoid carcinoma cells. Nature 309:418–425

Ullrich A, Schlessinger J (1990) Signal transduction by receptors with tyrosine kinase activity. Cell 61:203–212

Verstovsek G, Byrd A, Frey MR, Petreli NJ, Black JD (1998) Colonocyte differentiation is associated with increased expression and altered distribution of protein kinase C isoenzymes. Gastroenterol 115:75–85

Venkateswarlu S, Dawson DM, St Clair P, Gupta A, Willson JK, Brattain MG (2002) Autocrine heregulin generates growth factor independence and block apoptosis in colon cancer cells. Oncogene 21:78–86

Woodburn JR (1999) The epidermal growth factor receptor and its inhibition in cancer therapy. Pharmacol Ther 82:241–250

Yamamoto T, Kamata N, Kawano H, Shimiziu S, Kuroki T, Toyoshima K, Rikimaru K, Nomura N, Ishizaki R, Pastan I, Gamon S, Shimizu N (1986) High incidence of amplification of the EGF receptor gene in human squamous carcinoma cell lines. Cancer Res 46:414–416

Yasui W, Sumiyoshi H, Hata J, Kameda T, Ochiai A, Ito H, Tahara E (1988) Expression of epidermal growth factor in human gastric and colonic carcinomas. Cancer Res 48:137–141

Yonemura Y, Takamura H, Ninomiya I, Fushida S, Tsugawa K, Kaji M, Nakai Y, Ohoyama S, Yamaguchi A, Miyazaki I (1992) Interrelationship between transforming growth factor alpha and epidermal growth factor receptor in advanced gastric cancer. Oncology 49:157–161

Original Papers 2

Minimal Residual Disease in Bone Marrow and Peripheral Blood of Patients with Metastatic Breast Cancer

Joachim Bischoff, Robert Rosenberg, Michael Dahm, Wolfgang Janni, Klaus Gutschow

J. Bischoff (✉)
Department of Gynaecology, Onkologische Fachklinik Bad Trissl,
83080 Oberaudorf, Germany

Abstract.

The presence of occult micrometastases in bone marrow (BM) of patients with early breast cancer increases the risk of relapse. Detection of circulation tumor cells in peripheral blood (PB) may also influence the patient's prognosis. Few data are available on the correlation between tumor cell dissemination in BM and PB in solid epithelial tumors. Twenty-milliliter blood samples were collected from PB of 42 patients with advanced breast cancer and centrifuged using the density gradient OncoQuick (OncoQuick Greiner BioOne, Frickenhausen, Germany). The BM aspirates available from 11 of the 42 patients were centrifuged using density centrifugation Ficoll. Tumor cell detection was performed by microscopy after cytospin preparation and immunocytochemical staining with the monoclonal antibody A45-B/B3. Cytokeratin-positive cells were detected in 23 patients (55%) in the PB and in three patients (27%) in the BM. A cohort with bone lesions as the only metastatic side showed a correlation as follows: 7 of the 11 patients (64%) had negative findings in BM and PB, whereas cytokeratin-positive cells in PB were present in 3 of these 11 patients (27%). The presence of visceral metastases was associated with the detection of cytokeratin-positive cells in the PB in 20 of the 31 patients (65%) in this subgroup. The density gradient OncoQuick in combination with immunocytochemical staining allows the detection of cytokeratin-positive cells in PB of patients with advanced breast cancer. The immunocytochemical detection of cytokeratin-positive cells in PB seems to be associated with the site of metastatic manifestation.

Introduction

Despite apparently curative surgery, more than 50% of women with breast cancer relapse within 5 years of diagnosis. Early hematogenous dissemination is the most frequent means of systemic tumor spread. Therefore minimal residual disease is an important factor limiting improvement of breast cancer mortality rates. This occult tumor cell shedding is usually undetected by standard staging methods. However, since the development of monoclonal antibodies to epithelial membrane antigens, immunocytochemical detection of these micrometastases in secondary organs such as bone marrow (BM), peripheral blood (PB), and lymph nodes (LN) is possible (Pantel et al. 1994). Cytokeratin (CK)-specific antibodies in particular have been used for this purpose, because CK-polypeptides are expressed by normal or transformed epithelial cells, but not BM cells (Kasper et al. 1987; Stigbrand et al. 1998).

Several studies have shown that the presence of CK-positive cells in BM of breast cancer patients is associated with poor prognoses and furthermore is an independent predictor of early tumor relapse (Braun et al. 2000).

Thus, immunocytochemical assays might be useful to improve current tumor staging and to allow an early prediction of therapeutic effects. In order to monitor the course of individual patients at the level of isolated tumor cells (ITCs), a better accessible compartment would be favorable such as PB. Former techniques failed to detect a significant rate of circulating TCs in PB because of insufficient tumor cell (TC) enrichment. OncoQuick, a new density gradient centrifugation device, is able to enrich ITCs in PB with a factor up to 3.7 log, associated with a TC recovery of 72% in spiking experiments. Investigations employing OncoQuick and cultured TC from human lung, breast, prostate, colon and pancreas confirmed the spiking data. Combination of the density gradient device with detection methods such as immunocytochemistry, PCR, or flow cytometry allows the identification of TC. However, the biological role of circulating ITCs in PB has not yet been determined.

Patients and Methods

Patient Characteristics

The study group consisted of 42 patients with metastatic breast cancer who were admitted to the gynecological department of the hospital Bad Trissl between November 2000 and February 2001. All of the women were postmenopausal and received hormonal treatment, chemotherapy, or chemoendocrine therapy and bisphosphonates. Eleven patients had malignant bone lesions as the only metastatic site.

Bone Marrow Aspiration and Immunocytochemistry

After informed consent from all patients, a standard BM puncture was performed in all 11 of the patients who had malignant bone metastasis as the only metastatic site. Five milliliters of BM were obtained, and the two specimens from each patient were pooled before further processing. Mononuclear cells were isolated by density gradient centrifugation by Ficoll. The mononuclear cells were spun onto glass slides by cytocentrifugation. The cytospins were fixed and then stained using the pancytokeratin monoclonal antibody A45-B/B3 (Micromet, Germany). For visualization of the antibody binding, the APAAP technique was used (Ross et al. 1991). For each patient, five slides containing a total of 2×10^6 mononuclear cells were evaluated by two independent observers.

Peripheral Blood Samples and Immunocytochemistry

Twenty-milliliter blood samples were collected from the peripheral antecubital vein of all 42 patients. These patients had evidence of visceral and partial bone metastases. The blood sample from each patient was processed using an optimized density gradient centrifugation system, OncoQuick (Greiner BioOne, Germany), which can achieve an improved relative TC enrichment compared to the standard density gradient centrifugation systems. Mononuclear cells were isolated from the total blood by OncoQuick density gradient centrifugation and spun onto glass slides by cytocentrifugation. Epithelial cells were stained using the monoclonal antibody A45-B/B3 and the APAAP technique (Cordell et al. 1984). Due to the improved depletion of mononuclear blood cells using OncoQuick compared to Ficoll, all mononuclear cells were spun on a median number of two glass slides containing a total of 2×10^6 mononuclear cells, which were also microscopically evaluated by two independent observers.

Results

CK-Positive Cells in BM and PB

CK-positive cells were detected in the PB of 21 patients and in the BM of three patients. The number of such cells detected in PB was between 1 and more than 20 per 10^6 cells. One CK-positive cell per 1×10^6 mononucleated interface cells was found in the three positive-BM patients. Seven patients had negative findings in BM and PB. Three patients were CK-positive in PB and negative in BM, whereas in two patients, CK-positive cells were detected in BM but not PB.

CK-Positive Cells and Metastatic Site

Positive PB findings were observed in 9 of the 14 patients with liver metastases, in only five of the 16 patients with bone metastases, and three of the seven women with pulmonary metastatic sites. These data show a significant difference concerning the detection rate of CK-positive cells in PB in breast cancer patients with hepatic tumor spread in comparison to other metastatic manifestations. No clear correlation could be found between the number of detected cells and metastatic site.

CK-Postive Cells and Survival

Fifteen of the 42 enrolled patients died within a follow-up interval of 9 months; all died of cancer-related causes. Eleven of the 15 patients had positive findings in PB; eight of these women had liver metastases. These data revealed that the presence of CK-positive cells in PB is associated with the clinical outcome.

Discussion

The individual course of malignant diseases depends on the complex interaction of tumor-related factors. The multiplicity of interactions correlates with the steadily increasing number of prognostic markers (Henderson 1991). Although many of these factors have been proven to be of prognostic significance in single-center studies, they failed to be accepted as solid tumor prognostic factors by the College of American Pathologists Conference XXXV (Hammond et al.. 2000) because of the lack of large multicenter studies. Detection of isolated tumor cells (ITCs) in BM is reported to be an independent predictor of relapse in solid tumors such as breast cancer (Harbeck et al. 1994, Diel et al. 1996), colorectal cancer (Lindemann et al. 1992), gastric cancer (Heiss et al. 1995, Jauch et al. 1996), and non-small-cell lung cancer (Pantel et al. 1996). Few data exist regarding the value of minimal residual disease for identifying patients who would benefit from adjuvant chemotherapy or for measuring the response of multimodal treatment protocols.

Since analytic methods have been standardized and specificity is determined using monoclonal antibodies directed against CKs (Pantel et al. 1994), the detection of CK-positive cells in BM represents the gold standard for the detection of minimal residual disease. The phenomenon of dormant tumor cells which were detected, but have no clinical impact, influences the prognostic value. As a consequence, not all detected CK-positive cells have the potential to lead to clinically apparent metastases. Thus, there is a need to obtain more information on the biological properties and to evaluate disseminated tumor cells in other mesenchymal organs. A more accessible compartment than BM is PB. In earlier studies, detection rates of disseminated tumor cells in peripheral circulation were very low (Redding et al. 1983). In vivo experiments in rodents showed that only less than 0.1% of circulating tumor cells in PB survive the blood passage and spread to secondary organ (Fidler and Hart 1982). These findings have been interpreted as indicating that circulating ITCs in blood are of minor prognostic impact compared to those in bone marrow. First evidence of a prognostic impact of circulating ITCs in PB was obtained in a recent study of colorectal cancer patients, which detected significantly higher rates of CK-positive cells in Duke's stage C/D compared to earlier tumor stages, using immunomagnetic separation combined with an RT-PCR technique (Denis et al. 1997). According to the data reported by Denis et al., 21 of 34 patients with various advanced carcinomas including colorectal and breast cancer were CK-positive in PB after magnetic cell sorting (Martin et al. 1998). Telomerase activity, absent in normal epithelial cells, is another molecular marker for cancer cells. Soria et al. (1999), using telomerase-PCR-ELISA after magnetic cell harvest, found that 85% of their patient population with metastatic breast cancer were telomerase-positive. Our results confirm the high rate of circulating ITCs in PB of patients with advanced malignant disease.

Moreover, we found that TC detection depends on metastatic site and influences overall survival of women with breast cancer. This has not yet been described by other investigators, but is congruent to clinical experience wherein patients with bone metastasis have a better prognosis than those with visceral, especially liver, metastasis. Thus, our data reveal that liver metastasis is associated with the detection of ITCs, and the detection of ITCs in PB seems to correlate with worse prognosis. It is hoped that the further follow-up of our patients with bone metastasis and no evidence of ITCs in PB and BM will give more information about the biological role of ITCs. Further studies should also try to differentiate irrelevant circulating cells from those with metastatic potency by assessment of molecular methods such as phenotyping.

We can conclude that the density gradient OncoQuick in combination with immunocytochemical staining allows the identification of ITCs in PB of patients with advanced breast cancer. Our results support the hypothesis that the detection of ITCs in BM and PB represent comparable approaches to monitor minimal residual disease. Clinical trials with larger patient cohorts and longer follow-up periods must be held to evaluate the prognostic value of circulating ITCs.

References

Braun S, Pantel K, Müller P, Janni W, Hepp F, Kentenich C, Gastroph S, Wischnik A, Dimpfl T, Kindermann G, Riethmüller G, Schlimok G (2000) Cytokeratin-positive cells in the bone marrow and survival of patients with stage I, II or III breast cancer. N Engl J Med 342:525–33

Cordell JL, Falini B, Erber WN, et al (1984) Immunoenzymatic labeling of monoclonal antibodies using immune complexes of alkaline phosphatase and monoclonal anti-alkaline phosphatase: APAAP-complexes. J Histochem Cytochem 32:219–29

Cote RJ, Beattie EJ, Chaiwun B, et al (1995) Detection of occult bone marrow micrometastases in patients with operable lung carcinoma. Ann Surg 222:415–423

Denis MG, Lipart C, Leborgne J, Lehur PA, Galmiche JP, Denis M, Ruud E, Truchaud A, Lustenberger P (1997) Detection of disseminated tumor cells in peripheral blood of colorectal cancer patients. International Journal of Cancer 74:540–544

Diel D, Kaufmann M, Costa SD, Holle R, Minckwitz VG, Solomayer EF, Kaul S, Bastert G
(1996) Micrometastatic breast cancer cells in bone marrow at primary surgery:prognostic
value in comparison with nodal status. J Natl Cancer Inst 88:1652–8

Fidler IJ, Hart IR (1982) Biological diversity in metastatic neoplasms: origin and implications. Science 217:998–1003

Hammond ME, Fitzgibbons PL, Compton CC, Grignon DJ, Page DL, Fielding LP Bostwick D,
Pajak TF (2000) College of American Pathologists Conference XXXV: Solid tumor prognostic factors – which, how and so what? Arch Pathol Lab Med 124:958–965

Harbeck N, Untch M, Pache L, Eiermann W (1994) Tumor cell detection in the bone marrow
of breast cancer patients at primary therapy: results of 3-year median follow-up. Br J Cancer 69:566–71

Heiss MM, Allgayer H, Grützner KU, Funke I, Babic R, Jauch KW, Schildberg FW (1995) Individual development and uPA-receptor expression of disseminated tumor cells in bone
marrow: a reference to early systemic disease in solid cancer. Nat Med 1:1035–1039

Henderson IC (1991) Prognostic factors. In: Harris JR, Hellmann S, Kinne DW (eds) Breast
diseases. pp 332–346

Jauch KW, Heiss MM, Gruetzner U (1996) Prognostic significance of bone marrow micrometastases in patients with gastric cancer. J Clin Oncol 14:1810–1817

Kasper M, Stosiek P, Typlt H, Karsten U (1987) Histological evaluation of three new monoclonal anti-cytokeratin antibodies. 1. Normal tissues. Eur J Cancer Clin Oncol 23:137–147

Lindemann F, Schlimok G, Dirschedl P, Witte J, Riethmüller G (1992) Prognostic significance
of micrometastatic tumor cells in bone marrow of colorectal cancer patients. Lancet
340:685–689

Martin VM, Siewert C, Scharl A, Harms T, Heinze R, Ohl S, Radbruch A, Miltenyi S, Schmitz J
(1998) Immunomagnetic enrichment of disseminated epithelial tumor cells from peripheral blood by MACS. Exp Hematol 26:252–264

Pantel K et al (1996) Frequency and prognostic significance of isolated tumor cells in bone
marrow of patients with non-small-cell-lung cancer without overt metastases. Lancet
347:649–653

Pantel K, Schlimok G, Angstwurm M, Weckermann C, Schmaus W, Gath H Passlick B,
Izbicki J, Riethmüller G (1994) Methodological analysis of immunocytochemical screening for disseminated epithelial tumor cells in bone marrow. J Hematother 3:165–173

Redding HW, Coombes RC, Monagham P, Clink HM D, Imrie SF, Dearnaley DP,
Ormerod MG, Sloane JP, Gazet JC, Powles TJ, Neville AM (1983) Detection of micrometastases in patients with primary breast cancer. Lancet i:1271–1274

Ross AA, Cooper BW, Lazarus HM, Mackay W, Moss TJ, Ciobanu N, Tallmann MS,
Kennedy MJ, Davidson NE, Sweet D, Winter C, Adard L, Janse J, Copelan E, Meagher RC,
Herzig RH, Klumpp TR, Kanh DG, Warner NE (1991) Detection and viability of tumor
cells in peripheral blood stem cell collections from breast cancer patients using immunocytochemical and clonogenic assay techniques. Blood 82:2605–2610

Soria JC, Gauthier LR, Raymond E, Granotier C, Morat L, Armand JP, Boussin FD, Sabatier L
(1999) Molecular detection of telomerase-positive circulating epithelial cells in metastatic
breast cancer patients. Clin Cancer Res 5:971–975

Stigbrand T, Andrés C, Bellanger L, et al (1998) Epitope specificity of 30 monoclonal antibodies against cytokeratin antigens: the ISOBM TD5-1 Workshop. Tumor Biol 19:132–152

Estrogen Receptor Expression Profile of Disseminated Epithelial Tumor Cells in Bone Marrow of Breast Cancer Patients

Nina Ditsch, Barbara Mayer, Michaela Rolle, Michael Untch, Friedrich Wilhelm Schildberg, Ilona Funke

I. Funke (✉)
Department of Surgery, Ludwig-Maximilians-University Munich, Klinikum Großhadern, Marchioninistrasse 15, 81377 Munich, Germany

Abstract

The estrogen receptor (ER) status in primary breast cancer represents an important prognostic factor and has a profound impact on therapeutic decisions. However, ER expression profile on disseminated breast cancer cells is largely unknown, although these cells are one of the main target structures in adjuvant therapy after local curative resection (R0) achieved in most breast cancer patients. Thus, the present pilot study was designed to evaluate the ER expression profile on disseminated epithelial cells in bone marrow, one of the preferential organs for manifestation of distant metastases in breast cancer. Using the alkaline phosphatase anti-alkaline phosphatase-immunogold double staining procedure, in a panel of 17 breast cancer patients, epithelial cells (mab CK2) detected in bone marrow were analyzed for ER expression (mab 1D5) and compared with ER expression in the corresponding primary tumors. Whereas eleven of the 17 patients (64.7%) were ER-positive in primary carcinomas, only two patients (11.8%) revealed ER-positive epithelial cells in bone marrow. In addition, one of these two patients demonstrated a heterogeneous ER expression pattern, with both ER-positive and ER-negative epithelial cells in bone marrow. Although in both of these cases the ER-positive epithelial cells in bone marrow derived from ER-positive primary tumors, in this small patient cohort none of the prognostic relevant clinical and pathological factors tested, i.e., TNM-classification, grading, and ER status in primary breast cancer, correlated with the ER status in bone marrow. The striking discrepancy between ER expression in primary breast cancers and the corresponding disseminated epithelial cells in bone marrow suggests either the selective dissemination of ER-negative tumor cells into the bone marrow or a negative impact of the bone marrow microenvironment on epithelial ER expression. This phenomenon might influence therapeutic effects of antihormonal treatment.

Introduction

Estrogen receptor (ER) status has an important impact on the management of primary breast cancer [1, 2]. Negative ER status in primary breast cancer is associated with poor prognosis [3]. Due to the hormone-dependent growth of breast cancer, pre- and postmenopausal patients with a positive ER status in primary breast cancer are treated with antihormonal therapies. Another prognostic factor recently identified in breast cancer is the bone marrow status. The presence of epithelial cells in bone marrow indicating systemic disease at time of primary surgery correlates with poor prognosis [4–6]. However, only a subset of breast cancer patients with disseminated tumor cells in bone marrow develop bone metastases, suggesting that the molecular equipment of these cells is crucial for the formation of solid metastases. Therefore, antigenic characterization of the disseminated epithelial cells in bone marrow, including therapeutically relevant molecules such as ER expression, is an important prerequisite for the development of effective therapeutic strategies.

Patients and Methods

Patients

Seventeen breast cancer patients with positive bone marrow status were characterized for ER expression on both primary tumors and epithelial cells in bone marrow, and a number of clinical and pathological data were evaluated. The perioperative staging of the patients included chest radiography, abdominal ultrasound, and bone scintigraphy to evaluate distant metastases. Tumors were classified according to the UICC and TNM classifications [7]. Cellular differentiation was described by tumor grading.

Evaluation of ER Status in Disseminated Epithelial Cells in Bone Marrow

Bone marrow aspirates were taken from both spinae iliacae anteriores superiores during surgery of the primary tumor. After density gradient centrifugation through Ficoll/Hypaque (Pharmacia Freiburg, Germany), mononuclear cells were harvested from the interface of the Ficoll gradient, washed twice in phosphate-buffered saline (PBS) pH 7.4, and cytocentrifuged on glass slides. The calculated cell number was 5×10^5 cells per slide. ER expression on epithelial cells in bone marrow was immunocytochemically analyzed combining the alkaline phosphatase anti-alkaline phosphatase (APAAP) method with the immunogold staining procedure [8]. Briefly, after acetone fixation and incubation with 10% human AB-serum (Biotest Dreieich, Germany), the slides were washed in PBS and incubated with the monoclonal antibody (mab) 1D5 (IgG1, Dako Hamburg, Germany) directed against human ER. The slides were

Table 1. Characteristics of breast cancer patients with CK18-positive bone marrow status

Patient	ER status primary tumor	Grading	pT stage	pN stage	M stage
1	Positive	3	1c	1a	0
2	Positive	3	1c	0	0
3	Positive	3	1c	0	0
4	Positive	2	2	0	0
5	Positive	2	2	0	0
6	Positive	3	1b	0	0
7	Positive	2	1c	0	0
8	Positive	2	3	1biii	1
9	Positive	3	2	1biii	0
10	Positive	a	2	1bii	0
11	Positive	a	a	a	a
12	Negative	–	DCIS	0	0
13	Negative	3	1c	1biii	1
14	Negative	2	1c	0	0
15	Negative	1	1b	0	0
16	Negative	3	2	0	0
17	Negative	3	4c	1biv	1

[a] Data not available.

washed in PBS again, and gold-conjugated goat-anti-mouse IgG (Amersham Buckinghamshire, England) was added. After incubation with 5% mouse serum, the biotinylated mab CK2 (IgG1, Boehringer Mannheim, Germany) directed against cytokeratin component number 18 to identify the epithelial cells was applied. After a wash in PBS, alkaline-phophatase-conjugated streptavidin (Dianova Hamburg, Germany) was incubated. The reaction was developed with a substrate solution containing 5% neufuchsin, 3.8 mmol/l naphtol AS-BI phosphate, and 10 mmol/l sodium nitrite in 0.1 mol/l Tris-buffer at pH 9.4. After washing the slides in PBS, the immunogold staining was developed with the Intense TM Silver Enhancement Kit (Amersham) according to the manufacturer's instructions. The myeloma protein MOPC-21 (Sigma, Deisenhofen, Germany) was used as isotype control. A mixture of mononuclear cells and the ER-positive breast cancer cell line MCF-7 (HTB-22, American Type Culture Collection, Manassas, Va., USA) was used as tumor control.

Evaluation of ER Status in Primary Breast Cancer

In primary tumors, ER status was evaluated either immunohistochemically according to the score of Remmele and Stegner [9] or with a quantitative enzyme immunoassay (Abbott, Ludwigshafen, Germany) performed according to the manufacturer's instructions. The immunohistochemical data were kindly provided by the Institute of Pathology (Prof. U. Löhrs, Munich, Germany).

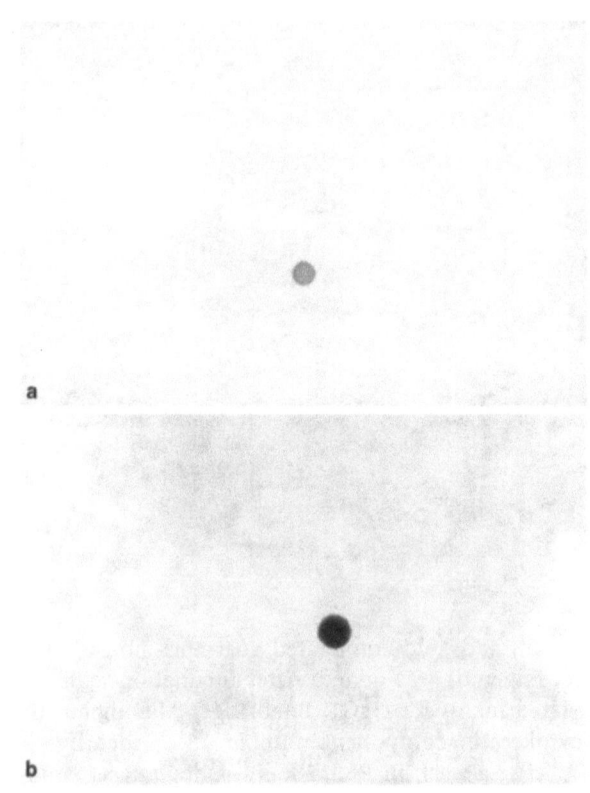

Fig. 1a, b. ER expression on epithelial cells in bone marrow of breast cancer patients detected with the APAAP-immunogold double staining procedure. **a** In most patients, epithelial cells (CK18⁺) revealed an ER-negative phenotype (*red cells*). **b** An individual CK18⁺ cell showing a positive ER phenotype (*black*). ×320

Statistical Evaluation

Correlations between ER expression on epithelial cells in bone marrow and various clinical and pathological parameters were assessed using the two-tailed Fisher's exact probability test. P values below 0.05 were considered significant.

Results

Disseminated epithelial cells (CK18⁺) cells in bone marrow of patients with primary breast cancer were immunocytochemically analyzed for ER expression using the APAAP-immunogold double staining procedure. Seventeen patients with a defined ER status in primary tumors and a positive bone marrow status

Table 2. ER status on epithelial cells in bone marrow correlated with the ER status in the corresponding primary breast carcinomas

ER status on CK18⁺ cells in bone marrow	ER status in primary breast carcinomas			
	ER-negative ($n=6$)		ER-positive ($n=11$)	
$CK18^+/ER^-$	6	(100%)	9	(81.8%)
$CK18^+/ER^-$ and ER^+	0	(0%)	1	(9.1%)
$CK18^+/ER^+$	0	(0%)	1	(9.1%)

were included in the present pilot study. The most important clinical and pathological factors of the patients are listed in Table 1. In most of the patients, epithelial cells in bone marrow revealed an ER-negative phenotype ($CK18^+/ER^-$, Fig. 1a). Only two patients (11.8%) showed ER-positive epithelial cells in bone marrow. Thus, in one patient (Table 1, patient 1), the individual epithelial cells detected in bone marrow simultaneously expressed ER ($CK18^+/ER+$, Fig. 1b), whereas the other patient (Table 1, patient 2) revealed a heterogeneous ER expression profile; i.e., both $CK18^+$ ER^- cells and $CK18^+/ER^+$ cells were present in bone marrow. Correlation of the ER status on epithelial cells in bone marrow with that in the corresponding primary tumors showed that in both patients, ER-expressing epithelial cells in bone marrow derived from ER-positive primary tumors (Table 2). However, most of the epithelial cells in bone marrow originated from an ER-positive primary tumor revealed an ER-negative phenotype. In addition, all patients ($n=6$) with ER-negative breast carcinomas likewise had $CK18^+/ER^-$ cells in bone marrow (Table 2). Correlation of the ER status on disseminated epithelial cells in bone marrow with other prognostic relevant clinical and pathological characteristics of the primary tumors, i.e., grading, pT, pN, and M stage, revealed no statistical significance (data not shown).

Discussion

Antihormonal therapy is the standard adjuvant treatment for breast cancer patients with a positive ER status in primary tumors. However, after complete removal of the primary tumor (R0 resection), which is achieved in most breast cancer patients, efficiency of the antihormonal therapy depends on the ER status on disseminated tumor cells remaining in the patient. In the present pilot study of 17 primary breast cancer patients with a positive bone marrow status, ER expression on epithelial cells disseminated into the bone marrow was immunocytochemically determined and compared with the ER profile in the corresponding primary tumors. ER expression was observed in 64.7% of the primary breast carcinomas, a percentage similar to that reported in large clinical trials. In striking contrast, only two patients (11.8%) revealed ER-positive epithelial cells in bone marrow. This low frequency suggests that ER-negative epithelial cells selectively disseminate in the bone marrow. Another explanation is a negative impact of the mesenchymal microenvironment resulting in the loss or down-regulation of the ER expression on disseminated epithelial cells. In addition, in one patient a heterogeneous ER profile on epithelial cells in bone marrow was observed, reflecting heterogeneity of ER expression reported in primary breast cancer [10]. Heterogeneity of antigen expression in minimal residual disease was reported for a number of molecules, such as MHC class I antigens, adhesion molecules, growth factor receptors. and proliferation-associated markers [8, 11–15]. Independently from the speculated mechanisms, the negative ER status described on epithelial cells disseminated in bone marrow might have therapeutic consequences, i.e., ER-negative disseminated tumor cells might escape from antihormonal therapy. However, the data of the pilot study presented here must be confirmed in an larger patient cohort.

References

1. Paech K, Webb P, Kuiper GGJM, Nilsson S, Gustafsson JA, Kushner PJ, Scanlan TS (1997) Differential ligand activation of estrogen receptors ER-alpha and ER-beta at AP1 sites. Science 277:1508–1510
2. Key TJ, Wang DY, Brown JB, Hermon C, Allen DS, Moore JW, Bulbrook RD, Fentiman IS, Pike MC (1996) A prospective study of urinary estrogen excretion and breast cancer risk. Br J Cancer 73 12:1615–1619
3. McPherson LA, Baichwal VR, Weigel RJ (1997) Identification of ERF-1 as a member of the AP2 transcription factor family. Proc Natl Acad Sci USA 94:4342–4347
4. Funke I, Schraut W (1998) Meta-analyses of studies on bone marrow micrometastases: an independent prognostic impact remains to be substantiated. J Clin Oncol 16:557–566
5. Braun S, Pantel K, Müller P, Janni W, Hepp F, Kentenich CR, Gastroph S, Wischnik A, Dimpfl T, Kindermann G, Riethmüller G, Schlimok G (2000) Cytokeratin-positive cells in the bone marrow and survival of patients with stage I, II, or III breast cancer. N Engl J Med 342:525–533
6. Funke I, Schraut W, Untch M, Schlimok G, Jauch KW, Schildberg FW (2001) Prognoserelevanz disseminierter Tumorzellen im Knochenmark: Prospektive Studie an 1045 Mammakarzinom-Patientinnen im Stadium I–III. Langenbecks Arch Surg 30:547–5497
7. UICC (1997) TNM classification of malignant tumors, 5th edn. Wiley-Liss, New York
8. Zia A, Schildberg FW, Funke I (2001) MHC class I negative phenotype of disseminated tumor cells in bone marrow is associated with poor survival in R0M0 breast cancer patients. Int J Cancer 93:566–570
9. Remmele W, Stegner HE (1987) Recommendation for uniform definition of an immunoreactive score (IRS) for immunohistochemical estrogen receptor detection (ER-ICA) in breast cancer tissue. Pathologe 8:138–140
10. Andersen J, Orntoft T, Skovgaard Poulsen H (1986) Semiquantitative estrogen receptor assay in formalin-fixed paraffin sections of human breast cancer tissue using monoclonal antibodies. Br J Cancer 53:691–694
11. Wasserman L, Dreilinger A, Easter D, Wallace A (1999) A seminested RT-PCR assay for Her-2/neu: initial validation of a new method for the detection of disseminated breast cancer cells. Mol Diagn 4:21–28
12. Gebhardt F, Zanker KS, Brandt B (1998) Differential expression of alternatively spliced c-erbB-2 mRNA in primary tumors, lymph node metastases, and bone marrow micrometastases from breast cancer patients. Biochem Biophys Res Commun 247:319–323
13. Braun S, Pantel K (1998) Prognostic significance of micrometastatic bone marrow involvement. Breast Cancer Res Treat 52:201–216

14. Hazan RB, Norton L (1998) The epidermal growth factor receptor modulates the interaction of the E-cadherin with the actin cytoskeleton. J Biol Chem 273:9078–9084
15. Pantel K, Schlimok G, Kutter D, Schaller G, Genz T, Wiebecke B, Backmann R, Funke I, Riethmüller G (1991) Frequent down-regulation of major histocompatibility class I antigen expression on individual micrometastatic carcinoma cells. Cancer Res 51:4712–4715

Detection of Circulating Tumor Cells in Blood Using an Optimized Density Gradient Centrifugation

Ralf Gertler, Robert Rosenberg, Katrin Fuehrer, Michael Dahm, Hjalmar Nekarda, Joerg Ruediger Siewert

R. Gertler (✉)
Chirurgische Klinik und Poliklinik,
Klinikum rechts der Isar der Technischen Universität München,
81675 Munich, Germany

Abstract

The aim of the study was to compare the new density gradient centrifugation system OncoQuick with the standard density gradient centrifugation system Ficoll for improved tumor cell enrichment in blood of tumor patients. Evaluation of OncoQuick and Ficoll density gradient centrifugation was performed by flow-cytometry and immunocytochemistry using 10 ml unspiked and tumor cell-spiked blood samples of tumor-free probands. From 10 ml blood, OncoQuick density gradient centrifugation separated a cell fraction which consisted of a mean cell number of 9.5×10^4 mononuclear cells compared to 1.8×10^7 cells by Ficoll. Density gradient centrifugation of tumor cell-spiked blood samples with OncoQuick and Ficoll led to similar tumor cell recovery rates, between 70% and 90% for both methods. The improved depletion of mononuclear blood cells by OncoQuick simplified further immunocytochemical evaluation of the enriched cell fraction, which could be spun onto 1–2 glass slides by cytocentrifugation. In comparison, the mononuclear cells separated by Ficoll had to be spun onto more than 50 glass slides for complete immunocytochemical evaluation. Consequently, tumor cell density on each cytospin was higher after OncoQuick preparation compared to Ficoll. Density gradient centrifugation with OncoQuick results in higher relative tumor cell enrichment than Ficoll density gradient centrifugation. This simplifies further immunocytochemical tumor cell detection and is a promising tool for the detection of circulating tumor cells in blood of tumor patients.

Introduction

Tumor recurrence in cancer patients after curative tumor resection can be explained by the presence of minimal residual disease (MRD). Disseminated tumor cells, which are not detectable by routine histopathology methods, are located at the three different compartments of MRD: bone marrow, lymph nodes, and blood (Pantel and Riethmüller 1995; Soeth et al.1997). Several authors have reported on the prognostic value of detected disseminated tumor cells correlating either with worse prognosis of the patients or advanced tumor stages. However, few data are available on the value of circulating tumor cells in blood, although blood represents the easiest accessible compartment of MRD (Weitz et al.1998).

Monitoring of the different blood compartments, which can be divided in portal-venous, central-venous, arterial, and peripheral-venous blood areas, may help to further understand the complexity of hematogenous tumor cell dissemination in patients with gastrointestinal carcinoma (von Knebel-Doeberitz et al. 2001). The frequency of circulating tumor cells in the different blood compartments or the presence of intermittent tumor cell shedding has not yet been determined. Limitations in sensitivity and specificity of MRD analysis are mainly due to unspecific markers for tumor cell detection, the presence of contamination or illegitimate transcription, and the phenomenon of dormant cells, which do not lead to metastatic disease (Jung et al. 2001).

Methods for MRD detection are immunocytochemistry (ICC) and reverse-transcriptase polymerase chain reaction (RT-PCR) (Pantel et al. 2000). A prerequisite for both MRD detection methods, however, is a special preparation of whole blood to separate the few expected tumor cells from the large number of normal blood cells. We evaluated the new density gradient centrifugation system OncoQuick in comparison to the standard method with Ficoll for improved relative tumor cell enrichment in blood.

Methods

All experiments were performed with peripheral venous blood samples, which were drawn from tumor-free probands. For tumor cell spiking experiments, the colon carcinoma cell line HT-29 was used.

Density Gradient Centrifugation

Mononuclear cells (MNCs) were separated from total blood by Ficoll (Biochrom, Germany) and by OncoQuick (Hexal Gentech) density centrifugation as further described.

OncoQuick

Density gradient centrifugation for separation of MNCs by OncoQuick (Greiner BioOne, Germany) was performed in 50-ml centrifugation tubes containing a porous barrier at the 15-ml line, separating a lower from an upper compartment. Pre-cooled, blood-filled OncoQuick tubes containing 15 ml OncoQuick separation medium were centrifuged at 1,600 g for 20 min at 4°C in a swing-out rotor (Hettich, Germany). After centrifugation, most blood cells were pelleted out in the lower compartment. In the upper compartment, an interphase of mononuclear cells formed between the upper plasma and the lower separation medium. To avoid any loss of cells, the entire contents of the upper compartment containing the interphase were poured into a fresh centrifugation tube. The porous barrier prevented any contamination of the separated MNCs with the fraction of pelleted blood cells. After the cells were washed at 500 g for 12 min at 4°C, the supernatant was aspirated. The pelleted cells were used for further evaluation.

Ficoll

Density gradient centrifugation for separation of MNCs by Ficoll was also performed in 50-ml centrifugation tubes with a porous filter disc at 15 ml (Leucosep) containing 15 ml of Ficoll. Blood-filled tubes were centrifuged at 1,000 g for 10 min at room temperature. To harvest the MNCs, gathered in a layer between plasma and Ficoll-Isopaque and well visible due to the considerable number of enriched cells, again, the entire contents of the upper compartment of the Leucosep tubes were poured into a fresh 50-ml centrifugation tube. The porous filter prevented any contamination of the separated MNCs with the pelleted cell fraction. The cells were washed at 500 g for 15 min at 4°C. The supernatant was aspirated without disturbing the pelleted cells, which were used for further detection of disseminated tumor cells.

Flow Cytometry

The mononuclear cell fractions separated by Ficoll and OncoQuick density centrifugation were isolated and analyzed by flow cytometry to determine the depletion of the different blood cell fractions. The difference in cell count between unspiked and tumor cell-spiked blood samples was used as a measure of tumor cell recovery.

Immunocytochemistry

The total number of separated MNCs with and without spiked tumor cells was microscopically determined using a Neubauer chamber. For immunocytochemical evaluation, a maximum of 200,000 cells was spun onto each glass slide. Cytokeratin-positive cells were identified using the mouse anticytokeratin monoclonal antibody (MAb) A45-B/B3 (Micromet, Germany). The reaction was developed using the alkaline phosphatase anti-alkaline phosphatase (APAAP) technique. The number of cytokeratin-positive cells was evaluated by two independent observers.

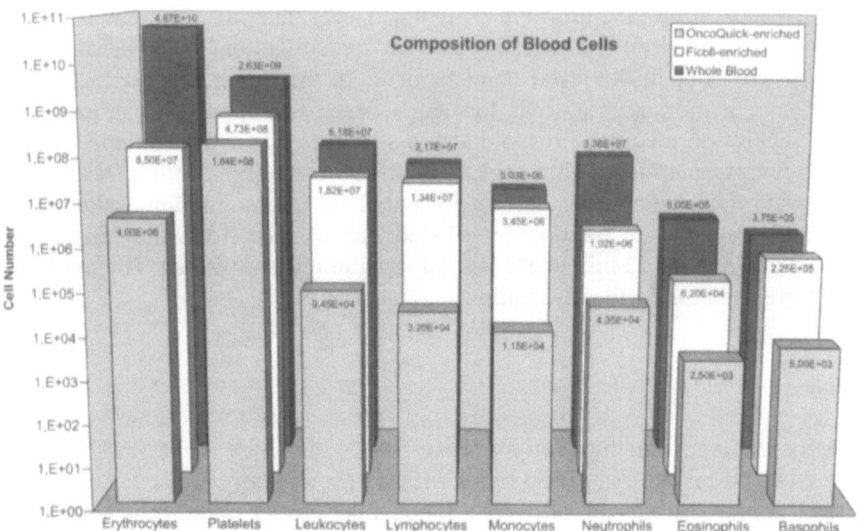

Fig. 1. Composition of the blood cell fractions of 10 ml total blood before and after density centrifugation using Ficoll or OncoQuick

Results

Depletion of Blood Cells with OncoQuick or Ficoll

Ten-milliliter blood samples were processed with the density gradient centrifugation systems OncoQuick and Ficoll. The mononuclear cell fraction, located in the interphase, was isolated and analyzed by flow cytometry to determine the depletion of the different blood cell fractions. Whereas OncoQuick revealed a mean total amount of 9.5×10^4 mononuclear cells, Ficoll enriched a mean of 1.8×10^7 mononuclear cells. OncoQuick reduced the white blood cell fraction to less than 1% of the original white blood cell count (Fig. 1). In comparison, after Ficoll centrifugation, 30% of the original white blood cells were still found. Analysis of the white blood cell differential revealed depletion factors of about 100-fold to 850-fold for lymphocytes, monocytes, neutrophils, eosinophils, and basophils after OncoQuick density gradient centrifugation.

Tumor Cell Recovery After OncoQuick or Ficoll

To determine the rate of recovered tumor cells after density gradient centrifugation with Ficoll or OncoQuick, we performed spiking experiments using the colorectal carcinoma cell line HT-29. From 10 tumor-free probands, 40 ml blood was drawn and divided in four 10 ml aliquots. Two aliquots of each proband were spiked with 2.7×10^6 or 2.7×10^5 tumor cells, and the remaining two aliquots were preserved unspiked. After centrifugation with OncoQuick or Fi-coll, tumor cell recovery was determined by flow cytometry. Both systems had a high tumor cell recovery of about 70%–90% of the spiked tumor cells. Whereas the spiked tumor cells were detected among a large number of mononuclear cells (1.8×10^7 cells) after Ficoll preparation, the spiked tumor cells were found in significantly less mononuclear cells (9.5×10^4 cells) after OncoQuick preparation.

Detection of Disseminated Tumor Cells by Immunocytochemistry

To evaluate the immunocytochemical detection rate of tumor cells in blood after density gradient centrifugation with Ficoll or OncoQuick, 10-ml blood samples of tumor-free probands were spiked with 100 and 1,000 tumor cells. Microscopical quantification of the separated MNCs using a Neubauer cell chamber revealed a mean amount of 2×10^5 mononuclear cells after Onco-Quick centrifugation and 1×10^7 cells after Ficoll centrifugation. For further ICC evaluation, a maximum cell number of 2×10^5 cells was spun on each cy-tospin and stained with a pancytokeratin antibody. Consequently, all MNCs separated by OncoQuick could be spun onto 1–2 glass slides, whereas about 50 cytospins were necessary for evaluation of all MNCs separated by Ficoll.

With 100 and 1,000 tumor cells spiked in 10 ml total blood, a mean recovery rate of 42% (range 25%–70%) was determined by ICC regardless of the enriched system used. After Ficoll centrifugation, only 1%–2% of the spiked tumor cells were detected per slide, whereas OncoQuick allowed the detection of 25%–50% of the spiked tumor cells per slide. Tumor cell density on immunocytochemical glass slides was significantly higher for OncoQuick preparations compared to Ficoll samples (Fig. 2).

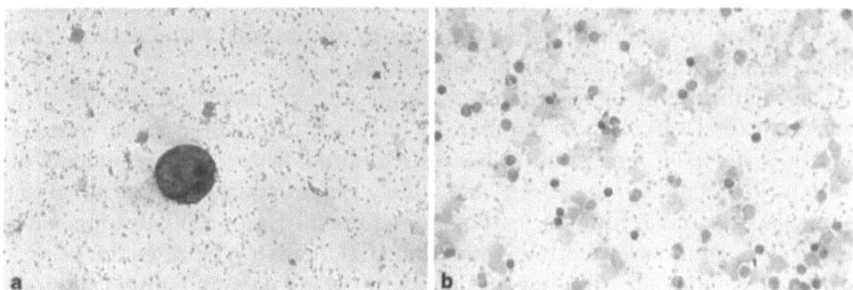

Fig. 2a, b. Immunocytochemical staining of tumor cell-spiked blood samples after density gradient centrifugation and preparation of cytospins (40-fold enlargement). **a** After OncoQuick preparation. **b** After Ficoll preparation

Discussion

Our validation study revealed that the optimized density gradient centrifugation with OncoQuick is a reliable system for the enrichment of disseminated tumor cells in blood. Advantages of OncoQuick are the improved depletion of mononuclear blood cells in the enriched cell fraction with comparable tumor cell recovery compared to Ficoll density gradient centrifugation.

Quantification of the enriched cells with both flow cytometry and microscopy showed a more than 100-fold better depletion of all blood cell fractions with OncoQuick compared to Ficoll. The more effective depletion of blood cells by OncoQuick simplified further immunocytochemical preparation of the separated cells. After OncoQuick centrifugation, the entire recovered cell fraction from 10 ml of whole blood could be spun on one or two slides, whereas more than 50 slides were necessary for complete immunocytochemical analysis of the cell fraction separated by Ficoll. Therefore, less material is required for the staining process of the glass slides, and the reduced number of cytospins, which must be evaluated by microscopy, saves time. Immunocytochemical analysis after OncoQuick centrifugation has proved to be extremely time- and cost-saving compared to Ficoll preparations.

Experiments with tumor cell-spiked blood samples showed comparable tumor cell recovery rates for both density gradient centrifugation methods. Depending on the number of spiked tumor cells and the analysis method used, tumor cell recovery rates of 25%–70% and 70%–90% were observed. Given the expected small number of circulating tumor cells in tumor patients, the loss of tumor cells during blood preparation should be further minimized. Nevertheless, the recovery rates may well be sufficient for the detection of circulating tumor cells in a clinical setting.

The combination of comparable tumor cell recovery and improved blood cell depletion resulted in an increased relative tumor cell enrichment using the density gradient centrifugation OncoQuick. Thus, OncoQuick preparations resulted in a higher tumor cell density on immunocytochemical glass slides, simplifying the detection of tumor cells.

The identification of disseminated tumor cells in blood of patients with gastrointestinal carcinoma is limited by the lack of tumor-specific markers (Bostik et al. 1998; Jung et al. 2001). Cytokeratins, which are components of the cytoskeleton of epithelial cells and widely expressed in gastrointestinal tumor cells, are used as indirect markers for epithelial tumor cell detection. Currently, cytokeratins represent the most sensitive markers for detection of disseminated tumor cells, although specificity of the cytokeratin family is limited by the expression of cytokeratins in mesenchymal cells, which might lead to "false-positive detection." The reduction of the mononuclear cell fraction by OncoQuick density gradient centrifugation does not completely rule out the risk of "false-positive" detection, but might well reduce unspecific detection. Molecular detection methods like RT-PCR may profit even more from the improved depletion of "contaminating" blood cells by OncoQuick density gradient centrifugation.

In summary, density gradient centrifugation with OncoQuick leads to improved depletion of blood cells with comparable tumor cell recovery, resulting in a higher relative tumor cell enrichment than that achieved with Ficoll density gradient centrifugation. This advantage simplifies further immunocytochemical tumor cell detection, limits the risk of false-positive results, and is a promising tool for the detection of circulating tumor cells in blood of tumor patients.

References

Bostik PJ, Chatterjee S, Chi DD, Huynh KT, Giuliano AE, Cote R, Hoon DS (1998) Limitations of specific reverse-transcriptase polymerase chain reaction markers in the detection of metastases in the lymph nodes and blood of breast cancer patients. J Clin Oncol 16:2632–2640

Jung R, Soondrum K, Krüger W, Neumaier M (2001) Detection of micrometastasis through tissue-specific gene expression: its promise and problems. Rec Res Cancer Res 158:32–39

von Knebel Doeberitz M, Koch M, Weitz J, Herfarth C (2001) Diagnostik und Bedeutung der "Minimal Residual Disease" bei Patienten mit kolorektalem Karzinom. Zentralbl Chir [Suppl 1]:15–19

Pantel K, Riethmüller G (1995) Methods for detection of micrometastatic carcinoma cells in bone marrow, blood and lymph nodes. Onkologie 18:394–401

Pantel K, von Knebel Doeberitz M (2000) Detection and clinical relevance of micrometastastic cancer cells. Curr Opin Oncol 12:95–101

Soeth E, Vogel I, Roder C, Juhl H, Marxen J, Kruger U, Henne-Bruns D, Kremer B, Kalthoff H (1997) Comparative analysis of bone marrow and venous blood isolates from gastrointestinal cancer patients for the detection of disseminated tumor cells using reverse transcription PCR. Cancer Res 57:3106–3110

Weitz J, Kienle P, Lacroix J, Willeke F, Benner A, Lehnert T, Herfarth C, v. Knebel Doeberitz M (1998) Dissemination of tumor cells in patients undergoing surgery for colorectal cancer. Clin Cancer Res 4:343–348

Antitumoral and Antimetastatic Effects of Continuous Particle-Mediated Cytokine Gene Therapy

Arne Dietrich, Katja Kraus, Ute Brinckmann, Christoph Stockmar, Anke Müller, Uwe Gerd Liebert, Manfred Schönfelder

A. Dietrich (✉)
Clinic for General Surgery, Surgical Oncology and Thoracic Surgery, Leipzig University, 04103 Leipzig, Germany

Abstract

We established a mice tumor model to investigate the effects of continuous cancer gene therapy, including antigen-presenting cell (APC) engineering and local stimulation of the immune system. B16 melanoma or Lewis lung carcinoma cells were injected intradermally on the back of C57/BL6 mice. The overlaying dermis or the tumor was shot with a gene gun (particle-mediated gene transfer) starting 8 days after tumor implantation in the case of the melanoma (Lewis lung carcinoma start day 7), continuing every fourth day thereafter until death. Control groups were mice without any therapy (A) or gene therapy with the empty plasmid (B). Therapy groups (Melanoma) received the genes as follows: group C – day 8, IL-12; day 12, IL-2...; group D – day 8, IFN-γ/B7.1; day 12, IFN-γ/B7.1...; group E – day 8, IFN-γ/B7.1; day 12, IL-12, day 16, IL-2.... Melanoma: Mean survival time was enhanced in all therapy groups significantly, whereby the greatest survival time was found in group C. Tumor growth was reduced in all therapy groups similarly (C and D significant). Lewis Lung: Only mice of group C had an enhanced survival and reduced tumor growth (both significant). An antimetastatic effect was seen in all therapy groups.

Introduction

Locally advanced and metastatic malignant disease continue to have a poor prognosis, and there is a certain need for new therapies. At present, gene therapy appears to be able to play a role in the interdisciplinary approach of cancer treatment. Cytokine gene transfer into tumor cells is known to initiate tumor regression and to have antimetastatic effects [1, 2, 4, 11–15]. Systemic side effects of the gene products or vector do not usually appear. Previous experiments in cytokine gene therapy proved combinations of two different genes to be superior compared to single therapies [1, 4, 10, 15, 19]. Thomas [17] described the importance of MHC I and B7.1 for sufficient systemic therapy with IL-12 and IL-2 in a mice tumor model using MHC I- and B7.1-positive or -negative cell lines. We established a mice tumor model to investigate the effects of continuous cancer gene therapy, including antigen-presenting cell (APC) engineering and local stimulation of the immune system. We aimed to achieve a strong T cell- mediated antitumoral effect. Therefore, we chose the genes coding for IFN-γ and B7.1 (i.e., APC engineering), in addition to IL-12 and IL-2 (i.e., stimulation of the immune system).

MHC I and the costimulatory molecule B7.1 (CD80) are both essential for the antigen presentation for CD8$^+$ cytotoxic T cells. The antigen presentation for CD8$^+$ cytotoxic T cells is only possible via MHC I. IFN-γ is able to upregulate MHC I in almost any cell line. B7.1 is only expressed on native APCs [2, 4, 6, 7, 11, 13, 14, 19].

T lymphocyte activation requires both an antigen-specific signal delivered through the T cell receptor and an unspecific costimulatory signal delivered by accessory receptors following their engagement by ligands expressed on APCs. In the absence of such costimulatory molecules, T-cell activation is impossible. Furthermore, it may lead to T-cell clonal anergy or apoptosis. B7.1 is one of the most studied costimulatory signal molecules. The interaction of B7.1 on APCs with its counterreceptor CTLA-4 and/or CD28 on T and NK cells results in proliferation and increased production of several cytokines such as IL-2, IFN-γ, TNF-α and GM-CSF. CD28 costimulation is important for the activation and proliferation of both T helper cells and CD8$^+$ cytotoxic T cells [9, 19].

The local stimulation of the immune system and the ability to induce antitumor immunity with various cytokines is well documented. IL-12 and/or IL-2 gene therapy has been described to be most effective. IL-12 is a proinflammatory cytokine secreted by macrophages, dendritic cells, and neutrophils. The major biological activity of IL-12 is on T and natural killer (NK) cells, in which it increases cytokine production, particularly IFN-γ, proliferation, and cytotoxicity. It induces type 1 response, that is, the differentiation of CD4$^+$ and CD8$^+$ type 1 cells, by both direct and indirect actions, promoting specific cytotoxic T cell responses and inhibiting the generation of Th2 cells. It also boosts the shift to antibody IgG subclasses.

IL-2 (T cell growth factor) enhances both nonspecific immune responses such as NK cells and lymphokine-activated killer (LAK) cells as well as MHC-restricted cytotoxic T-cell responses. It is a well established antitumoral agent. However, systemic administration is limited due to side effects [1, 4, 10, 12, 14–16, 18, 19].

Material and Methods

Mouse Tumor Model

Experiments were performed in C57/BL6 mice (Center for Experimental Medicine, Leipzig University). The Lewis lung carcinoma and the B16 melanoma cell line (chemically induced autologous cell lines of the C57/BL6 mice; Deutsche Tumorbank, Heidelberg, Germany) were cultured in RPMI 1640 medium supplemented with 10% fetal calf serum, 2 mM L-glutamine, 100 U/ml penicillin, and 100 µg/ml streptomycin. The mice were shaved on the back using a long hair cutter, and remaining hair was then removed with Pilcaderm Cream (ASID BONZ, Böblingen, Germany). Then, 5×106 Lewis Lung cells (or 5×105 B16 melanoma cells) in 25 µl PBS were injected intradermally on the back.

The overlaying dermis or the tumor was shot with the Helios Gene Gun (Bio-Rad, Munich, Germany) starting 8 days after tumor implantation for the B16 melanoma (after 7 days for the Lewis lung carcinoma), and then every fourth day until death.

Therapy groups are shown in Table 1. Control groups were mice without any therapy or gene therapy as described above, with the empty pRSC plasmid.

We used 10 animals (5 male, 5 female), 10 weeks old, per group. Tumor growth and body weight were monitored every second day until death. A tumor sample was taken from four mice per group for histological examination 18 and 33 days following tumor implantation. A postmortem examination with histological examination of the lung and liver was performed on all animals.

Statistical Analysis

Evaluation of statistical differences in data obtained regarding tumor size and survival time was performed with Student's t-test.

Table 1. Therapy groups. B16 melanoma, gene therapy started 8 days after tumor implantation; Lewis lung carcinoma, always 1 day earlier

Group/day	8	12	16	20	24	28	32	36
A (Control)	–	–	–	–	–	–	–	–
B (pRSC)	pRSC	pRSC	pRSC	pRSC	pRSC	pRSC	pRSC	...
C (IL12/IL2)	IL12	IL2	IL12	IL2	IL12	IL2	IL12	...
D (IFN/B7)	IFN/B7	IFN/B7	IFN/B7	IFN/B7	IFN/B7	IFN/B7	IFN/B7	...
E (IFN/B7/IL12/IL2)	IFN/B7	IL12	IL2	IFN/B7	IL12	IL2	IFN/B7	...

Expression Plasmid

Cloning of mIL-12p35 and mIL-12p40 into One Expression Plasmid

PBluscript SK vectors containing the cDNA for mIL-12p40 or mIL-12p35 were obtained from the American Type Culture Collection (ATCC, Rockville, MD). The pRSC expression plasmid, a plasmid with two multiple cloning sites, was generously provided by Dr. E. Hersh (Arizona Cancer Center, University of Arizona, Tucson). The mIL-12p40 gene was cloned into the first multiple cloning site driven by the RSV promotor, whereas IL-12p35 was cloned into the second multiple cloning site driven by the CMV promoter. The correct cloning was confirmed by sequencing.

Cloning of mB7.1 and mIFN-γ into One Expression Plasmid

The cDNA from the mB7.1 (CD80) molecule was cloned into the CMV-driven cloning site of the pRSC plasmid. The puc19 mB7.1 plasmid was generously provided by Prof. T. Blanckenstein (Max Delbrück Zentrum, Berlin, Germany). The DNA coding for mIFN-γ was received from Hoffmann La Roche (Basel, Switzerland) in a pMugamma PL plasmid and cloned into the RSV-driven cloning site. The correct cloning was confirmed by sequencing.

Expression Plasmid for mIL-2

The expression plasmid pLTR-mIl-2 containing the cDNA for mIL-2 was also obtained from Prof. T. Blanckenstein.

Cloning, preparation and cleaning of all DNA was performed as described in [8].

Cytocine and Flow Cytometry Analysis

We performed an enzyme-linked immunosorbent assay (ELISA) to prove sufficient cytokine secretion and flow cytometry for expression of the surface molecules of the transfected tumor cells in vitro. Cells were prepared as described in "In Vitro Transfection."

ELISA

ELISA was performed as described in [5]. MIL-12p75, mIL-2, and mIFN-γ concentrations were determined by sandwich ELISA systems with unlabeled capture antibodies and labeled detection antibodies (SEROTEC ELISA Kit for IL-2 and IFN-γ (SEROTEC, Biozol, Eching). For detection of mIL-12p75, a self-made ELISA was used with a rat anti-mouse Ab specific for heterodimeric mouse IL-12p75 (Hofmann-LaRoche).

Flow Cytometry

Flow cytometry analysis was gently performed by Dr. U. Sack at the Institute for Immunology of the Leipzig University. Melanoma cells were shot (see "In Vitro Transfection") with the plasmid coding for mB7.1 and mIFN-γ. Control groups were native B16 melanoma cells and melanoma cells shot with the empty pRSC plasmid. Cells were stained with anti-CD 80 PE and anti-H2Db Fitc for analysis.

Bio-ELISA for Biological Active mIL-12p75

Native mice spleen cells were incubated with the supernatants of mIL-12p75 transfected melanoma cells for 48 h. Supernatants were tested for IFN-γ. The positive control group was incubated with mIL-12p75 protein 500 pg/ml, and the negative control was incubated with supernatants from B16 melanoma cells transfected with the empty pRSC plasmid.

In Vivo and In Vitro Gene Transfer

The helium-driven Helios Gene Gun (particle-mediated gene transfer) was used for gene transfer. Plasmid DNA was precipitated onto 0.6-μm gold particles for in vitro gene transfer and onto 1.6-μm gold particles (Bio-Rad, Munich) for in vivo gene transfer. DNA and gold were mixed up to a gold-DNA loading rate of 0.5 mg gold and 1 μg plasmid DNA per shot. Particles were resuspended in absolute ethanol (99.996% ethanol, Merck, Darmstadt, Germany) for in vitro transfer and in a solution of 0.01 mg PVP (polyvinyl pyrolidone, Sigma, Deisenhofen, Germany) per ml in absolute ethanol for in vivo transfection. The DNA-gold-particle solution was coated onto the inner surface of a Tefzel tube (Bio-Rad, Munich) using the Bio-Rad tubing loader. The tubing was cut into 0.5-inch segments, the bullets ready to go for the Helios Gene Gun.

In Vitro Transfection

Here, 5×106 B16 melanoma cells in 20 μl complete RPMI 1640 were stretched out in a circle of 1.5 cm in diameter in a six-well plate and shot with a 200 psi helium pulse. Two milliliters complete RPMI 1640 was added, and supernatants were collected after 48 h for ELISA or cells for flow cytometry.

In Vivo Transfection

The tumor or the overlaying dermis was shot with a 400 psi helium pulse.

Histopathological Analysis

Organs or tumor samples were fixed in 10% buffered formalin, paraffinized, and stained with hematoxylin and eosin for histopathological analysis. Tumor samples were used to evaluate the immigration of various immunocompetent cells. Lung and liver were investigated for metastasis.

Immunohistochemistry

CD4$^+$ and CD8$^+$ T cells were stained in frozen tissue sections as described in [8] (using rat monoclonal anti-CD8 or anti-CD4 antibodies (Pharmingen, San Diego, CA) and a peroxidase-based detection kit (Vector AEC Substrate Kit for Peroxidase, Vector Laboratories, Burlingame, CA). Mouse spleen was used as a positive control tissue. Positive cells were counted.

Results

In Vitro Experiments

In order to prove the function of the plasmid constructs, we used the B16 melanoma cell line for in vitro investigations. This is due to the fact that the in vitro transfection rate of the melanoma is three to four times higher, in comparison to the Lewis lung carcinoma (data not shown). Cells were shot in vitro with the according expression plasmid and resuspended in 2 ml culture media. Supernatants were collected after 48 h for ELISA and contained up to: mIL-12, 29.6 ng/ml; mIL-2, 53.8 ng/ml; and IFN-γ, 0.23 ng/ml. Control groups (B16 cells alone or transfected with the empty pRSC plasmid) did not show any cytokine levels.

The Bio-ELISA for biologically active mIL-12p75 was positive (IFN-γ 1.1 ng/ml), the negative control was negative (less than 0.016 ng/ml IFN-γ), and the positive control was positive (IFN-γ 1 ng/ml).

In flow cytometry, 15% of the B7.1/IFN-γ transfected cells were positive for both MHC I and B7.1; 82% were positive for only MHC I and 3% remained negative for both.

Control groups (B16 cells alone and B16 cells shot with the empty pRSC plasmid) did not express MHC I or B7.1.

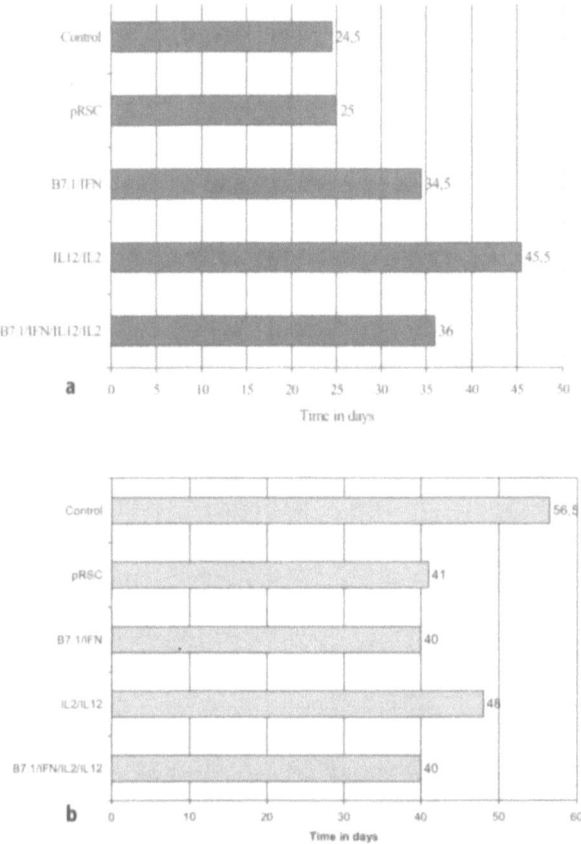

Fig. 1a, b. Median survival following tumor implantation. **a** B16 melanoma. Median survival time following tumor implantation, Student's *t*-test: control groups vs. B7/IFN (*p*<0.04), IL12/IL2 (*p*<0.01), and B7/IFN/IL12/IL2 (*p*<0.04). **b** Lewis lung carcinoma. Median survival time following tumor implantation. Student's *t*-test: pRSC vs. IL-12/IL-2 (*p*<0.001)

In Vivo Experiments

B16 Melanoma

Here, 5×10^5 B16 melanoma cells were injected intradermally on the back of C57/Bl6 mice. Within 8 days, the tumors grew to a size of 3 to 8 mm in diameter. One to two mice per group were excluded due to no tumor growth or tumor growth of more than 8 mm in diameter. Animals were treated as shown in Table 1.

The median survival is shown in Fig. 1a. Median survival differences of all therapy groups versus control groups are significant. The greatest survival was seen in the group receiving gene therapy with the genes coding for IL-12

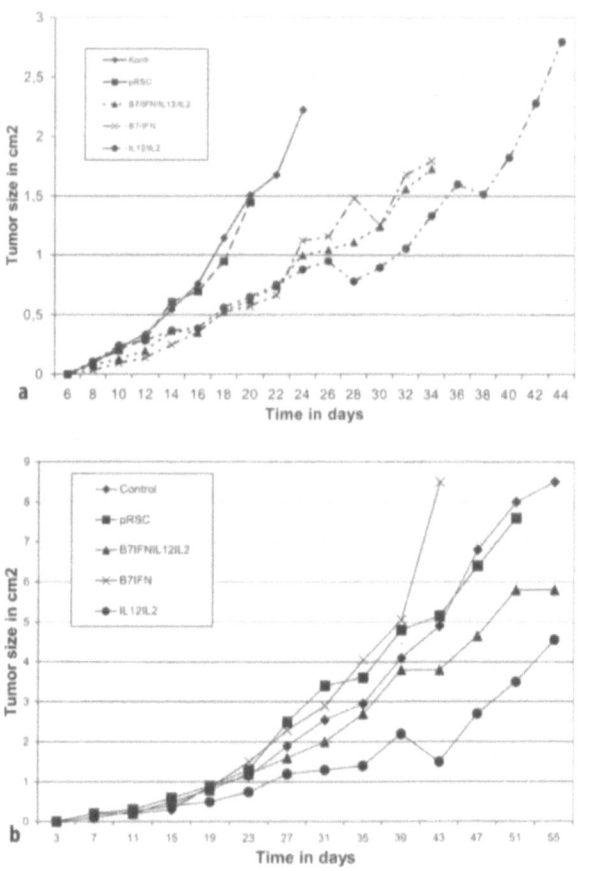

Fig. 2a, b. Tumor growth. **a** Mean tumor sizes, B16 melanoma. Calculations were stopped when the number of survivors dropped below five per group (starting number=10). Student's *t*-test, day 20: control groups vs. therapy groups B7/IFN and IL12/IL2 (*p*<0.03). **b** Mean tumor sizes, Lewis lung carcinoma. Calculations were stopped when the number of survivors dropped below five per group (starting number=10). Student's *t*-test, day 35: pRSC vs. the therapy group IL12/IL2 (*p*=0.003)

and IL-2. However, the difference compared to the other two therapy groups is not significant.

Treatment led to reduced tumor growth in all three therapy groups, with no significant differences between them (mean tumor size, see Fig. 2a). The two control groups showed similar tumor growth and median survival rates. There were no effects of the gene therapy with the empty pRSC plasmid compared to the control group, without any therapy clinically.

The body weight (data not shown) did not show any differences among the groups and was almost constant during the entire experiment. Mice became more and more cachectic with the progression of the tumors.

No side effects of the gene therapy were visible. In a similar experiment (data not shown), the serum levels of mIL-12p40 and mIL12-p75 were tested. Both were not detectable.

Tumor samples indicated a higher rate of an inflammatory response in all three therapy groups. Immunohistochemistry for $CD4^+$ and $CD8^+$ cells did show an increased number of both peri- and intratumoral $CD4^+$ and $CD8^+$ T cells in all therapy groups (data not shown).

A postmortem examination was performed on all animals. Liver and lung were searched for metastatic lesions semiquantitatively. There was a lower rate of pulmonary secondaries in all therapy groups and the pRSC control group at the time of death (data not shown). The rate of liver metastasis did not show significant differences.

Lewis Lung Carcinoma

We injected 5×106 Lewis Lung cells intradermally on the back of C57/Bl6 mice. Within 7 days, the tumors grew to a size of 3–8 mm in diameter, and the overlaying dermis or the tumor was shot every fourth day with the gene gun.

All animals receiving gene transfer with the gene gun suffered tissue loss of the tumor and a certain amount of bleeding due to the soft consistency of the Lewis lung carcinoma. The resulting chronic anemia would potentially cause an earlier death in all groups, and thus, the pRSC group is the real control group with regard to the effects of the cytokine gene therapy.

The median survival was only enhanced in the IL-12/IL-2 group (Fig. 1b). The greatest average survival was seen in the group with no gene transfer. However, the oldest individual was in the IL-12/IL-2 group (77 days). The median survival difference between the IL-12/IL-2 group and the pRSC control group is significant (p <0.04). There were no obvious effects in the IFN-γ / B7.1 group and the IFN-γ /B7.1/IL-12/IL-2 group.

Treatment also led to significant reduced tumor growth in the IL-12/IL-2 group (compared to the pRSC group, day 35, p <0.001). All other groups were almost the same in this regard. The mean tumor size is shown in Fig. 2b. The two control groups showed similar tumor growth. Tumor diameters were measured at skin level, and there were no effects of the gene transfer regarding tumor growth.

The body weight (data not shown) did not show any differences among the groups and was almost constant during the entire experiment. No side effects of the gene products and vector components were seen.

Tumor samples showed a higher rate of an inflammatory response in all three therapy groups. There was an increased number of peritumoral granulocytes and macrophages. More T cells and plasma cells were seen intratumoral.

Immunohistochemistry for CD4$^+$ and CD8$^+$ cells did not show major differences among all of the groups (data not shown). However, there was a tendency to an increased number of both peri- and intratumoral CD4$^+$ and CD8$^+$ T cells in the IL-12/IL-2 and IFN-γ/B7.1/IL-12/IL-2 groups.

A postmortem examination was performed on all animals. Liver and lung were searched for metastatic lesions semiquantitatively. There was a high rate of both pulmonary and liver secondaries in the control group not receiving any gene transfer. They had the longest average survival, and were therefore most likely to suffer an increased rate of metastasis over time. However, compared to the pRSC group, all therapy groups had an equivalent or lower rate of secondaries, except for the IL-12/IL-2 group with more lung metastasis (at an advanced age).

There was no metastasis at all in the IFN-γ/B7.1 group.

The data suggest, in addition to the reduced tumor growth and enhanced survival, an antimetastatic effect.

Discussion

Most of the animal experiments and human trials in cancer gene therapy have used only one (cytokine) DNA. Clary [4] (IL-2+IFN-γ), Zitvogel [19] (IL-12+B7.1), Nagai [10] (IL-12 and IL-18), and Addison [1] (IL-12 and IL-2) demonstrated combination therapies to be superior to single therapies. Publications regarding the use of three or four genes in cancer gene therapy are not currently known.

Continuous therapy with the Gene Gun is easy to handle and showed promising clinical data in mice [18]. It is suitable for repeated gene transfers and there are no additional effects of antigenic viral vectors.

The combination of APC-engineering and local stimulation of the immune system seems to be logical to achieve the highest possible specific immune response. However, artificial APC engineering will never be a substitute for the complex function of native APCs.

The combination therapy of all four genes did result in reduced tumor growth and enhanced survival in the melanoma group. However, therapy with genes for IL-12 and IL-2 was superior compared to additional genes for IFN-γ/B7.1 or IFN-γ/B7.1 alone. In case of the Lewis lung carcinoma, the IL-12/IL-2 group was the only one with a clinical effect. Obviously, APC-engineering is less efficacious in the case of the B16 melanoma and Lewis lung carcinoma, both known to be poor antigenic tumors.

The activities of B7.1 in the presence of IL-12 are discussed with much controversy. Rudy [14] found experimental evidence of an inhibitory effect of IL-12 via secretion of IFN-γ (the inhibitory effect of IL-12 was blockable by an anti-IFN-γ Ab) in vitro. This is consistent with our data. Zitvogel [19] countered the study by describing a synergistic effect of IL-12 and B7.1 in vivo. Albertini [2] used the technique of dual particle-mediated gene transfer of B7.1 and IFN-γ for dual expression of HLA molecules and the costimulatory molecule B7.1, a simple method of APC engineering. Rees [13] focuses on the importance of MHC for antigen presentation.

Thomas [17] found the combination of IL-12 and IL-2 superior compared to the single treatment. He also described the importance of the B7.1 costimulatory molecule in addition to the cytokine therapy proven in CD80-negative and CD80-positive subclones of a tumor cell line in mice. Rees found similar data with the IL-12/IL-2 treatment in IFN-γ knockout mice.

We did not have control groups with single cytokine gene therapy, assuming combination therapies to be better (see above), and to reduce the number of animals to a certain necessary minimum. In opposition to this, Rakhmilevich [12] reported similar results in the B16 melanoma with a single cytokine gene therapy. That study showed that they could significantly inhibit the tumor growth using the same model with a more extended, more frequent, and earlier-starting therapy with IL-12 only.

An antimetastatic effect was seen in all therapy groups. However, there was always also a lower rate of metastasis in the pRSC control group. The etiology therefore remains to be determined. This could be attributed to the semiquantitative examination, since the data of tumor growth and survival suggest that there are no effects of the empty plasmid.

The Lewis lung carcinoma is only suitable for ballistic gene transfer. Repeated bleedings due to the soft consistency of the tumor decrease the animals' lifespan.

Results of gene gun-mediated in vivo delivery of cytokine cDNA suggest further development and clinical testing as an approach to human cancer gene therapy. Clinical phase I studies with IL-12 [16], IFN-γ [11], and IL-2 [15] were completed successfully. Improved vectors or a more frequent gene transfer may also lead to further improvement.

References

1. Addison CL, Bramson JL, Hitt MM, Muller WJ, Gauldie J, Graham FL (1998) Intratumoral coinjection of adenoviral vectors expressing IL-2 and IL-12 results in enhanced frequency of regression of injected and untreated distal tumors. Gene Ther 5:1400–1409
2. Albertini MR, Emler CA, Schell K, Tans KJ, King DM, Sheehy MJ (1996) Dual expression of human leukocyte antigen molecules and the B7.1 costimulatory molecule (CD80) on human melanoma cells after particle-mediated gene transfer. Cancer Gene Ther 3:192–201
3. Carr-Brendel V, Markovic D, Smith M, Tayler-Papadimitriou J, Cohen EP (1999) Immunity to breast cancer in mice immunized with X-irradiated breast cancer cells modified to secrete IL-12. J Immunother 22:415–422
4. Clary MB, Coveney EC, Blazer DG, Philip R, Lyerly HK (1996) Active immunotherapy of pancreatic cancer with tumor cells genetically engineered to secrete multiple cytokines. Surgery 120:174–181
5. Decken K, Köhler G, Palmer-Lehmann K, Wunderlich A, Mattner F, Gately MK, Alber G (1998) Interleukin-12 is essential for a protective Th1 response in mice infected with Cryptococcus neoformans. Infect-Immun 66:4994–5000

6. Hiura M, Hashimura T, Watanabe Y, Kuribayashi K, Yoshida O (1994) Induction of specific anti-tumour immunity by interferon-γ gene-transferred murine bladder carcinoma MBT-2. Folia Biologica 40:49–61
7. Katsanis E, Xu Z, Bausero MA, Dancisak BB, Gorden KB, Davis G, Gray GS, Orchard PJ, Blazar BR (1995) B7-1 expression decreases tumorigenicity and induces partial systemic immunity to murine neuroblastoma deficient in major histocompatibility complex and costimulatory molecules. Cancer Gene Ther 2:39–46
8. Kraus K (2001) Der Partikel-vermittelte Gentransfer einer Kombination der Gene für Interleukin 12, Interleukin 2, Interferon γ und B7-1 zur Therapie solider maligner Tumore am Modell des murinen B16-Melanoms. Thesis, Leipzig University, Leipzig, pp 5–40
9. Meyer GC, Batrla R, Rudy W, Meuer SC, Wallwiener D, Gückel B, Moebius U (1999) Potential of CD80-transfected human breast carcinoma cells to induce peptide-specific T lymphocytes in an allogeneic human histocompatibility leukocyte antigens (HLA)-A2.1+-matched situation. Cancer Gene Ther 6:282–288
10. Nagai H, Hara I, Horikawa T, Fujii M, Kurimoto M, Kamidono S, Ichihasshi M (2000) Antitumor effects on mouse melanoma elicted by local secretion of interleukin-12 and their enhancement by treatment with interleukin-18. Cancer Invest 18:206–213
11. Nemunaitis J, Bohart C, Fong T, Meyer W, Edelmann G, Paulson RS, Orr D, Jain V, ÓBrien J, Kuhn J, Kowal KJ, Burkeholder S, Bruce J, Ognoskie N, Wynne D, Martineau D, Ando D (1998) Phase I trial of retroviral vector-mediated interferon (IFN)-gamma gene transfer into autologous tumor cells in patients with metastatic melanoma Cancer Gene Ther 5:292–300
12. Rakhmilevich AL, Turner J, Ford MJ, McCabe D, Sun WH, Sondel PM, Grota K, Yang NS (1996) Gene gun-mediated skin transfection with interleukin 12 gene results in regression of established primary and metastatic murine tumors. Proc Natl Acad Sci 93:6291–6296
13. Rees RC, Mian S (1999) Selective MHC expression in tumors modulates adaptive and innate antitumor responses. Cancer Immunol Immunother 48:374–381
14. Rudy W, Guckel B, Siebels M, Lindauer M, Meuer SC, Moebius U (1997) Differential function of CD80- and CD86-transfected human melanoma cells in the presence of IL-12 and IFN-gamma. Int immunol 9:853–860
15. Schreiber S, Kämpgen E, Wagner E, Pirkhammer D, Trcka J, Korschan H, Lindemann A, Dorffner R, Kittler H, Kastelitz F, Küpcü Z, Sinski A, Zatloukal K, Buschle M, Schmidt W, Birnstiel M, Kempe RE, Voigt T, Weber HA, Pehamberger H, Mertelsmann R, Bröcker EB, Wolff K, Stingl G (1999) Immunotherapy of metastatic malignant melanoma by a vaccine consisting of autologous interleukin 2-transfected cancer cells: outcome of a phase I study. Human Gene Ther 10:983–993
16. Sun Y, Jurgovsky K, Moller P, Alijagic S, Dorbic T, Georgieva J, Wittig B, Schadendorf D (1998) Vaccination with IL-12 gene-modified autologus melanoma cells: reclinical results and a first clinical phase I study. Gene Ther 5:481–490
17. Thomas GR, Chen Z, Enamorado I, Bancroft C, Van Waes C (2000) IL-12 and IL-2-induced tumor regression in a new murine medel of oral squamous-cell carcinoma is promoted by expression of the CD80 co-stimulatory molecule and IFN-gamma. Int J Cancer 86:368–374
18. Wang C, Quevedo ME, Lannutti BJ, Gordon KB, Guo D, Sun W, Paller AS (1999) In vivo gene therapy with interleukin-12 inhibit primary vascular tumor growth and induces apoptosis in a mouse model. J Invest Dermatol 122:775–781
19. Zitvogel L, Robbins PD, Storkus WJ, Clarke MR, Maeurer MJ, Campbell RL, Davis CG, Tahara H, Schreiber RD, Lotze MT (1996) Interleukin-12 and B7.1 co-stimulation cooperate in the induction of antitumor immunity and therapy of established tumors. Eur J Immunol 26:1335–1341

Genetic Subtyping of Renal Cell Carcinoma by Comparative Genomic Hybridization

Kerstin Junker, Gregor Weirich, Mahul B. Amin, Petr Moravek, Winfried Hindermann, Joerg Schubert

K. Junker (✉)
Department of Urology, Friedrich-Schiller University, 07743 Jena, Germany

Abstract

The prognosis of renal cell carcinoma (RCC) varies dependent on histologic tumor subtypes. However, differentiation between RCC types may sometimes be difficult on histologic grounds alone. Furthermore, the prognostic value of histologic parameters for the individual prognosis is limited. Additional information on the molecular level seems necessary to obtain more certainty in diagnostic and prognostic evaluation. By investigating genetic alterations in different RCC subtypes, we sought to obtain a genotype-phenotype correlation. Eighty-two clear-cell, 53 papillary, 23 chromophobe RCCs and 26 renal oncocytomas were investigated. Comparative genomic hybridization (CGH) was performed on DNA from paraffin-embedded tissue samples. DNA was isolated from tumor areas by microdissection and amplified by degenerated oligonucleotide primed polymerase chain reaction (DOP-PCR). CGH was performed according to standard protocols. We were able to detect specific alterations in each RCC subtype: clear cell RCC showed –3p, +5/5q, -8p, -9, -14, -18; papillary (chromophilic) RCC gains of chromosomes 7, 17, 16, 3, 12; chromophobe RCC loss of chromosomes 1, 2, 6, 10, 13, 17, 21; renal oncocytomas loss of chromosomes 1/1p and 14. Furthermore, for clear cell RCC, it was possible to define alterations which are associated with metastatic disease: loss of 9, 10, 14. Our results demonstrate that each RCC subtype is characterized by distinct genetic alterations. The definition of genetic alterations seems helpful for a tumor typing especially when morphology is equivocal. Therefore, genetic analyses represent a powerful diagnostic and prognostic tool for RCC.

Introduction

Tumors of the kidney account for 3% of all human neoplasms. The majority of these tumors are renal cell carcinomas (RCCs). RCCs are characterized by

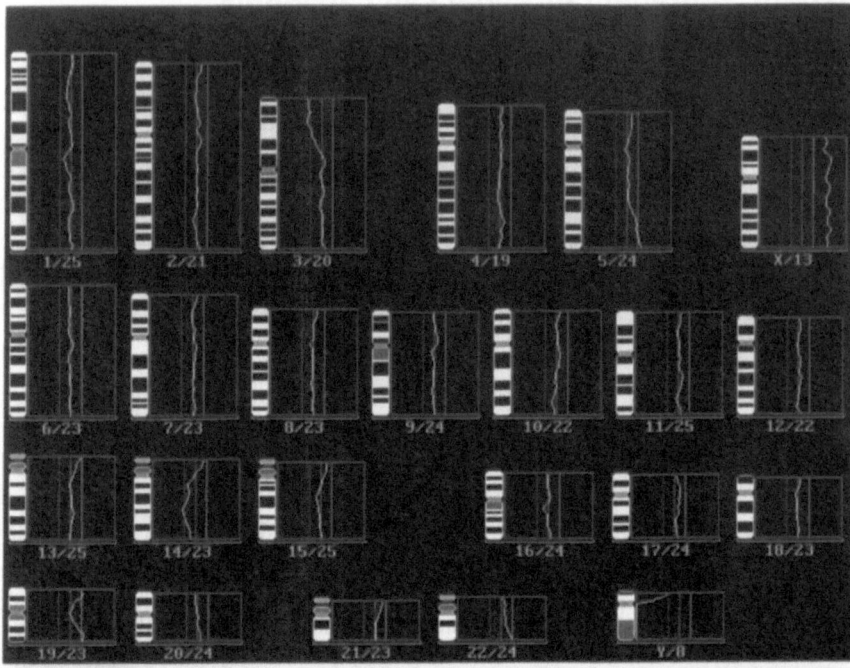

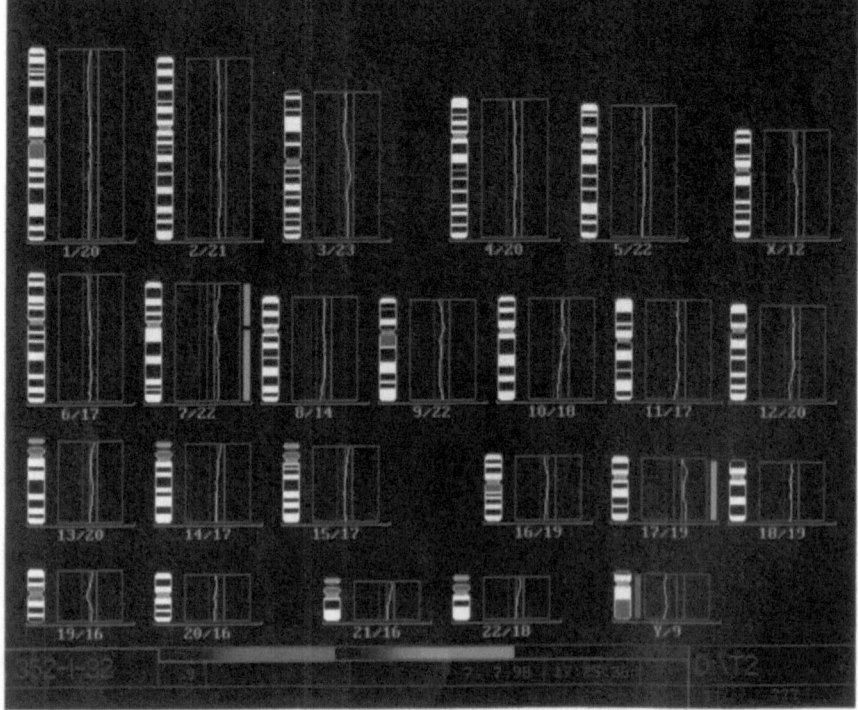

Fig. 1a–d. CGH profiles for each RCC tumor type. **a** Clear cell RCC with loss on chromosomes 3 and 14 and gain on chromosome 5. **b** Papillary (chromophilic) RCC with gains of chromosomes 7 and 17 as well as loss of the Y chromosome. **c** Chromophobe RCC with loss of chromosomes 1, 2, 6, 10, 13, 17 and 21. **d** Renal oncocytoma with loss of chromosomes 1 and 14

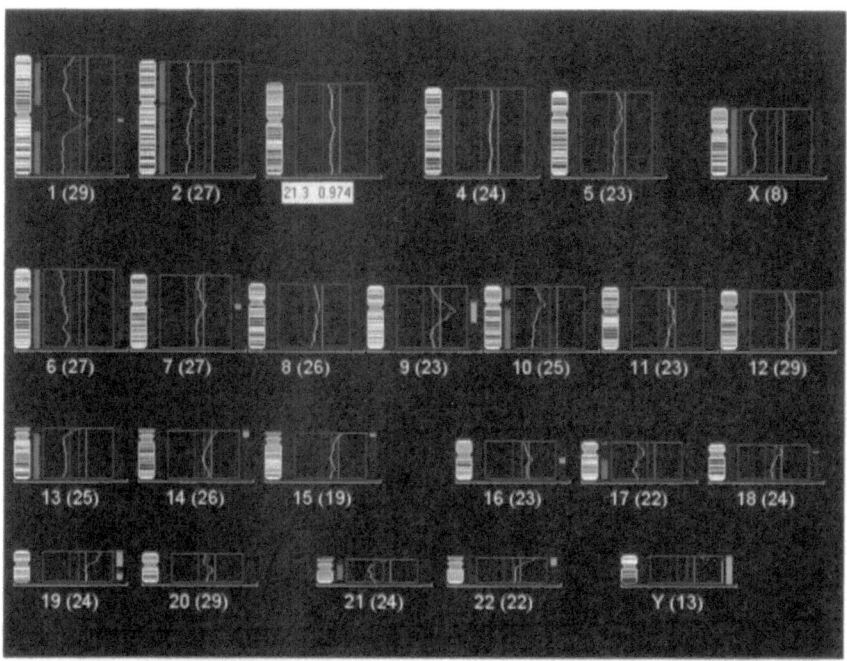

c

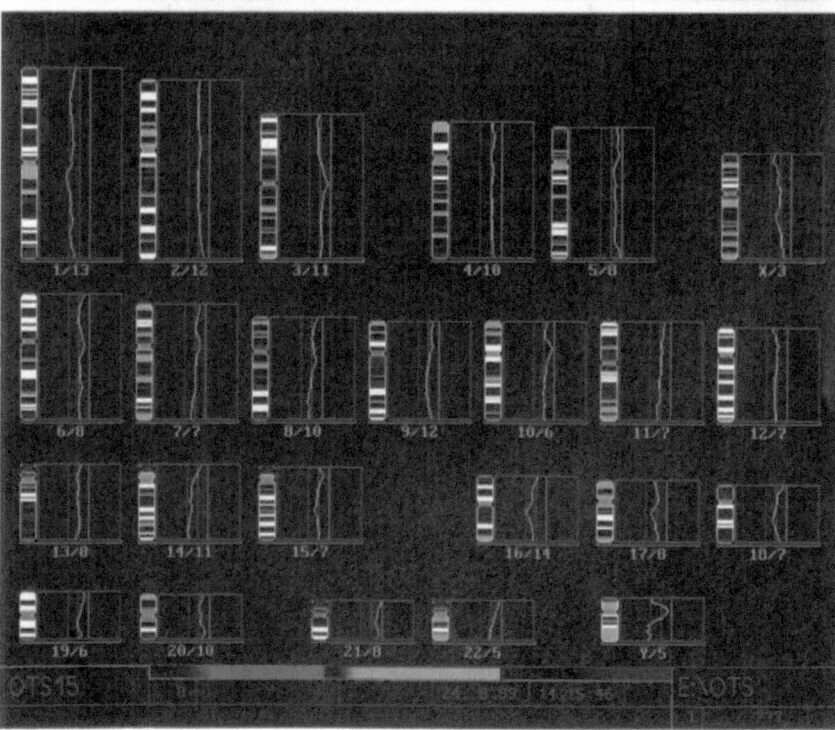

d

high resistance to chemo-, radio-, and immunotherapy. Metastatic disease represents the major prognostic factor in RCC patients. At the moment, no parameters are available for individual prognostic evaluation including response to therapy.

The classification system introduced by Thoenes et al. in 1986 led to a practicable clinically relevant subtyping of RCC [1]. The system is based on histologic and histochemical features. At present, three benign and six malignant renal tumor types are included in the Thoenes classification, which was the basis for the WHO classification of RCC in 1998 (UICC; Fig. 1) [2]. The UICC system has partly been corroborated by immunohistochemical and genetic investigations, which have shown that morphologically different RCC types are based on different genetic alterations.

The diagnostic practice of tumor typing relies primarily on morphology using UICC criteria. In some cases, however, tumor histology remains equivocal, and morphology alone cannot predict a metastatic potential. Therefore, additional information on the molecular level is necessary to obtain more certainty in diagnostic and prognostic evaluation. We have subjected four major subtypes of renal epithelial neoplasms (clear cell RCC, papillary RCC, chromophobe RCC, renal oncocytoma) to comparative genomic hybridization (CGH) analysis in order to establish genetic fingerprints which may serve as a reliable supplement for RCC diagnosis and patient management.

Materials and Methods

DNA was isolated from 5–10 frozen or formalin-fixed paraffin-embedded tissue sections. For CGH, normal DNA was isolated from blood cells collected from normal individuals using a commercial kit (Qiagen).

In order to obtain sufficient amounts of tumor DNA for CGH analysis, DNA was amplified according to a modified protocol for DOP-PCR [3]. This protocol employs Sequenase during the first eight cycles of nonspecific PCR, followed by 30 additional cycles under specific conditions using TaqPolymerase (Stoffel fragment). Labeling of tumor DNA and normal DNA was achieved by 20 PCR cycles using biotin-16dUTP and digoxigenin-11dUTP, respectively.

One microgram of both tumor DNA and normal DNA was hybridized to 50 μg Cot-1 DNA on normal metaphases at 37°C for 48 h. Detection of fluorescent signals was carried out with avidin-FITC (tumor DNA) and anti-digoxigenin-rhodamine (normal DNA). DAPI/Antifade was used for chromosome counterstaining. Fifteen metaphases were analyzed in each case using an Axioplan-Microscope (Zeiss, Germany) and a computer system from Metasystems (Altlussheim, Germany). Chromosomal alterations were defined as shifts to the red (loss of chromosomal region in the tumor DNA) or the green borderline (gain of chromosomal region in the tumor DNA).

Table 1. Frequency of genetic alterations in different RCC tumor types

Clear cell RCC	Papillary (chromophilic) RCC	Chromophobe RCC	Oncocytomas
Loss of 3p: 97%	Gain of 7: 84%	Loss of 1: 87%	Loss of 1/1p: 79%
Loss of 9: 34%	Gain of 17: 55%	Loss of 10: 69%	Loss of 14: 16%
Gain of 5: 32%	Gain of 16: 20%	Loss of 6: 56%	
Loss of 14: 25%	Gain of 12: 18%	Loss of 2: 50%	
Loss of 10: 18%	Gain of 3: 16%	Loss of 17: 56%	
	Loss of Y: 16%	Loss of 13: 44%	
		Loss of 21: 38%	

Results

In total, 174 tumors were analyzed by CGH including 82 clear cell, 53 papillary, 23 chromophobe RCC, and 26 renal oncocytomas. In 161 tumors, genetic alterations were detected by CGH (93%). Clear cell RCCs were characterized by total or partial loss of chromosomes 3p, 6, 9, 10, 1 and 4 and gain of chromosome 5/5q. In papillary RCC, we frequently found gains of chromosomes 7, 17, 16, 12, and 3 as well as loss of Y chromosome. The typical alteration of chromophobe RCC was combined losses of chromosomes 1, 2, 6, 10, 13, 17, and 21. Loss of chromosome 1 and less frequently loss of chromosome 14 occurred in renal oncocytomas. The results are presented in detail in Table 1. A representative CGH profile for each tumor type is given in Fig. 1.

Considering staging and metastases, in clear cell RCC, we found an association between progression of disease and losses of chromosomes 9, 10, and 14. Unfortunately, the number of cases was too small for correlation analyses in all other subtypes.

Discussion

The UICC classification system for renal tumors (Table 2) supports the concept that each RCC subtype represents an independent tumor entity. Several immunohistochemical and genetic investigations have supported this concept. A tumor-specific genetic fingerprint may be helpful as a diagnostic tool in

Table 2. UICC classification system, 1998 (adapted from [9])

Renal cell adenoma	Renal cell carcinoma
Metanephric	Clear cell
Papillary	Papillary
Oncocytic	Chromophobe
	Collecting duct
	Neuroendocrine
	Unclassified

cases where morphology remains equivocal. Clinical and histological data alone are insufficient for a prediction of individual outcome. There are many data regarding genetic alterations in clear cell RCC, fewer data about papillary RCC, and only some reports about rare tumor types like chromophobe and oncocytic RCC.

The aim of our study was to ascertain a standardized genetic fingerprint of each of the four major renal epithelial tumors using CGH. CGH allows for the analysis of chromosomal imbalances, i.e., losses or gains of whole chromosomes or parts of chromosomes. The advantage of CGH is the applicability to archival material; thus artifacts generated by cultured tumor cells can be avoided.

Applying CGH to DNA derived from formalin-fixed paraffin-embedded tissues, we were able to demonstrate a specific pattern of genetic alterations for each of the four tumor types. In clear cell RCC, we frequently found deletions on chromosome arm 3p. The high frequency (97%) indicates that loss of 3p is an early event in tumor development of clear cell RCC, independent of tumor stage or grade. This is in concordance with results reported by other groups [4–7]. Loss of chromosomes 9, 10, and 14 as well as gain of chromosome 5/5q were detected with lower frequencies. Alterations of chromosomes 9, 10, and 14 were associated with tumor progression (more frequently in higher stage and grade as well as in metastatic disease). On the other hand, gain of chromosome 5 was more common in clear cell RCC from patients with better outcome. Therefore, CGH-generated genetic data yielded valuable information about individual prognosis in clear cell RCC. The genetic pattern of papillary RCC is completely different from that of clear cell RCC. In papillary tumors, gains of chromosomes 7 and 17 as well as loss of the Y chromosome were frequently observed, whereas gains of chromosomes 16, 12, and 3 were not consistently found. Loss of 3p was not detected. Results are in concordance with published results from other groups [5, 8, 9]. There are only some reports concerning genetic alterations of chromophobe RCC. We detected combinations of losses of chromosomes 1, 2, 6, 10, 13, 17, and 21 as a typical feature of this tumor type. The only frequent genetic alteration of renal oncocytomas was loss of chromosome 1/1p. Based on loss of chromosome 1 in oncocytomas and chromophobe RCC, Störkel proposed a genetic relationship between both tumors [1]. However, this hypothesis should be corroborated by additional analyses.

No alterations were detected in 23 tumors, and in single tumors fingerprints other than those mentioned above were detected. Performing CGH, it is possible to detect only losses and gains of chromosomal regions but not balanced translocations, which have previously been identified for some tumors. Furthermore, deleted or amplified regions can only be detected by CGH if they are larger than 10–20 Mb.

Our results demonstrate that clear cell RCC, papillary RCC, chromophobe RCC, and renal oncocytomas are each characterized by a distinct fingerprint of genetic alterations which can be ascertained using CGH. The definition of genetic alterations seems helpful for a reliable RCC subtyping, especially when histopathological features of a given tumor are equivocal. The use of CGH may also help to improve individual prognosis prediction, as was shown for a subset of clear cell RCC.

References

1. Guinan P, Sobin LH, Algaba F, Badellino F, Kameyama S, MacLennan G, Novick A (1997) TNM staging of renal cell carcinoma: Workgroup No. 3. Union International Contre le Cancer (UICC) and the American Joint Committee on Cancer (AJCC) Cancer 80:992-933
2. Storkel, S (1999) [Epithelial tumors of the kidney. Pathological subtyping and cytogenetic correlation]. Urologe A 38:425-432
3. Chudoba IHT, Senger G, Claussen U, Haas OA (1997) Comparative genomic hybridization using DOP-PCR amplified DNA from a small number of nuclei. Cs Pediat 52:519-521
4. Kovacs G (1994) The value of molecular genetic analysis in the diagnosis and prognosis of renal cell tumours. World J Urol 12:64-68
5. van den Berg E, van der Hout AH, Oosterhuis JW, Storkel S, Dijkhuizen T, Dam A, Zweers HM, Mensink HJ, Buys CH, de Jong B (1993) Cytogenetic analysis of epithelial renal-cell tumors: relationship with a new histopathological classification. Int J Cancer 55:223-227
6. Velickovic M, Delahunt B, Grebe SK (1999) Loss of heterozygosity at 3p14.2 in clear cell renal cell carcinoma is an early event and is highly localized to the FHIT gene locus. Cancer Res 59:1323-1326
7. Bernues M, CasadevallC, Miro R, Caballin MR, Gelabert A, Ejarque MJ, Chechile G, Egozcue J (1998) Analysis of 3p allelic losses in renal cell carcinomas: comparison with cytogenetic results. Cancer Genet Cytogenet 107:121-124
8. Kattar MM, Grignon DJ, Wallis T, Haas GP, Sakr WA, Pontes JE, Visscher DW (1997) Clinicopathologic and interphase cytogenetic analysis of papillary (chromophilic) renal cell carcinoma. Mod Pathol 10:1143-1150
9. Kovacs G, Fuzesi L, Emanual A, Kung HF (1991) Cytogenetics of papillary renal cell tumors. Genes Chromosomes Cancer 3:249-255

Telomere Length and hTERT Expression in Patients with Colorectal Carcinoma

Robert Rosenberg, Ralf Gertler, Dominik Stricker, Silke Lassmann, Martin Werner, Hjalmar Nekarda, Joerg Ruediger Siewert

R. Rosenberg (✉)
Chirurgische Klinik und Poliklinik, Klinikum rechts der Isar, Technische Universität München, 81675 Munich, Germany

Abstract

The stabilization of telomere length by telomerase activation is an important step in carcinogenesis. Quantification of the catalytic telomerase subunit hTERT (human Telomerase Reverse Transcriptase) is a new indirect measure for telomerase. Telomere length and hTERT expression in cancer tissue and corresponding normal mucosa of 57 patients with completely resected colorectal carcinoma (UICC stage I-IV, R0) were determined for correlation with histopathological parameters and survival. Telomere lengths were measured using Southern Blot and hTERT-encoding mRNA was quantified by real-time RT-PCR. Telomere length and hTERT expression were significantly correlated in normal mucosa and cancer tissue ($p<0.001$).Telomere length and hTERT expression decreased with ageing only in normal mucosa. Cancer tissue had significantly shorter telomeres ($p<0.001$) and significantly lower hTERT expression levels ($p<0.001$) than corresponding normal mucosa. UICC stage I tumors showed significantly shorter telomeres than UICC stage II–IV tumors ($p<0.002$). Telomere length and hTERT expression were significantly correlated with overall survival. Telomere length and hTERT expression play an important role in ageing and carcinogenesis. Both parameters were identified as prognostic factors in patients with colorectal carcinoma.

Introduction

Telomeres consist of a high number of small, tandemly repeated DNA sequences. Located at the end of eukaryotic chromosomes, they prevent end-to-end fusion, irregular recombination, and other events that are normally lethal to a cell (Blackburn 1991). As DNA polymerase is unable to replicate the very ends of linear DNA, every replication cycle leads to a progressive shortening of the telomeric ends in normal somatic cells (Harley 1990; Hastie 1990). This phenomenon appears to be linked to the limited proliferative capacity of normal somatic cells (Hoos 1999). Telomerase, a ribonucleoprotein, catalyzes the addition of TTAGGG repeats to the ends of chromosomes (Morin 1989). Escaping from the proliferative limitations of cellular senescence, telomerase reactivation seems to be a prerequisite for the development of immortalized malignant tumor cells from mortal somatic cells (Feng 1995).

The human telomerase complex consists of the human Telomerase-associated RNA (hTR), providing the template for telomeric repeat synthesis (Nakamura 1997), and the human telomerase reverse transcriptase (hTERT), representing the catalytic subunit of the complex (Lustig 1999).

In the present study, we measured telomere length using Southern Blot and quantified hTERT-encoding mRNA by real-time RT-PCR in cancer tissue and corresponding adjacent mucosa of 57 patients with colorectal carcinoma. We report on the carcinogenetic relevance of both parameters in curatively (R0) resected colorectal carcinoma patients.

Methods

We examined 57 curatively resected colorectal carcinoma patients, who underwent surgery between 1993 and 1996. From the resected specimen of each patient, matched samples from the cancer tissue and the adjacent normal mucosa were obtained. All tissue samples were shock-frozen in liquid nitrogen within 1 h of resection and stored at –80°C until use.

Genomic DNA and total RNA were extracted from cryostat sections of all samples using the QIAamp DNA Mini Kit (Qiagen, Hilden, Germany) and the High Pure RNA Tissue Kit (Roche Diagnostics, Mannheim, Germany), respectively. Telomere lengths were determined by a modified TeloQuant Telomere Length Assay Kit (Pharmingen, San Diego, Calif., USA) protocol by Southern blot technique. Kinetic PCR quantification of hTERT-encoding mRNA was performed in a real-time RT-PCR using the LightCycler TeloTAGGG hTERT Quantification Kit (Roche Diagnostics, Germany). The quantities of hTERT-mRNA were expressed as the ratio of mRNA-copy numbers of hTERT to mRNA-copy numbers of the house-keeping gene PBGD.

Results

Median telomere lengths (TL) in cancer tissues and adjacent mucosa of all 57 patients were 5.7 kbp (range 4.1–7.6) and 6.9 kbp (range 5.5–8.6 kbp), respectively. Median hTERT expression levels were 23.2 (range 4.6–214.3) in cancer tissues and 41.4 (range 12.5–209.9) in adjacent mucosa samples (Fig. 1). Patient-by-patient comparison of matched tissue samples showed that cancer tissue had significantly shorter telomeres and significantly lower hTERT expression levels than adjacent mucosa ($p < 0.001$).

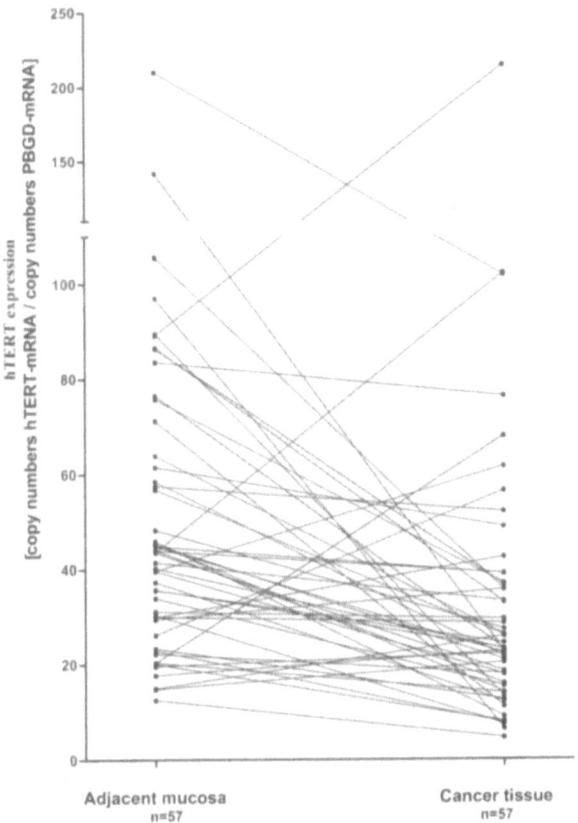

Fig. 1. hTERT-mRNA expression in matched samples of cancer tissue and adjacent mucosa of 57 completely resected colorectal carcinoma patients. *Connecting lines* illustrate that 45 patients (78.9%) had lower and 12 patients (21.1%) had higher hTERT-mRNA levels in the cancer tissue compared to the adjacent mucosa

Only in adjacent mucosa did both telomere length and hTERT expression decrease with ageing. In cancer tissue, regulation of both parameters were independent of age. To adjust this age-dependent variation and to outline the individual differences between cancer tissue and adjacent mucosa, the ratios of cancer tissue to adjacent mucosa for both telomere length and hTERT expression were calculated for each patient. The telomere length ratio showed a median of 0.8 (range 0.5–1.2), the hTERT ratio a median of 0.5 (range 0.1–3.3).

The correlation with histopathological parameters revealed a significant correlation between the degree of tumor infiltration (pT category) and telomere length in cancer tissue (Table 1). pT1 and pT2 tumors (n=18) showed significantly shorter telomeres compared to pT3 and pT4 tumors (n=39; p<0.02). Levels of hTERT expression were not correlated with pT category.

Table 1. Telomere length (TL) and hTERT expression (hTERT) in noncancer and cancer tissue for both parameters of 57 patients with colorectal carcinoma

	n	Noncancer		Cancer	
		TL	hTERT	TL	hTERT
		Median	Median	Median	Median
Patients	57 (100%)	6.9	49.6	5.7	32.5
pT					
pT 1–2	18 (32%)	6.7	48.1	5.3	23.3
pT 3–4	39 (68%)	6.9	50.3	6.0	36.7
p value		n.s.	n.s.	<0.02	n.s.

For survival analysis, optimal cut-offs for telomere lengths and hTERT expression levels were calculated by log-rank statistics for our study group of 57 patients. Thirty-five patients with telomeres longer than 5.4 kbp in the carcinoma tissue had a significantly worse overall survival, with a 5-year survival of 52% compared to 86% for 22 patients with telomere lengths of 5.4 kbp or less ($p<0.03$). For hTERT expression, 13 patients with hTERT expression levels greater than 37 showed a tendency towards shorter overall survival compared to 44 patients with hTERT expression levels of 37 and less ($p=0.056$).

Discussion

In most matched tissue samples, the histologically normal adjacent mucosa had longer telomeres than the corresponding colorectal cancer tissue. Reflecting the phenomenon of replication-dependent telomere losses, the observed reduction of telomere length during the process of carcinogenesis from normal mucosa to cancer tissue underlines the high proliferative capacity of tumor cells. Shortened telomeres in most cancer tissues also suggest that compensation for replication-dependent telomere losses occurs, if at all, late in tumorigenesis.

For the first time, it was shown that hTERT-mRNA was expressed in all colorectal cancer tissues and their adjacent mucosa samples. Thus, the detection pattern of hTERT-mRNA differed considerably from that of telomerase activity which was reportedly found in colorectal carcinomas but remained undetectable in normal colorectal mucosa using the TRAP assay. While hTERT-mRNA has been identified as a determining factor for telomerase activity in cancer tissues like colorectal carcinoma (Nakamura 1999; Niyama 2001; Tahara 1999), our data now suggest that hTERT-mRNA expression might not be sufficient for telomerase activation in noncancer tissues. As earlier proposed by Nakamura et al., who found lower telomerase activity levels than expected from hTERT-mRNA expression levels in cancerous and noncancerous gastric and colorectal tissue, telomerase activity might not only be controlled by transcription of hTERT, but could additionally be influenced at the posttranscriptional, translational, and posttranslational level or by telomerase inhibitors (Nakamura 1999).

The present study illustrates the well-known phenomenon of telomere length shortening with ageing in normal somatic cells (Harley 1990), including normal colorectal mucosa (Hastie 1990; Nakamura 2000) as a result of accumulated cell cycles. We now could additionally show that hTERT-mRNA expression also decreased with ageing in normal colorectal mucosa. In cancer tissue, however, we found no correlation with age for either telomere length or hTERT expression. Therefore, the hypothesis that telomere reduction occurs in parallel between cancer tissue and adjacent mucosa in patients with colorectal carcinoma as suggested by Nakamura et al. could not be supported by our results.

During the process of carcinogenesis, colorectal carcinomas seem to escape age-related telomere length and hTERT expression control. Telomere length and expression of hTERT-mRNA in cancer tissue even appear to be specific characteristics of each individual tumor at that time of age. The ratios of cancer tissue to adjacent mucosa for both parameters thus reflect the ability of the tumor to stabilize or even elongate its telomeres by hTERT expression. In this context, successful stabilization of telomeres by hTERT expression and consecutive telomerase activation appears to be a prerequisite for indefinite and aggressive tumor progression finally resulting in poor prognosis of the patients. The newly introduced ratios for telomere length and hTERT expression might thus have potential for clinical use as markers for proliferative capacity and aggressiveness of tumors.

References

Blackburn EH (1991) Structure and function of telomeres. Nature 350:569–573

Feng J, Funk WD, Wang SS, Weinrich SL, Avilion AA, Chiu CP, Adams RR, Chang E, Allsopp RC, Yu J (1995) The RNA component of human telomerase. Science 269:1236–1241

Harley CB, Futcher AB, Greider CW (1990) Telomeres shorten during ageing of human fibroblasts. Nature 345:458–460

Hastie ND, Dempster M, Dunlop MG, et al (1990) Telomere reduction in human colorectal carcinoma and with ageing. Nature 346:866–868

Hoos A, Nekarda H (1999) Telomerase – Potential und Grenzen der klinischen Anwendbarkeit. Dtsch Med Wochenschr 124:223–230

Lustig AJ (1999) Crisis intervention: the role of telomerase. Proc Natl Acad Sci USA 96:3339–3341

Nakamura TM, Morin GB, Chapman KB, et al (1997) Telomerase catalytic subunit homologs from fission yeast and human. Science 277:955–959

Nakamura Y, Tahara E, Tahara H, et al (1999) Quantitative reevaluation of telomerase activity in cancerous and noncancerous gastrointestinal tissues. Mol Carcinog 26:312–320

Nakamura KI, Furugori E, Esaki Y, et al (2000) Correlation of telomere lengths in normal and cancer tissue in the large bowel. Cancer Lett 158:179–184

Niyama H, Mizumoto K, Sato N, et al (2001) Quantitative analysis of hTERT mRNA expression in colorectal cancer. Am J Gastroenterol 96:1895–1900

Morin GB (1989) The human telomere transferase enzyme is a ribonucleoprotein that synthesizes TTAGGG repeats. Cell 59:521–529

Tahara H, Yasui W, Tahara E, et al (1999) Immunohistochemical detection of human telomerase catalytic component, hTERT, in human colorectal tumor and non-tumor tissue sections. Oncogene 18:1561–1567

Estimation of Concentration of Chosen Adhesive Factors in Suprarenal Tumours of "Incidentaloma" Type

Krzysztof Kołomecki, Henryk Stępień, Tomasz Stępień, Zbigniew Pasieka, Krzysztof Kuzdak

T. Stępień (✉)
Department of Endocrinological and General Surgery,
Institute of Endocrinology, Medical University of Łódź,
91-425 Łódź, Poland

Abstract

The role of adhesive molecules in the pathogenesis of adrenal gland tumours formation remains unclear. Here we present the concentrations of soluble vascular cell adhesion molecule-1 (sVCAM-1) and soluble intracellular adhesion molecule-1 (sICAM-1) in the blood of patients with adrenal "incidentaloma". We found that the mean concentrations of sVCAM and sICAM in the serum of the patients with adrenocortical cancers were significantly higher than those of the patients with benign adenomas or control cases. These results suggest that the levels of adhesion molecules may be a marker of malignancy of adrenal incidentalomas.

Introduction

In recent times the involvement of adhesive molecules in the development of many neoplasms and noncancer diseases such as atherosclerosis, asthma, kidney and hepatic diseases, and others has been widely discussed. The role of adhesive molecules has been studied most thoroughly in inflammatory reactions. It seems that neoplastic cell invasion is a process similar to transmigration of leucocytes to an inflammatory focus, and thus comparative examination of adhesive receptors present on normal and neoplastic cells is very important for research, and possibly also for diagnostic and therapeutic purposes [1, 2].

There are three types of adhesive molecules: selectins, integrins, and the immunoglobin (Ig) superfamily: vascular cell adhesion molecule (VCAM) and intracellular adhesion molecule (ICAM) [1]. The Ig superfamily receptors are composed of a variable number of repeated immunoglobulin-like domains [3]. These molecules, expressed generally in endothelium, interact with integrins and selectins and control firm adherence of cells, for example leucocytes

[4]. Cellular adhesion molecules VCAM-1 and ICAM-1 have been implicated in tumour progression and metastasis in malignant melanoma, renal cell carcinoma, glioblastoma, and others [5–7].

A significant clinical problem which still awaits solution is determining whether the character of the tumour is benign or malignant, which is particularly difficult in hormonally inactive adrenal tumours of "incidentaloma" type. In our earlier reports we demonstrated the role of proangiogenic factors in the development of suprarenal tumours, which makes it possible to use them as markers of malignancy of these neoplasms [8, 9]. Recent reports show that adhesive factors affect the process of angiogenesis in a significant way [10].

Aim of Study

The aim of this work was to evaluate the concentrations of the soluble forms of VCAM-1 and ICAM-1 (sVCAM-1 and sICAM-1) in the blood at the patients with tumour of suprarenal glands inactive hormonally like malignant or benign "incidentaloma".

Material and Methods

The study comprised 29 patients with hormonally inactive suprarenal tumours of "incidentaloma" type treated in the Clinic of General and Endocrinological Surgery, Medical University of Łódź, between 1999 and 2001. In ten patients (six women and four men, mean age 57 years), cancer of adrenal glands was diagnosed. In seven of these patients, the tumour was removed with the adrenal gland, and pathological examination using histochemical tests revealed the malignant character of the tumour. In three cases the tumour was inoperative (T4N1M1), as numerous distant metastases were present, together with infiltration in neighbouring tissues, including blood vessels, and neoplastic cachexia. The diagnosis was based on clinical symptoms, fine needle aspiration biopsy (BACC), and computed tomography (CT) with CT densitometry. In 19 patients (12 women and seven men, mean age 43 years) adenoma corticis glandulae suprarenalis was revealed by histopathology after removal of the tumour.

The control group comprised ten healthy persons (five women and five men, mean age 48 years).

In all patients, serum concentrations of sVCAM-1 and sICAM-1 were determined by the ELISA method using kits from R&D Systems (Minneapolis, Mich., USA).

Statistical evaluation was carried out using Student's t-test.

Table 1. Concentrations of sVCAM-1 and sICAM-1 in the serum of studied patients

	sVCAM-1	sICAM-1
Control group	642.0 (SD=91.7)	301.0 (SD=38.1)
Adrenocortical carcinoma	1147.0 (SD=410.9)	561.0 (SD=179.0)
	$p<0.01$	$p<0.01$
Adrenocortical adenoma	581.3 (SD=147.0)	407.8 (SD=131.6)
	$p>0.05$	$p=0.02$
	$p1<0.01$	$p1=0.01$

p, Significance of difference between the values of studied and control cases; $p1$, significance regarding the values for patients with malignant or benign tumours.

Table 2. Concentrations of sVCAM-1 and sICAM-1 in the serum of patients with inoperative and inoperative adrenal cortex cancers

	sVCAM	sICAM
Control group	642.0 (SD=91.7)	301.0 (SD=38.1)
Operated patients (7 cases)	1283.0 (SD=393.7)	539.0 (SD=213)
	$p<0.01$	$p<0.01$
Inoperative patients (3 cases)	828.0 (SD=278.8)	614.0 (SD=55.5)
	$p>0.05$	$p<0.01$

p, Significance of difference between the values of studied and control cases.

Results

The obtained values of concentration of the studied factors are presented in Tables 1 and 2. All values are expressed in "ng/ml".

In eight patients (80%) with adrenocortical cancer, the normal range of concentration of studied adhesion molecules was exceeded; these values were as high in only two patients (10.5%) with benign adrenocortical tumour.

Discussion

There are more and more reports suggesting the possibility of a practical application of molecular markers in the diagnostics of solid tumours, including tumours of endocrine glands, which are hormonally inactive. Preoperative diagnostics of these tumours, and thus qualification for surgery, is a complex problem because due to a lack of hormonal activity of these tumours, hormonal tests are of no value. Imaging studies may not be sufficient for correct evaluation of the character of these tumours. In our studies we have demonstrated that the mean concentrations of soluble receptors of sVCAM and sICAM in the serum of patients with adrenocortical cancers is significantly higher than those of patients with benign adrenocortical adenomas or of control cases. From the clinical point of view, the observation that in 80% of cancer patients the level of these parameters is significantly increased (compared to only 10.5% of patients with benign tumours) is of even greater importance. According to the rule of three standard deviations, the determined range of normal values covers 97% of the whole population, and thus these range values may be accepted as the norm. If we can demonstrate that the value of a given parameter is significantly increased in the majority of patients with a given disease, then this parameter may be regarded as a marker.

Our results are consistent with observations of other authors. Karayiannakis found that serum concentrations of VCAM-1 and ICAM-1 may reflect tumour progression and metastasis in colorectal cancer. He also observed that serum levels of these molecules decreased significantly after radical resection of the tumour, which confirms the fact that these molecules are connected with the presence of the tumour [12]. Similar results were obtained by Yoo in patients with stomach cancer [13], by Liu in patients with head and neck carcinoma [14], and by Dosquet in patients with renal cancer [15]. Verhaegh demonstrated that the expression of these molecules is not increased in basal cell carcinoma, which is related to low effect of cell-mediated immunity being an important mechanism in limiting basal cell carcinoma tumour spread [16]. However, Regidor showed significantly higher concentrations of VCAM-1 and ICAM-1 in the cytosol of breast cancer tissue compared to benign breast tissue and corresponding sera [17]. Thus, according to the majority of authors, blood concentrations of VCAM-1 and ICAM-1 may be regarded as markers of malignancy of many tumours, but the small number of these reports precludes clinical application of these observations.

Another interesting observation is that the concentration of one of these adhesion molecules (VCAM-1) in patients with inoperative adrenocortical cancer was not significantly elevated compared to the control group. The small number of observations does not allow drawing final conclusions, but this observation is consistent with our earlier results of studies on the concentrations of proangiogenic cytokines and metalloproteinases in these patients. We have observed that in patients with inoperative adrenal cortex cancer, some of these factors are not elevated in comparison with patients from the control group with benign tumours [8]. It is possible, thus, that malignant primary tumours produce substances which inhibit the development of the tumour itself and the process of metastasising. Compounds such as endostatin and angiostatin inhibit angiogenesis, which is necessary for tumour development [18, 19]. Cellular adhesion molecules are newly identified mediators of angiogenesis. It seems that they stimulate endothelial cells' migration and growth, and formation of new vessels in the extracellular matrix, similarly to other proangiogenic factors. Adhesion molecules also enable migration of metastasising neoplastic cells through blood vessel walls [7, 15, 20, 21].

Conclusions

The concentrations of sVCAM and sICAM in the blood serum of patients with hormonally inactive adrenal cortex cancers are significantly higher than in patients with hormonally inactive benign adrenal cortex adenoma. This suggests that the concentrations of these adhesion molecules in the blood may be a marker of malignancy of adrenal tumours of the "incidentaloma" type.

References

1. Korczak-Kowalska G, Matysiak W, Górski A (1997) Adhesive molecules – current concepts in medicine. Med Sci Monit 3:431–436
2. Hogg N, Berlin C (1995) Structure and function of adhesion receptors in leukocyte trafficking. Immunol Today 16:327–330
3. Williams AF, Barclay AN (1988) The immunoglobulin superfamily. Annu Rev Immunol 6:381–387
4. Dunon D, Piali L, Imhof A (1996) To stick or not to stick: the leukocyte homing paradigm. Curr Opin Cell Biol 8:714–723
5. Johnson JP (1999) Cell adhesion molecules in the development and progression of malignant melanoma. Cancer Metastasi Rev 18(3):345–357
6. Hemmerbin B, Scherbening J, Kugler A, Radzum HJ (2000) Expression of VCAM-1, ICAM-1, E- and P-selectin and tumour-associated macrophages in renal cell carcinoma. Histopatology 37:78–83
7. Salmaggi A, Eoli M, Frigerio S, Ciusani E, Silvani A, Boiardi A (1999) Circulating intercellular adhesion molecule-1 (ICAM-1), vascular cell adhesion molecule-1 (VCAM-1) and plasma thrombomodulin levels in glioblastoma patients. Cancer Lett 146:169–172
8. Kołomecki K, Stępień H, Narębski JM (2000) Vascular endothelial growth factor and basic fibroblast growth factor in blood serum of patients with hormonally active and inactive adrenal gland tumours. Cytobios 101:55–64
9. Kołomecki K, Stępień H, Bartos M, Narębski J (2001) Evaluation of MMP-1, MMP-8, MMP-9 serum levels in patients with adrenal tumours prior and after surgery. Neoplasma 48:116–121
10. Drixler TA, Voest E, van Vroonhoven TJ, Rinkes IH (2000) Angiogenesis and surgery: from mice to man. Eur J Surg 160:435–446
11. Blalock HM (1960) Social statistics. Mc Graw-Hill, New York
12. Karayiannakis AD, Syrgios KN, Zbar A, Kremmyda A, Bramis I, Tsigric C (2001) Serum levels of E-selectin, ICAM-1 and VCAM-1 in colorectal cancer patients: correlations with clinicopathological features, patient survival and tumour surgery. Eur J Cancer 37:2392–2397
13. Yoo NC, Chung HC, Park JO, Rha SY, Kim JH, Roh JK, Min JS, Kim BS, Noh SH (1998) Synchronous elevation of soluble intercellular adhesion molecule-1 (ICAM-1) and vascular cell adhesion molecule-1 (VCAM-1) correlates with gastric cancer progression. Yonsei Med J 39:27–36
14. Liu CM, Sheen TS, Ko JY, Shun CT (1999) Circulating intercellular adhesion molecule (ICAM-1), E-selectin and vascular cell adhesion molecule-1 (VCAM-1) in head and neck cancer.Br J Cancer 79:360–362
15. Dosquet C, Coudert MC, Lepage E, Cabane J, Richard F (1997) Are angiogenic factors, cytokines and soluble adhesion molecules prognostic factor in patients with renal cell carcinoma? Clin Cancer Res 3:2451–2458
16. Verhaegh M, Beljaards R, Veraart J, Hoekzema R, Neumann M (1998) Adhesion molecule expression in basal cell carcinoma. Eur J Dermatol 8:252–255
17. Regidor PA, Callies R, Regidor M, Schindler AE (1998) Expression of the cell adhesion molecules ICAM-1 and VCAM-1 in the cytosol of breast cancer tissue, benign breast tissue and corresponding sera. Eur J Gynaecol Oncol 19:377–383
18. O'Reilly MS, Holmgren L, Shing Y (1994) Angiostatin: a novel angiogenesis inhibitor that mediates the suppression of metastases by a Lewis lung carcinoma. Cell 79:315–328

19. O'Reilly MS, Boehm T, Shing Y, Fukai N, Vasios G, Lane WS, Flynn E, Birkhead JR, Olsen BR, Folkman J (1997) Endostatin: an endogenous inhibitor of angiogenesis and tumour growth. Cell 88:277–285
20. Verkarre V, Patey-Mariand de Serre N, Vazeux R, Teillac-Hamel D, Chretien-Marquet B, LeBihan C, Leborgne M, Fraitag S, Brousse N (1999) ICAM-3 and E-selectin endothelial cell expression differentiate two phases of angiogenesis in infantile hemangiomas. J Cutan Pathol 26:17–24
21. Kuehn R, Lelkes PI, Bloechle C, Nindorf A, Izbicki JR (1999) Angiogenesis, angiogenic growth factors and cell adhesion molecules are upregulated in chronic pancreatic diseases: angiogenesis in chronic pancreatitis and in pancreatic cancer. Pancreas 18:96–103

Evaluation of the Levels of bFGF, VEGF, sICAM-1, and sVCAM-1 in Serum of Patients with Thyroid Cancer

Zbigniew Pasieka, Henryk Stępień, Jan Komorowski, Krzysztof Kołomecki, Krzysztof Kuzdak

Z. Pasieka (✉)
Clinic of General and Endocrinological Surgery, Institute of Endocrinology, Medical University of Łódź, Pabianicka St. 62, 93513 Łódź, Poland

Abstract

Tumour growth and development depend on a complex cascade of angiogenic factors. The aim of the study is evaluation of the level of growth factors VEGF and bFGF, and adhesion molecules sICAM-1, sVCAM-1 in the serum of patients with papillary thyroid cancer. The study comprised 35 patients aged 21–68 years (mean age 46±14) who had papillary thyroid cancer diagnosed on the basis of thin needle aspiration biopsy, and were qualified for operative treatment. This group comprised 28 women and seven men. The control group was 26 healthy individuals. Serum concentrations of bFGF, VEGF, sICAM-1, and sVCAM-1 were evaluated by the enzyme-linked immunosorbent assay (ELISA) method. We have observed significantly higher mean concentrations of bFGF, VEGF, and sICAM-1 in the serum of patients with thyroid cancer compared with the control group. There was no significant difference between the sVCAM-1 concentrations of the thyroid cancer group and the control group.

Introduction

Formation of blood vessels, which deliver oxygen and energetic substances, is the main factor necessary for the development of neoplastic tumour. This process is described as angiogenesis, a cascade of events dependent on angiogenic and antiangiogenic factors released by the tumour cells and also by native endothelial, epithelial, and mesothelial cells, and leucocytes. Angiogenesis is initiated as a result of imbalance between the activity of pro- and antiangiogenic factors [1]. The multistage phenomenon of epithelial cell invasion, their migration, proliferation, and differentiation depends not only on the activity of extracellular matrix enzymes, growth factors, and expression of their receptors, but is also regulated by adhesion molecules. Among growth factors, special roles in angiogenesis are played by fibroblast growth factor (bFGF) and vascular endothelial growth factor (VEGF).

VEGF is a potent mitogen for endothelial cells of the arteries, veins, and lymphatic vessels, but also for other types of cells [2, 3]. This factor is produced by cells of many neoplasms, such as glioblastoma multiforme and haemangioblastoma, neoplasms of the gastrointestinal tract, kidney cancer, urinary bladder cancer, and other cancers with significant necrosis [4–6].

bFGF is one of the family of heparin-binding growth factors and may be acidic (aFGF) or basic (bFGF) [7]. This factor plays an important role in the neoangiogenesis of solid tumours [8].

Adhesion molecules are also involved in the pathogenesis of malignant solid tumours and their capability of forming distant metastases.

The term cellular adhesion molecules (CAM) denotes surface cellular receptors and their ligands, which enable contact and communication between the cell and extracellular matrix, and also between cells. The family of adhesion molecules comprises five main groups: selectins, integrins, cadherins, immunoglobulin-like molecules, and isoforms of molecule CD44. Adhesion molecules participate in the differentiation of cells, inflammatory processes, graft rejection reaction, and neoplastic dissemination [9–11]. The family of immunoglobulin-like molecules includes, among others, intercellular adhesion molecules (ICAM-1) and vascular adhesion molecules (VCAM-1). ICAM-1 and VCAM-1 are glycoproteins present as transmembrane proteins and as soluble molecules. Constitutional presence of ICAM-1 was demonstrated on thyrocytes in papillary thyroid cancer [12]. VCAM-1 plays an important role in the process of tissue differentiation, activation of T cells, and neoplastic dissemination [13, 14].

The roles of the discussed angiogenic factors in various types of neoplasms have been well studied and documented; however, there are few reports dealing with angiogenesis of endocrine glands, in particular the thyroid. The aim of the present study was evaluation of peripheral blood serum concentrations of bFGF, VEGF, soluble ICAM-1 (sICAM-1), and sVCAM-1 in patients with papillary thyroid cancer.

Material and Methods

The study comprised 35 patients aged 21–68 years (mean age 46±14) who had papillary thyroid cancer diagnosed on the basis of thin needle aspiration biopsy, and who qualified for operative treatment. There were 28 women and seven men. The studied patients were in euthyreosis, which was confirmed by preoperative clinical examination, evaluation of free thyroid hormones in the serum (fT_3, fT_4), and thyrotropic hormone TSH. Blood for tests was sampled form a peripheral vein on the day before operation. Material obtained during operation was fixed in 10% neutralised formalin and used for routine histopathological examination (macroscopic evaluation, preparation of paraffin sections, and fixing in haematoxylin and eosin) for final verification of diagnosis. The control group comprised 26 healthy persons. Serum concentrations of bFGF, VEGF, sICAM-1, and sVCAM-1 were evaluated by the enzyme-linked immunosorbent assay (ELISA) method. The study was approved by the Ethical Committee for Research Studies of the Medical University of Łódź. The obtained results are expressed as means ± standard error. The differences between the study and control groups were assessed by analysis of variance (ANOVA) and lowest statistical difference (LSD) test.

Results

We observed significantly higher mean concentrations of bFGF in the serum of patients with thyroid cancer compared with the control group (12.76±1.74 vs. 5.52±0.77 pg/ml, $p<0.05$.) and significantly higher mean concentrations of VEGF in the serum of patients with thyroid cancer compared with the control group (281.37±31.45 vs. 61.99±14.08 pg/ml, $p<0.05$; Fig. 1).

We also observed significantly higher mean concentration of sICAM-1 in the serum of patients with thyroid cancer compared with the control group (455.23±28.66 vs. 299.62±11.54 ng/ml, $p<0.05$).

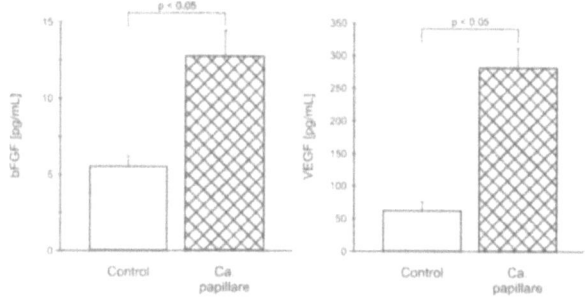

Fig. 1. The mean concentrations of bFGF and VEGF in the serum of patients with thyroid cancer and the control group

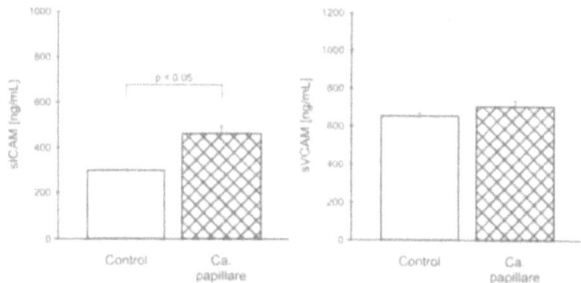

Fig. 2. The mean concentrations of sICAM-1 and sVICAM-1 in the serum of patients with thyroid cancer and the control group

There was no significant difference between the mean serum concentration of sVCAM between the thyroid cancer group and the control group (717.00 ± 50.56 vs. 644.58 ± 2, $p>7.30$ ng/ml; Fig. 2).

Discussion

The aim of the study was evaluation of the level of growth factors and adhesion molecules in the serum of patients with diagnosed papillary thyroid cancer. These factors play an important role in the processes of neoangiogenesis, tumour growth, and distant metastases formation. Evaluation of neoangiogenesis, level of angiogenic factors and their inhibitors in the serum, and body fluids of their tissue expression may be useful for determining the advance of neoplastic process, presence of distant metastases, efficacy of applied treatment, and prognosis. This fact has been well documented in the literature; however, the problem of angiogenesis in endocrine glands, including thyroid cancer, has not been well described. Angiogenesis in thyroid cancer was thus the subject of our investigation. We present first results of studies devoted to evaluation of the levels of bFGF, VEGF, sICAM-1, and sVCAM-1 in peripheral blood serum of patients with papillary thyroid cancer. We found significant elevation of the levels of bFGF, VEGF, and sICAM-1 in the serum of patients with papillary thyroid cancer compared with the control group. The level of sVCAM-1 did not differ significantly between the study and control groups. Our observations are consistent with those of other authors who evaluated these parameters in peripheral blood serum in various types of cancer. Significant elevations of VEGF and bFGF were observed in the serum of patients with soft tissue sarcoma [15]. The level of bFGF was significantly increased in the serum of patients with various forms of lung cancer, compared with the control group [16]. In multiple myeloma, the serum level of bFGF was significantly increased [17]. Also, in malignant melanoma significant increases of VEGF and bFGF in blood serum were reported [18]. Additionally, in the case of head and neck cancers, significant increases of VEGF and bFGF and their prognostic value were stressed [19]. VEGF and bFGF were significantly elevated in the serum of patients with large intestine cancer, and the level of VEGF correlated closely with the presence of liver metastases [20]. Assessment of the levels of adhesion molecules has also been well described. Increased concentrations of sICAM-1 and sVCAM-1 in peripheral blood serum have been reported in many forms of cancer. Significant elevation of sICAM-1was documented in the serum of patients with ovarian cancer [21]. The levels of sVCAM-1 and sICAM-1 are significantly higher in the serum of patients with nasal-pharyngeal cancer. In laryngeal cancer, the level of sVCAM-1 is significantly elevated, whereas the level of sICAM-1 is similar to that of the control group. In oral cavity cancer, the levels of sICAM-1 and sVCAM-1 were not increased significantly [22]. In cervical cancer, significantly high levels of sICAM-1 were seen in comparison with both the control group and a benign cervical neoplasms group [23]. In primary liver cancer, an elevated level of sICAM-1 was described compared with the control group, as well as in comparison with benign liver tumours [24]. In primary liver cancers, there was a significant correlation between the level of sICAM-1 and cancer advance, and the presence of distant metastases, efficacy of treatment, and postoperative recurrence [25]. In lung cancer, the level of sICAM-1 was significantly increased in comparison with healthy persons [26]. Metastatic tumours showed a higher level of this factor, compared with primary tumours; however, there was no correlation between the level of sICAM-1 and prognosis [27]. Stomach cancer is connected with an increase of both sICAM-1 and sVCAM-1. The levels of these parameters were higher in patients with distant metastases, and in patients with inoperative advanced stomach cancer [28]. Elevated levels of sICAM-1 and sVCAM-1 were described in cancer of colon and rectum; it was connected with the presence or absence of distant metastases [29]. In women with breast cancer, an increased level of sVCAM-1 was noted, as well as a positive correlation between the level of this parameter and vascular density factor, disease progression, and postoperative recurrence [30]. Taking these reports into consideration, we conclude that papillary thyroid cancer is one of the neoplastic processes where angiogenic factors play a significant role. Whether or not the levels of these parameters are connected with disease advance and the presence of distant metastases and what their prognostic value is will be the subjects of further studies.

References

1. Fidler IJ, Ellis LM (1994) The implications of angiogenesis to the biology and therapy of cancer metastasis. Cell 79:185–188
2. Ferrara N, Henzel WJ (1989) Pituitary follicular cells secrete a novel heparin-binding growth factor specific for vascular endothelial cells. Biochem Biophys Res Commun 161:851–859
3. Ploüet J, Schilling J, Gospodarowicz D (1989) Isolation and characterization of a newly identified endothelial cell mitogen produced by at T20 cells. EMBO J 8:3801–3807
4. Brown LF, Berse B, Jackman RW, Tognazzi K, Mansean EJ, Dvorak HF, Senger DR (1993) Increased expression of vascular permeability factor (vascular endothelial growth factor) and its receptors in kidney and bladder carcinoma. Am J Pathol 143:1255–1262
5. Brown LF, Berse B, Jackman RW, Tognazzi K, Mansean EJ, Senger DR, Dvorak HF (1993) Expression of vascular permeability factor (vascular endothelial growth factor) and its receptor in adenocarcinomas of the gastrointestinal tract. Cancer Res 53:4727–4735
6. Shweioki D, Itin A, Soffer D, Keshet E (1992) Vascular endothelial growth factor induced by hypoxia may mediate hypoxia-initiated angiogenesis. Nature 359:843–845
7. Basilico C, Moscatelli D (1992) The FGF family of growth factors and oncogenes. Adv Cancer Res 59:115–1
8. Moscatelli D, Presta M, Joseph-Silverstein J, Rifkin DB (1986) Both normal and tumor cells produce basic fibroblast growth factor. J Cell Physiol 129:273–276
9. Edelman GM (1993) A golden age for adhesion. Cell Adhes Comm 1: 1–7
10. Springer TA (1990) Adhesion receptors of the immune system. Nature 346:425–434
11. McCormick BA, Zetter BR (1992) Adhesive interactions in angiogenesis and metastasis. Pharmacol Ther 53:239–260
12. Kawai K, Resetkova E, Enomoto T, Fornasier V, Volpe R (1998) Is human leukocyte antigen-DR and intercellular adhesion molecule-1 expression on human thyreocytes constitu-

tive in papillary thyroid cancer? Comparative studies of human thyroid xenografts in severe combined immunodeficient and nude mice. J Clin Endocrinol Metab 83:157–164

13. Garofalo A, Chirivi RG, Foglieni C, Pigott R, Mortarini R, Martin-Padura I, Anichini A, Gearing AJ, Sanchez-Madrid F, Dejana E (1995) Involvement of very late antigen 4 integrin on melanoma in interleukin 1-augmented experimental metastasis. Cancer Res 55:414–419
14. Fogler WE, Volker K, McCormick KL, Watanabe M, Ortaldo JR, Wiltrrout RH (1996) NK cell infiltration into lung, liver, and subcutaneous B16 melanoma is mediated by VCAM-1/VLA-4 interaction. J Immunol 156:4707–4714
15. Feldman AL, Pak H, Yang JC, Alexander HR, Libutti SK (2001) Serum endostatin levels are elevated in patients with soft tissue sarcoma. Cancer 15:1525–1529
16. Ueno K, Inoue Y, Kawaguchi T, Hosoe S, Kawahara M (2001) Increased serum levels of basic fibroblast growth factor in lung cancer patients: relevance to response of therapy and prognosis. Lung Cancer 31:213–219
17. Sezer O, Jakob C, Eucker J, Niemoller K, Gatz F, Wernecke K, Possinger K (2001) Serum levels of the angiogenic cytokines basic fibroblast growth factor (bFGF), vascular endothelial growth factor (VEGF) and hepatocyte growth factor (HGF) in multiple myeloma. Eur J Haematol 66:83–88
18. Ugurel S, Rappl G, Tilgen G, Reinhold U (2001) Increased serum concentration of angiogenic factors in malignant melanoma patients correlates with tumor progression and survival. J Clin Oncol 19:577–583
19. Dietz A, Rudat V, Conradt C, Weidauer H, Ho A, Moehler T (2000) Prognostic relevance of serum levels of the angiogenic peptide bFGF in advanced carcinoma of the head and neck treated by primary radiochemotherapy. Head Neck 22:666–673
20. Davies MM, Jonas SK, Kaur S, Allen-Mersh TG (2000) Plasma vascular endothelial but not fibroblast growth factor levels correlate with colorectal liver metastasis vascularity and volume. Br J Cancer 82:1004–1008
21. Darai E, Bringuier AF, Walker-Combrouze F, Feldman G (1998) Soluble adhesion molecules in serum and cyst fluid from patients with cystic tumours of the ovary. Hum Reprod 13:2831–2835
22. Liu CM, Sheen TS, Ko JY, Shun CT (1999) Circulating intercellular adhesion molecule 1 (ICAM-1) E-selectin and vascular cell adhesion molecule 1 (VCAM-1) in head and neck cancer. Br J Cancer 79:360–362
23. Okamoto Y, Tsurunaga T, Ueki M (1999) Serum soluble ICAM-1 levels in the patients with cervical cancer. Acta Obstet Gynecol Scand 78:60–65
24. Sun JJ, Zhou XD, Liu YK, Tang ZY, Feng JX, Zhou G, Xue Q, Chen J (1999) Invasion and metastasis of liver cancer. Expression of intercellular adhesion molecule 1. J Cancer Res Clin Oncol 125:28–34
25. Huang YS, Wu JC, Chan CY, Chao Y, Chang FY, Lee SD (1999) Circulating intercellular adhesion molecule-1 in chronic liver disease and hepatocellular carcinoma. Zhonghua Yi Xue Za Zhi (Taipei) 62:487–495
26. DeVita F, Infusino S, Auriemma A, Orditura M, Catalan AU (1998) Circulating levels of soluble intercellular adhesionmolecule-1 in non-small cell lung cancer patients. Oncol Rep 5:393–396
27. Grothey A, Heistermann P, Philippou S, Voigtman R (1998) Serum levels of soluble intercellular adhesion molecule-1 (ICAM-1, CD54) in patients with non small cell lung cancer: correlation with histological expression of ICAM-1 and tumour stage. Br J Cancer 77:801–807
28. Kaihara A, Iwagaki H, Gouchi A, Hizuta A, Isozaki H, Takakura N, Tanaka N (1998) Soluble intercellular adhesion molecule-1 and natural killer cell activity in gastric cancer patients. Res Commun Mol Pathol Pharmacol 100: 283–300
29. Kitagawa T, Matsumoto K, Iriyama K (1998) Serum cell adhesion molecules in patients with colorectal cancer. Surg Today 28:262–267
30. Byrne GJ, Ghellal A, Iddon J, Blann AD, Venizelos V, Kumar S, Howell A, Bundred NJ (2000) Serum soluble vascular cell adhesion molecule-1: role as a surrogate marker of angiogenesis. J Natl Cancer Inst 92:1329–1336

Molecular Whole-Body Cancer Staging Using Positron Emission Tomography: Consequences for Therapeutic Management and Metabolic Radiation Treatment Planning

Michael Schmücking, Richard P. Baum, Frank Griesinger, Norbert Presselt, Reiner Bonnet, Christian Przetak, Andreas Niesen, Jochen Leonhardi, Eric C. Lopatta, Bernhard Herse, Thomas G. Wendt

R.P. Baum (✉)
Klinik für Nuklearmedizin, Zentralklinik Bad Berka,
99437 Bad Berka, Germany

Abstract

A prospective analysis was performed in 124 non-small cell lung cancer patients to determine the role of F-18 fluorodeoxyglucose (FDG)-positron emission tomography (PET) for molecular (metabolic) staging (n=63), therapy monitoring after induction-chemotherapy (n=34), and conformal radiation treatment planning (n=27). Staging by FDG-PET was significantly more accurate than CT ($p < 0.001$) and changed therapeutic management in 52% of all patients. After induction-chemotherapy, patients with complete metabolic remission histologically did not show vital tumor cells in contrast to patients with metabolic partial remission or progressive disease. Metabolic radiation treatment planning by PET led to smaller planning target volumes (PTVs) for radiation therapy (between 3% and 21% in 25/27 patients), resulting in a reduction of dose exposure to healthy tissue. In two patients, PET-PTV was larger than CT-based PTV, since PET detected lymph node metastases smaller than 1 cm. FDG-PET provides clinically important information; changes therapeutic management, can predict noninvasively effectiveness of chemotherapy, and may lead to better tumor control with less radiation-induced toxicity.

Background

Radiation therapy is an important component of primary treatment in non-small cell lung cancer (NSCLC). For definitive radiation therapy of inoperable NSCLC, the Radiation Therapy Oncology Group (RTOG) studies from the era of two-dimensional (2D) radiotherapy document that the risk of intrathoracic first recurrences declines with increasing dose (64% with 40 Gy, 45% with 50 Gy, and 38% with 60 Gy) [18]. A detailed analysis shows that as many as 37% of the first recurrences in the thorax are outside the treatment volume. Recurrences within the treatment volume occur in only 26% of the cases.

These results suggest that more exact knowledge of the tumor extent combined with a further dose escalation might enhance the locoregional tumor control and thus improve patient survival.

As late as the early 1990s, it was still standard procedure to apply a radiation dose based on 2D radiotherapy plans. The target volume was drawn into representative computed tomography (CT) sections at the level of the central beam of the main tumor mass and at the level of the upper and lower field margins. The use of x-ray CT scans since the end of the 1970s had already improved tumor delineation, also avoiding damage to normal tissue (spinal cord, heart, healthy lung tissue). Consequently, the therapeutic ratio of radiation therapy improved. The introduction of 3D radiation treatment planning in the 1990s was a further major step forward [14, 15, 20]. This enabled the calculation of unconventional (e.g., noncoplanar) field configurations. In 3D conformal radiation therapy, the isodoses can maximally follow the target volume delineated. It is possible to increase the dose and – at the same time – avoid damage to normal tissue; the prerequisite is that the target volume is delineated with great precision.

The use of positron emission tomography (PET) with F-18 fluorodeoxyglucose (FDG) might improve 3D radiation therapy planning, as PET has higher specificity in detecting the primary tumor and higher sensitivity and specificity in detecting lymph node metastases compared to CT scanning. In addition, PET is more accurate for differentiating between tumor involvement and atelectasis or poststenotic inflammatory lesions [1, 23, 24].

Prior to treatment, it is possible to use PET for mediastinal staging [1–3, 22, 23] and to identify distant metastases, consequently altering the management of patients with NSCLC [1, 2, 21]. PET is increasingly used for monitoring chemotherapy, radiation therapy, and chemoradiation [8], but also for 3D radiation treatment planning [8, 12, 13].

The objective of the present prospective study was to examine whether the additional molecular (metabolic) information provided by FDG-PET: (1) alters the therapeutic management of patients with NSCLC; (2) alters the delineation of the target volume for NSCLC according to the International Commission on Radiation Units and Measurements, Report 50 [9]; (3) changes the dose exposure of the lung quantified by dose-volume histograms; and (4) may predict therapeutic outcome earlier compared to morphological imaging methods.

Material and Methods

Findings in 124 patients were analyzed prospectively in a routine clinical setting. Quantification of the glucose metabolism [standardized uptake values (SUVs)] and metabolic transverse diameter (MTD) as well as of the metabolic tumor index (MTI=SUV×MTD) was performed. The patients were examined with the following three aims:

1. Tumor staging in histologically confirmed NSCLC (n=63 patients)
2. Therapy monitoring after induction chemotherapy (n=34 patients)
3. 3D radiation treatment planning of teletherapy (n=27 patients)

First, 350–600 MBq F-18 FDG was injected 45 to 90 min before a transmission-corrected whole-body study was started. PET data (iterative reconstruction) were correlated with CT scans (by image fusion) and histological findings. Statistical analyses were done using the two-tailed McNemar test, Wilcoxon test, U-test (Mann-Whitney), and Mantel-Haenszel test. Actuarial survival was calculated by the Kaplan-Meier method.

Results

Tumor Staging

Nodal involvement and M-status differed in 52% and 27% of the patients, respectively, comparing the results obtained by F-18 FDG-PET and CT scan. Consequently, therapeutic management was changed in 52% of the patients. Based on histopathologic specimens obtained by surgery, PET correctly identified lymph node metastases with a sensitivity of 82% and a specificity of 94%. Overall diagnostic accuracy was 90%, with positive and negative predictive values of 82% and 94%, respectively. There were four false-positive findings (caused by anthracosilicotic nodules, nonspecific but tumor-related inflammatory changes, and lymphadenitis). None of the histologically proven pN1 lesions were detected by PET (due to micrometastases or intense FDG uptake in the primary tumor located close to the hilus). However, all pN2 and pN3 lesions were staged correctly.

Based on morphologic criteria (lymph node size), the sensitivity and specificity of CT were 76% and 47%, respectively (PET vs. CT, $p<0.0001$). Actuarial survival at 18 months was 51% for primary lesions with SUV>10 and 71% for SUV<10, respectively. Due to the small numbers of patients and a median follow-up period of only 8 months, the difference in survival between the two SUV groups (SUV<6 and SUV>6) shows only a trend (p=0.065).

Therapy Monitoring After Induction Chemotherapy

The patients with complete metabolic remission as demonstrated by FDG-PET showed histologically no vital tumor cells, whereas the histological specimens of the patients with partial response (PR) or progressive disease (PD) revealed by PET always showed vital tumor cells.

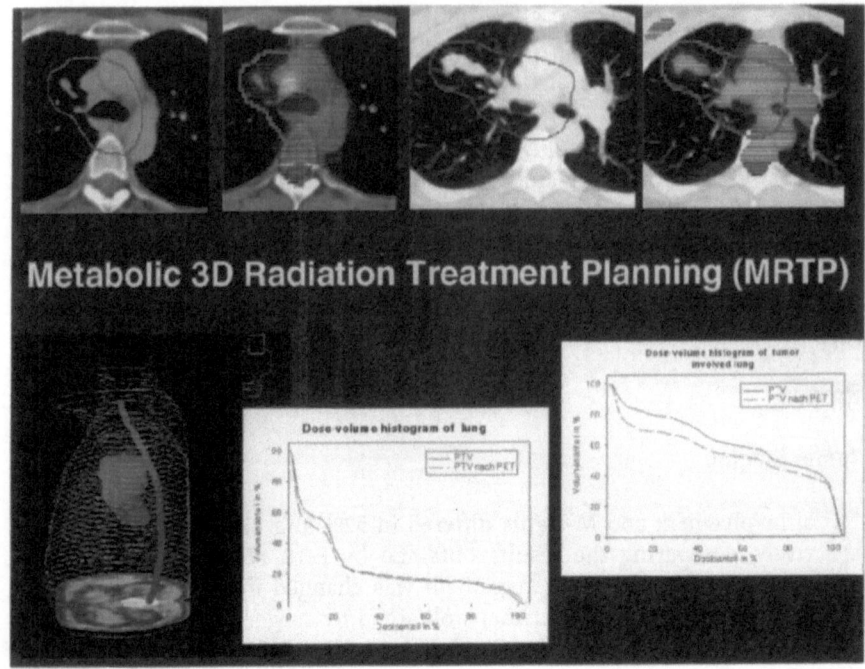

Fig. 1. Image fusion of PET and CT scan (using HERMES computer software) and calculation of the target volume (*red line*) based on the metabolic tumor activity as shown by FDG-PET. This target volume was subsequently imported into the HELAX radiation treatment planning system. In addition, a reduction of dose exposure to the lung is shown: DVH of a radiation treatment plan with a PTV based only on CT scan (*continuous black line*) or based on the additional metabolic information obtained by FDG-PET (*green broken line*)

3D Radiation Treatment Planning

The planning target volume (PTV) could be reduced in the range of 3% to 21% compared to conventional imaging modalities when PET results were also used for the 3D radiation treatment planning (applying image fusion of metabolic tumor volumes obtained by PET with morphologic tumor volumes by CT scan). For example, PET allowed differentiation between viable tumor and atelectasis, resulting in a smaller PTV. The dose-volume histograms (DVH) of the PET-based treatment plans showed a reduction of the dose to the organs at risk, i.e., lung, heart, and spinal cord.

The volume of lung tissue receiving more than 20 Gy (V_{lung} 20 Gy), could be reduced by 5% to 17% in boost therapy of NSCLC (Figs. 1, 2). In two patients, the treatment volume based on PET findings was larger than the one based on CT scan, since PET detected lymph node metastases of normal size (<1 cm in diameter) in CT.

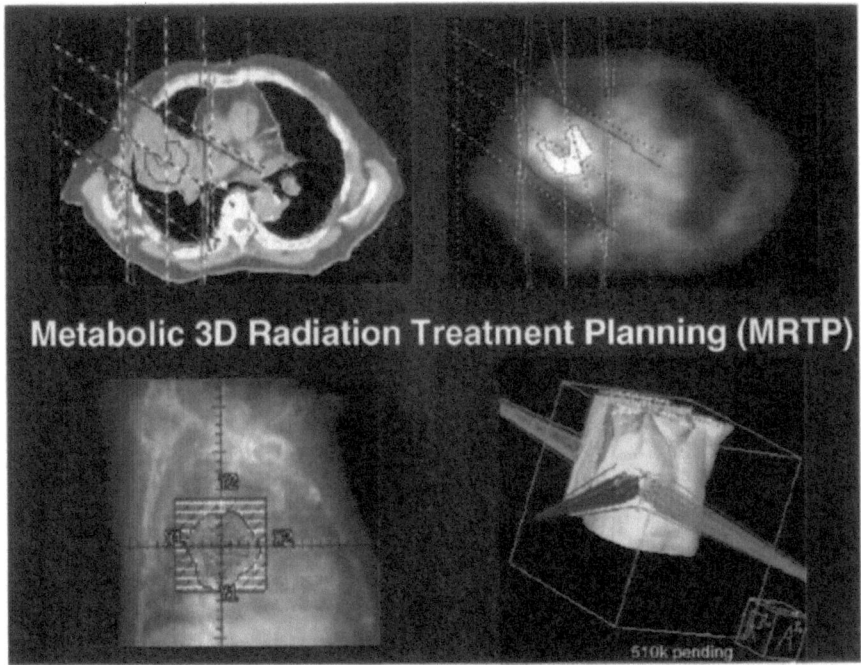

Metabolic 3D Radiation Treatment Planning (MRTP)

Fig. 2. The gross target volume (*GTV*) could be reduced substantially by using metabolic PET data (*right*) compared to anatomic CT data (*left*), resulting in smaller planning target volumes (*PTV*) for radiation treatment planning (latest version of the Pinnacle system)

Discussion and Conclusion

To our best knowledge, the present contribution is the first prospective study of patients with NSCLC describing the use of PET in 3D planning of radiation therapy and the consequent modifications of planning target volume and dose volume histogram using image fusion [19]. Retrospective studies published to date investigated the possible influence of PET in 2D [8, 12, 13, 16, 17] and 3D planning of radiation therapy [5, 6, 24]. Image fusion was not always performed and in some studies, PET was only visually compared with CT [6, 24].

Tumor Staging

Our data demonstrate that F-18 FDG PET as a noninvasive metabolic imaging technique provides clinically important and complimentary information compared to anatomic imaging by CT. Mediastinal (N2) lymph node metastases were staged correctly by F-18 FDG-PET with a sensitivity of 100%. The detection of N3 lesions and distant metastases (especially adrenal involvement) by whole-body PET changed the planned curative treatment to a palliative approach in 19% of all cases.

In patients with NSCLC and enlarged mediastinal lymph nodes or morphologically indeterminate extrathoracic lesions, FDG-PET has been included in our center as the diagnostic method of choice to aid the decision-making process regarding further clinical management. Correlation of clinical information with the SUV of the primary lesions may provide prognostic information independent of other clinical findings; these preliminary results, however, must be evaluated over a longer follow-up period with a large number of patients to obtain greater statistical validity.

Therapy Monitoring After Induction Chemotherapy

Molecular evaluation of tumors by FDG-PET after induction chemotherapy of stage III NSCLC can predict noninvasively and precisely the effectiveness of chemotherapy. PET precedes morphological imaging modalities in determining therapy response after neoadjuvant treatment and may be able to predict the pathologic and potentially the long-term therapeutic outcomes.

3D Radiation Treatment Planning

Our first results indicate that PET is an important complimentary tool for morphological imaging used for the exact localization of nodal tumor involvement and in some cases for determining the extent of the primary tumor.

Due to smaller PTV, radiation therapy could be delivered with less toxicity in most patients. As stated by Graham et al. [10, 11], the actuarial incidence of $\geq$grade 2 pneumonitis within 24 months after irradiation could be reduced up to 23%, if V_{lung} (20 Gy) will be reduced by 5%–17%.

Better tumor control with less radiation-induced toxicity and a higher therapeutic ratio of radiation therapy may be achieved by using PET and metabolic tumor localization in addition to anatomic tumor delineation by CT scan, applying image fusion.

References

1. Baum RP, Schmuecking M, Plichta K, Presselt N, Bonnet R, Lopatta E, Niesen A, Przetak C, Leonhardi J (2000) Staging of non small cell lung cancer (NSCLC) – is PET really clinically important or just a research tool? J Nucl Med 41:293P
2. Baum RP, Bonnet RB, Presselt N, Leonhardi J (2001) Positronenemissionstomographie (PET) mit F-18-FDG in der Diagnostik des Bronchialkarzinoms und zur Dignitätsabklärung von pulmonalen Raumforderungen. Nuklearmediziner 24:9–23
3. Baum RP, Rust M, Adams S, Strassmann G, Berekfeld J, Wagner R, Hertel A, Hör G (1996) Influence on patients' management by whole-body F-18 FDG PET for preoperative staging of non small cell lung cancer. J Nucl Med 37:121P

4. Byhardt RW, Martin L, Pajak TF, Shin KH, Emami B, Cox JD (1993) The influence of field size and other treatment factors on pulmonary toxicity following hyperfractionated irradiation for inoperable non-small lung cancer (NSCLC) – analysis of a Radiation Therapy Oncology Group (RTOG) protocol. Int J Radiat Oncol Biol Phys 27:537–544

5. Cai J, Chu JC, Recine D, Sharma M, Nguyen C, Rodebaugh R, Saxena VA, Ali A (1999) CT and PET lung imaging registration and fusion in radiotherapy treatment planning using the chamfer-matching method. Int J Radiat Oncol Biol Phys 43:883–891

6. Debois M, Fossard A, Vansteenkiste J, De Wever W, Verschakelen J, Bogaerts J, Gatti G, Stroobants S, Dupont P, Huyskens D, Kutcher J, Vanuytsel J (1998) Impact of PET scan on the target volume in lung cancer radiotherapy planning. Radiother Oncol 48:13S

7. Emami B, Lyman J, Brown A, Coia L, Goitein M, Munzenrider JE, Shank B, Solin LJ, Wesson M (1991) Tolerance of normal tissue to therapeutic irradiation. Int J Radiat Oncol Biol Phys 21:109–122

8. Erdi YE, Macapinlac H, Rosenzweig KE, Humm JL, Larson SM, Erdi AE, Yorke ED (2000) Use of PET to monitor the response of lung cancer to radiation treatment. Eur J Nucl Med 27:861–866

9. ICRU-Report 50, International Commission on Radiation Units and Measurements (1993) Prescribing, recording and reporting photon beam therapy. 1st edn. ICRU-Publications, Bethesda, Maryland USA

10. Graham MV, Purdy JA, Emami B, Harms W, Bosch W, Lockett MA, Perez CA (1999) Clinical dose-volume histogram analysis for pneumonitis after 3D treatment for non-small cell lung cancer (NSCLC). Int J Radiat Oncol Biol Phys 45:323–329

11. Graham MV, Jain NL, Kahn MG, Drzymala RE, Purdy JA (1996) Evaluation of an objective plan-evaluation model in the three-dimensional treatment of nonsmall cell lung cancer. Int J Radiat Oncol Biol Phys 34:469–474

12. Kiffer JD, Berlangieri SU, Scott AM, Quong G, Feigen M, Schumer W, Clarke CP, Knight SR, Daniel FJ (1998) The contribution of 18F-fluoro-2-deoxy-glucose positron emission tomographic imaging to radiotherapy planning in lung cancer. Lung Cancer 19:167–177

13. Kubota R, Yamada S, Kubota K, et al (1992) Intratumoral distribution of F-18 fluorodeoxyglucose in vivo: high accumulation in macrophages and granulation tissues studied by microautoradiography. J Nucl Med 33:1972–1980

14. Kutcher GJ, Leibel SA, Mohan R, Harrison LB, Armstrong JG, Zelefsky MF, LoSasso TJ, Burmann CM, Mageras GS, Chui CS, Brewster LJ, Masterson ME, Ling CC, Fuks Z (1993) Advances in precision treatment: Some aspects of 3D conformal radiation therapy. Front Radiat Ther Oncol 27:209–226

15. Kutcher GJ, Burman C, Brewster MS, Goitein M, Mohan R (1991) Histogram reduction method for calculating complication probabilities for three-dimensional treatment planning evaluations. Int J Radiat Oncol Biol Phys 21:137–146

16. Munley MT, Marks LB, Scarefone C, Sibley GS, Part EF, Turkington TG, Jaszczak RJ, Gilland DR, Anscher MS, Coleman RE (1999) Multimodality nuclear medicine imaging in three-dimensional radiation treatment planning for lung cancer: Challenges and prospects. Lung Cancer 23:105 114

17. Nestle U, Walter K, Schmidt S, Licht N, Nieder C, Motaref B, Hellwig D, Niewald M, Ukena D, Kirsch CM, Sybrecht GW, Schnabel K (1999) 18F-Deoxyglucose positron emission tomography (FDG-PET) for the planning of radiotherapy in lung cancer: High impact in patients with atelectasis. Int J Radiat Oncol Biol Phys 44:593–597

18. Perez CA, Stanley K, Rubin P, Kramer S, Brady LW, Marks JE, Perez-Tamayo R, Brown GS, Concannon JP, Rotman M, and the Radiation Therapy Oncology Group (1980) Patterns of tumor recurrence after definitive irradiation for inoperable non-oat cell carcinoma of the lung. Int J Radiat Oncol Biol Phys 6:987–994

19. Przetak C, Baum RP, Slomka PJ (2001) Image fusion raises clinical value of PET. Diagnostic Imaging Europe 17:10–15

20. Rosenmann J, Chaney EL, Sailer S, Sherouse GW, Tepper JE (1991) Recent advances in radiotherapy treatment planning. Cancer Invest 9:465–481

21. Schmuecking M, Plichta K, Lopatta E, Baum RP (1999) Wertigkeit der F-18 FDG-PET für das Therapie-Management und die Definition des PTV in der Strahlentherapie des Bronchialkarzinoms. Strahlenther Onkol 175:76 S
22. Ukena D, Rentz K, Leutz M, et al (1998) Evaluation of lung cancer with FDG-positron emission tomography (PET). Eur Resp J 12:393
23. Vansteenkiste JF, Stroobants SG, De Leyn PR, Dupont PJ, Bogaert J, Maes A, Deneffe GJ, Nackaerts KL, Verschakelen JA, Lerut TE, Mortelmans LA, Demedts MG (1998) Lymph node staging in non-small-cell lung cancer with FDG-PET scan: A prospective study on 690 lymph node stations from 68 patients. J Clin Oncol 16:2142–2149
24. Vanuytsel LJ, Vansteenkiste JF, Stroobants SG, De Leyn PR, De Wever W, Verbeken EK, Gatti GG, Huyskens DP, Kutcher GJ (2000) The impact of 18-F-fluoro-2-deoxy-D-glucose positron emission tomography (FDG-PET) lymph node staging on the radiation treatment volumes in patients with non-small cell lung cancer. Radiother Oncol 55:317–324

Recurrences of Thyroid Cancer After Radical Surgery and Complementary Treatment: Are Macroscopic, Microscopic, Scintigraphic, and Biochemical Criteria Sufficient in the Evaluation of Radicality of Primary Treatment?

Lech Pomorski, Jacek Cywiński, Krzysztof Kołomecki, Zbigniew Pasieka, Magdalena Bartos, Krzysztof Kuzdak

This paper presents our own experience in surgical treatment of thyroid cancer recurrences.

K. Kołomecki (✉)
Clinic of Endocrinological and General Surgery,
Medical University of Łódź, Pabianicka 62, 93513 Łódź, Poland

Abstract

From 1974 to 1999, 1,001 patients were operated on for thyroid cancer, including 778 (78%) for differentiated thyroid cancer and 223 (22%) for other thyroid malignant neoplasms. Radical operations were performed in 716 (92%) patients with differentiated thyroid cancer and in 85 (38%) patients with other thyroid malignant neoplasms. After surgery, all patients underwent various methods of complementary treatment, depending on cancer type and grading (levothyroxine, 131I, radiotherapy and/or chemotherapy). These patients had no evidence of persistent disease after finishing treatment (Tg, CEA, calcitonin, scintigraphy). We observed recurrences of thyroid cancer, although macroscopic, microscopic, biochemical, and scintigraphic criteria of radicality were present. At 18 months' to 24 years' follow-up, we observed recurrences in 94 (11.7%) of 801 patients treated radically, including in 53 (7.4%) of 716 patients with differentiated thyroid cancer and in 41 (48%) of 85 patients with other thyroid malignancies. Among 37 patients with thyroid bed recurrence, 18 (48.6%) underwent radical operations and 19 (51.4%) palliative ones. Of 33 patients with regional lymph node recurrence, radical operations were performed in 26 (78.8%) and palliative ones in seven (21.2%). Of 24 patients with distant metastases, four (17%) (with single metastasis) underwent surgery (three radical operations and one palliative one). Other methods of treatment were used in the remaining patients. Occurrence of thyroid cancer recurrences in the thyroid bed and lymph nodes indicates that macroscopic, microscopic, and scintigraphic criteria of radicality are not sufficient. Recurrences after radical surgery are more infrequent in patients with differentiated thyroid cancers than in those with other thyroid malignant neoplasms. In many pa-

204 Lech Pomorski et al.

tients, thyroid bed and lymph node recurrences can be removed radically during surgery.

Introduction

Thyroid cancer may recur in its primary localization, surrounding tissues, regional lymph nodes, and distant places, which results from a nonradical removal of cancer (residual disease) or metastasis that was not diagnosed and removed during a primary operation. In certain cases malignancy may occur de novo in tissue left or in a singular cell loaded by mutation – e.g., in patients with medullary thyroid carcinoma or in RET proto-oncogene mutation carriers after thyroidectomy. Incidence of disease recurrence after macroscopic and microscopic radical excision of a tumor indicates that not all cancer cells were removed during surgery.

Thyroid cancer mostly recurs in the regional lymph nodes and thyroid bed. It occurs in patients who underwent limited treatment (limited surgery and hormonotherapy) and in patients who had extensive treatment (total thyroidectomy, selective or elective regional lymphadenectomy, 131 I therapy, and suppressive hormonotherapy).

Aim

The aim of our study was to assess whether clinical, biochemical, and scintigraphic criteria are sufficient for the evaluation of treatment radicality in thyroid carcinoma patients and the risk of recurrence.

Material and Methods

From 1974 to 1999, 1,001 patients were operated on due to thyroid cancer (Table 1), including 835 women (83.4%) and 166 men (16.6%). The women-to-men ratio was 5:1 and the mean age 53.4 years. According to the WHO classification, differentiated thyroid carcinomas (DTC) were diagnosed in 778 patients (78%), and other thyroid malignant neoplasms (OTMN) in 223 (22%).

Radical operations were performed in 716 (92%) patients with DTC and palliative ones in 62 (8%). In the OTMN group, radical operations were performed in 85 (38%) patients and palliative ones in 138 (62%). All patients with

Table 1. Thyroid cancer: present study

	No.	%
Papillary carcinoma	473	47.3
Follicular carcinoma	305	30.5
Medullary carcinoma	56	5.6
Anaplastic carcinoma	110	10.9
Others	57	5.7
Total	1001	100.0

DTC advanced more than T1aNoMo underwent primary thyroidectomy with elective/selective modified lymphadenectomy and complementary treatment according to the following schedule: surgery, 131I, L-thyroxine, regardless of various tumor variants. The patients with papillary carcinoma of T1aNoMo grade had only L-thyroxine complementary treatment. Patients after nonradical operations were excluded from this study. Follow-up examinations were performed every 3 months in the first year and every 6 months in next years. The following examinations were performed: clinical examination, biochemical tests (thyroglobulin in DTC patients and calcitonin, CEA in patients with medullary carcinoma), chest X-ray, and ultrasonography. After radioiodine treatment, whole body scintiscan using 131I was performed after the first 6 months and afterwards at the 1st, 3rd, and 5th year, when the results of the other examinations were normal. Suppressive treatment with L-thyroxine was carried out under TSH level (TSH<0.1 μU/ml). Daily doses of L-thyroxine ranged from 1.8 to 4.34 μg/kg (average 2.96±0.53 μg/kg). We assumed the following criteria of health: no clinical symptoms of recurrence, thyroglobulin <1 ng/ml, calcitonin=5 ng/ml, CEA <4 μg/ml, normal chest X-ray, and no pathological uptake at scintiscan.

Results

At follow-up, which ranged between 1.8 and 24 years (average 8.9 years), we diagnosed recurrences in 94 (11.7%) of the 801 patients treated radically. This diagnosis was made after finishing a basic treatment, although there were no clinical, biochemical, and scintigraphic data of persisting disease. Recurrence was detected in 53 (7.4%) of 716 patients with DTC and in 41 (48%) of 85 patients with OTMN. The first test, which gave us a clue of recurrence, was: biochemical examination, 38 (40.4%); scintigraphy, 23 (24.4%); clinical examination, 14 (15.0%); and radiography, 9 (9.6%). In ten patients, recurrence was diagnosed on the basis of numerous tests, including ultrasound. Regional recurrence was detected in 70 of all patients (37, thyroid bed; 33, regional lymph nodes), whereas distant metastases were revealed in 24 patients; three of them also had regional recurrence. Regional recurrence was diagnosed in 38 (5.3%) of 716 patients with DTC and in 32 (37.6%) of 85 patients with OTMN.

Distant metastases were diagnosed in 13 (1.8%) patients with DTC and in 11 (12.9%) patients with OTMN.

Thirty-seven patients with thyroid bed recurrence were reoperated on. In 18 of these patients (48%), recurrent tumors were removed radically, whereas 19 (52%) underwent only a palliative operation. Of 33 patients with recurrence in lymph nodes, in 26 (78.8%) malignant tumors were removed, and in seven palliative operations were carried out. Of 24 patients with distant metastases, only four (17%) were operated on (they had a single metastasis). In three of them, the metastatic tumors were removed radically; two patients had metastases to ribs and one had a skin metastasis. The forth patient from this group had a metastatic tumor infiltrating both bottom and hip bones; this patient was treated palliatively. The other patients with metastases or regional recurrence were reoperated on nonradically and therefore they were treated using other methods of therapy.

Discussion

Recurrences may develop in a primary localization of cancer, in surrounding tissues, regional lymphatic nodes and distant places, which results from a nonradical removal of cancer (residual disease) or the occurrence of metastases that were not diagnosed during primary treatment [1].

Thyroid cancer of every type and grading may recur. At 15-year follow-up, Cady [2] described recurrences of DTC in 11% of patients from a low-risk group and in 24% of patients from a high-risk group. Noguchi et al. [3] from Japan and Hay et al. [4] describe recurrences in 1.3% and 6% of patients with papillary microcarcinoma, respectively. According to them, incidence of recurrence depend on the extent of primary thyroid tumor removal [3, 4] and complementary treatment [5]. Radical surgical treatment and various methods of complementary treatment applied in our center do not prevent the development of thyroid cancer recurrence, either. Effective lymphadenectomy performed by us in thyroid cancer patients does result, however, in lower incidence of lymph node recurrence in our clinic patients than in other centers. Nevertheless, in our experience, recurrence in the thyroid bed occurs more frequently than in regional lymph nodes – in 37% and 33% of patients, respectively. It may result from the removal of micrometastases in lymph nodes excised electively. We observed micrometastases in 11.8% of patients with papillary carcinoma, in 6.1% patients with follicular carcinoma, in 8.3% of patients with medullary carcinoma, and in 15.4% of patients with nondifferentiated cancer [6]. This radical treatment concerning regional lymph nodes is accepted by some authors in light of to the high percentage of metastasis [7, 8] but not recommended by others [9]. Every recurrence gives evidence of residual neoplasm cells left after primary treatment. Only in patients loaded by mutation does there exist probability of malignancy process de novo from every single thyroid cell left. This resulted in the concept of thyroid remnant ablation after prophylactic thyroidectomy in patients loaded by RET proto-oncogene mutation [9]. In our study, various accessible tests revealed no evidence of persisting disease in patients with thyroid cancer recurrence. Recurrences were more frequent in patients with OTMN than in those with DTC.

It turned out that thyroglobulin and scintigraphy are the most sensitive markers of recurrent process in patients with DTC, and calcitonin in patients with medullary carcinoma. It was also determined that ultrasound was highly sensitive for the diagnosis of regional lymph node metastasis.

Conclusions

Occurrence of thyroid cancer recurrences in the thyroid bed and lymph nodes indicate that macroscopic, microscopic, biochemical and scintigraphic criteria of radicality are not sufficient.

Recurrences after radical surgery are more infrequent in patients with differentiated thyroid cancers than in those with other thyroid malignant neoplasms.

In numerous patients, thyroid bed and lymph node recurrences can be removed radically during surgery.

References

1. Gagel RF, Goepfert H, Callender DL (1996) Chaining concepts in the pathogenesis and management of thyroid carcinoma. CA Cancer J Clin 46:261–283
2. Cady B (1981) Surgery of thyroid cancer. World J Surg 5:3–14
3. Noguchi S, Yamashita H, Murakami N, Nakayama I, Masakatsu T, Kawamoto H (1996) Small carcinomas of the thyroid. A long-term follow-up of 867 patients. Arch Surg 131:187–191
4. Hay ID, Grant CS, VanHeerden JA, Goellner JR, Ebersold JR, Bergstralh EJ (1992) Papillary thyroid microcarcinoma: a study of 535 cases observed in a 50-year period. Surgery 112:1139–1147
5. Ozaki O, Notsu T, Hirai K, Mori T (1983) Differentiated carcinoma of the thyroid gland. World J Surg 7:181–185
6. Pomorski L, Rybiński K (1996) Lymphadenektomie beim Schilddrüsenkarzinom-Staging und Therapie. Zentralbl Chirurg 121:455–458
7. Dralle H, Gimm O (1996) Lymphadenektomie beim Schilddrüsenkarzinom. Chirurg 67:788–806
8. Witte J, Schlotmann U, Simon D, Dotzenrath C, Ohman C, Goretzki PE (1997) Bedeutung der Lymphknotenmetastasen differenzierter Schilddrüsenkarzinome für deren Prognose-eine Metaanalyse. Zentralbl Chir 122:259–265
9. Kukora JS (1998) Thyroid cancer. In: Cameron JL (ed) Current surgical therapy, 6th edn. Mosby, St Louis, pp 592–598

Summary 3

Summary and Congress Report: Molecular Staging of Cancer – Concepts of Today, Therapies of Tomorrow

Heike Allgayer, Markus M. Heiss, Friedrich W. Schildberg

H Allgayer (✉)
Department of Surgery, Klinikum Grosshadern,
Ludwig Maximilians University of Munich, Marchioninistr. 15,
81377 Munich, Germany

An overwhelming wealth of information has been generated since scientists started to define the molecular events which describe the malignant transformation and progression of cells, and their development towards life-threatening metastatic disease. Some of these research results have already influenced the clinical diagnostic process and therapeutic strategies. It is strongly believed that this progressive development will accelerate and completely change our approach toward cancer. However, as of this writing, the transfer of molecular discoveries into new clinical applications has occurred in only a few examples.

The First International Congress on Molecular Staging of Cancer, held in Munich in December 2001, was a first attempt to establish an international platform of exchange among highly ranked molecular biologists, cell biologists, tumor immunologists, and clinical and surgical oncologists with the focus of the molecular staging of cancer. This translational approach should be fruitful for both clinical and experimental experts, and the beginning of an exciting network. The highlighted topics included tumor-associated proteolysis, minimal residual disease, new approaches for molecular diagnosis and targeting, and the resulting first molecular staging models. It also included a session focusing on technology transfer, opening up a new field of funding for innovative concepts. Finally, the existing and future impacts of molecular staging on clinical strategies were discussed.

The congress was organized at the Department of Surgery of the Ludwig Maximilians University (LMU) of Munich, under the auspices of the German Society of Surgery together with its Molecular Oncology Section, and the International Metastasis Research Society. The congress was opened with welcome addresses by the Secretary General of the German Society of Surgery, Prof. W. Hartel, Berlin, and the President of the Professional Board of German Surgeons, Prof. J. Witte, Berlin.

In his Presidential Address, included in this book as an Introduction, the Congress President Prof. F.W. Schildberg described the present gap between the wealth of molecular information gained with new technologies such as ge-

nomics and proteomics, and the transfer of that information into clinical diagnosis and therapy. There are few examples, such as hereditary colorectal
and breast cancers, in which this transfer in part has already occurred. For diverse cancer types such as gastric cancer, in which there are still significant
problems in defining an individual's prognosis with the established morphological criteria (pTNM) and conventional staging models – this in addition to
insufficient adjuvant therapeutic options of treatment – there is an urgent
need for new molecular staging models and therapies based on the individual's tumor biology.

The Scientific Program was opened with an Honorary Keynote Lecture of
an internationally renowned scientist whose career impressively illustrates the
journey from first molecular discoveries to broad innovative molecular
knowledge in tumor biology: Prof. Garth L. Nicolson, Irvine, California, USA.
In his keynote lecture, "Cycles in Cancer Research: The History of Cancer Cell
Membranes, Cancer-Associated Micro-organisms, and Gene Expression Research Comes Full Circle," Dr. Nicolson summarized the development of the
field since his description of the fluid mosaic model of the cell membrane,
which led to discoveries characterizing tumor cell membranes, the description
of new metastasis-related genes, the discovery of interactions between tumor
cells and microorganisms such as mycoplasmas and viruses, and increasing
knowledge about gene mutations and gene expression and their distinct roles
in cancer inception and cancer progression.

Session 1 of the Scientific Program focused on the topic of *tumor-associated
proteolysis*. An overview of existing protease subclasses with special emphasis
on their potential clinical relevance was given by Prof. Manfred Schmitt (Department of Gynecology, Technical University Munich, Germany). Of the protease classes which promote invasion and metastasis in various cancer types,
matrix metalloproteinases (MMPs), cathepsins, and the urokinase (u-PA) system have been shown to be prognostic for several cancer types and have been
targets for new therapeutic attempts. However, early efforts with first-genera-
tion MMP inhibitors did not succeed in clinical trials, and cathepsin inhibitors have not yet entered the clinical-trial stage. There are several promising strategies involving the u-PA system which in part have given good results
in in vivo models, some of which will soon be part of phase I–II trials. Such
trials of multifunctional inhibitors involving more than one protease system
are also underway. Prof. G. Hoyer-Hansen from the Finsen Laboratory, University of Copenhagen, Denmark, gave an excellent overview of the urokinase-
receptor (u-PAR) and u-PAR-isoforms, and the known data on its function in
invasion. She also introduced several monoclonal u-PAR antibodies targeting
different u-PAR subdomains, which will be valuable for diagnosis. Dr. J.
Aguirre-Ghiso of the group of Prof. Liliana Ossowski, Mount Sinai School of
Medicine, New York, gave a fascinating account of the finding that u-PAR is
far more than an invasion-promoting molecule, but rather plays important
roles in outside-in signaling, thus influencing tumor cell proliferation. When
u-PAR is physically interacting with integrins, an ERK signal is activated and
favors tumor cell proliferation. However, if u-PAR/integrin interaction is inter-

rupted (by an antibody developed byof G. Hoyer-Hansen), the p38 pathway is favored and the tumor cell is brought into dormancy. This may very well suggest a novel approach to treat minimal residual disease by inducing dormancy. Dr. Heike Allgayer gave an introduction to the transcriptional regulation of u-PAR overexpression in gastrointestinal cancer cells. Using the example of one AP-2/Sp1 motif mediating diverse means of u-PAR regulation including regulation by the *c-src* oncogene, it was illustrated that u-PAR-mediated proteolysis in tumor cells can be countered by direct inhibition at the transcriptional level, but also at the signal transduction level, when Src (which is overly active in more than 70% of colorectal and gastric cancers) is inhibited. Preliminary data suggest that subpopulations of patients can be identified in whom a tumor-specific regulation by this promoter element could occur, which suggests u-PAR and its molecular regulators as markers for new molecular staging models and individually designed novel therapies. The session was closed with an excellent overview by Prof. Keld Dano, Head of the Finsen Laboratory, University of Copenhagen, Denmark, about u-PAR and its interactions with other protease systems and with stromal cells, which can support tumor cell invasion by producing proteases in a potential paracrine fashion. In light of new data from the Finsen laboratory, it was concluded that the most promising therapeutic attempts will be to inhibit more than one protease system, and to include the stromal cell interaction in new strategies.

Session 2 was held on existing *molecular staging models* and potential new candidates as staging markers. Prof. H. Höfler and Dr. H. Vogelsang (Departments of Pathology and Surgery, respectively, of the Technical University Munich) gave their insights into molecular events of sporadic and hereditary gastric cancer. For sporadic cancers, the growth factor receptors ErbB-2 and K-Sam are prognostic for intestinal and diffuse-type cancers. Other molecules which have been shown to be of prognostic relevance include the u-PA system (u-PA and PAI-1), cyclin E (a cell-cycle regulator), EGF, E-cadherin and molecules involved in its signaling (beta-catenin), and the apoptosis suppressor bcl-2. Drs. Höfler and Vogelsang presented their own data regarding E-cadherin which suggest that this marker will be useful for an individualized diagnosis of diffuse-type gastric cancers, in particular. Of the hereditary gastric cancers, a diffuse-type syndrome, hereditary diffuse-type gastric cancer (HDGC) characterized by diverse E-cadherin mutations, is differentiated from gastric cancers, which parallel other hereditary cancer syndromes such as HNPCC, FAP, Peutz Jeghers syndrome, and Li Fraumeni syndrome, which are associated with mutations of mismatch repair genes APC, STK11, and p53, respectively. For E-cadherin mutation carriers, prophylactic gastrectomies are being considered, as these mutations are associated with a high lifetime risk for gastric cancer. Molecular methods which allow a safe screening for all mutations mentioned enable the identification of high-risk individuals for endoscopic surveillance. Dr. Markus M. Heiss (Department of Surgery, Klinikum Grosshadern, LMU Munich, Germany) introduced a first molecular staging model established by his group for sporadic gastric cancers. Considering the expression of the u-PA-protease system (PAI-1) and minimal residual disease in the bone marrow, subpopulations of patients were identified in whom the clinical outcome differed considerably from what would be expected from morphological/clinical staging parameters. For example, in early-stage tumors without macroscopic lymph node involvement (pN0), additional evidence of high PAI-1 expression and disseminated tumor cells in the bone marrow lowered the survival probabilities of these patients to those of patients with clinically evident lymph node disease (pN1). Prof. Gary E. Gallick (Department of Cancer Biology, M.D. Anderson Cancer Center, Houston, Texas, USA) introduced molecular markers from Src-mediated signal transduction cascades which might become prognostic, in addition to established markers such as the APC gene, p53, and Ras. His group showed that high Src activity which correlated with high u-PAR expression was independently predictive for a poor prognosis in colorectal cancers. Furthermore, Src-activated Akt might become a predictive marker for the success of signal transduction-based therapies. In addition, data suggest that TIAM-1, the guanine-nucleotide exchange factor for Rac, and the c-Met receptor are candidates for markers indicating tumor progression, the latter in addition being a target for ribozyme-based therapy. Prof. H. Schackert (Department of Surgical Research, University of Dresden, Germany) and Dr. G. Möslein (Department of Surgery, University of Düsseldorf, Germany) gave an overview of the molecular diagnosis and clinical implications of hereditary nonpolyposis colorectal cancer (HNPCC). HNPCC is one of the earliest examples of how predictive molecular diagnosis selects for a clinical surveillance program for affected individuals. The most common mutations concern the mismatch repair genes hMSH2 and hMLH1. Further mutations concern the genes hMSH6, hPMS1, and hPMS2. However, there are remaining issues which must be resolved regarding the clinical surveillance program, as well as the clinical consequences of prophylactic surgery. The main problem is the clinical heterogeneity of the disease. Criteria for an extensive prophylactic surgery as suggested are broad adenomas and de novo carcinomas, accelerated adenoma-carcinoma progression, and reduced compliance by the patient for frequent colonoscopies. Prof. Menashe Bar-Eli (Department of Cancer Biology, M.D. Anderson Cancer Center, Houston) and Prof. Judith P. Johnson (Institute of Immunology, LMU) gave insights into new molecular determinants of melanoma progression. Among them are adhesion molecules such as MCAM, tyrosine kinase receptors such as c-Kit, but potentially also transcriptional regulators such as AP-2 or mader. A newly discovered protein, PHLDA1, is downregulated during the progression from benign nevi to melanomas. Prof. A. Frilling (University of Essen, Germany) summarized the status of MEN type 2, in which the detection of mutated c-Ret is an indication for prophylactic thyroidectomy. Dr. T. Sutter (Department of Surgery, University of Halle, Germany) gave an introduction to cyclins and other cell-cycle regulators and their potential role as new staging markers. Lastly, Dr. M. Untch (Department of Gynecology, LMU) gave an overview of the molecular staging of breast cancer. For hereditary breast cancers, large clinical studies clearly indicate the predictive value of mutations in the tumor suppressor genes BRCA1 and BRCA2. Patients with BRCA1 mutations have a

45% risk until age 50 and an up to 85% risk until age 75 of getting breast cancer. A combination of BRCA1 and BRCA2 mutations predicts an especially poor prognosis for the individual patient. For sporadic breast cancers, again presence of the u-PA-protease system (u-PA and PAI-1) clearly predicts poor survival, and an overexpression of *c-erbB-2* is not only prognostic but has already led to established adjuvant clinical treatment concepts, including Herceptin.

A Lunch Session was held on the topic of technology transfer to companies. The forum was presented by Prof. H. Domdey (BioM, Munich), F. Schaebsdau (Bioscience Ventures, Munich), and Dr. M. Reymond (Department of Surgery, University of Magdeburg, Germany). The session was held as an open discussion, with the three panelists answering questions from the audience. The conclusion of the discussion was that institutions such as BioM Munich or Venture Capital Groups can provide much more than financing for new ideas, namely networking, free consulting, contacts to research peers and politics, and cooperation with other companies.

Scientific Session 3 concerned the topic *of minimal residual tumor disease as a new staging entity in solid carcinomas.* Data were introduced by Dr. Uwe Grützner (Department of Surgery, Klinikum Grosshadern, LMU) on disseminated tumor cells in a large series of colorectal cancer patients, by Prof. Dr. K. W. Jauch (Chair, Department of Surgery, University of Regensburg, Germany) on gastric cancer, by Dr. I. Funke (Department of Surgery, Klinikum Grosshadern, LMU) and Dr. Nadia Harbeck (Department of Gynecology, Technical University Munich) on large series of breast cancer patients, and Dr. R. Oberneder (Department of Urology, LMU) on urological cancers. The data were obtained using different methods (immunocytochemistry, PCR) and markers (cytokeratins, but also others such as CEA) of detection, but the consensus of all participants and chairs was that the mere qualitative detection of disseminated tumor cells in the bone marrow at the time of primary surgery cannot be regarded as a reliable prognostic parameter, since false positives caused by the surgical trauma and/or the presence of the primary tumor can obscure the detection of biologically relevant minimal residual disease. Prognostic relevance could be shown in some cases for subgroups. Strategies to circumvent this problem are the follow-up of these cells after curative tumor resection over time, and molecular phenotyping of the cells. Examples of the former strategy were given by Dr. Grützner regarding a colorectal study, and for the latter concerning the expression of MMP-7, u-PAR, *c-erbB-2*, and *c-met* in a gastric cancer study by Dr. Jauch, and regarding u-PAR, c-erbB-2, and EP-CAM in a breast cancer study by Dr. Harbeck. An interesting new method for a broad molecular phenotyping by comparative genome analysis and microarray analysis following single-cell PCR was introduced by Dr. C. Klein (Institute of Immunology, LMU). It is believed that such methodology will help to identify biologically and clinically critical subtypes of minimal residual disease which will support the development of powerful molecular staging models.

This conclusion was supported by the Keynote Lecture by Prof. G. Rieth-müller (Chair, Institute of Immunology, LMU), who gave an excellent over-view of the current status of methodological possibilities and actual studies on minimal residual disease. The perspective was supported by the second Keynote Lecture, by Prof. C. Herfarth (Chair, Department of Surgery, Heidel-berg, Germany), who outlined the importance of molecular methods and also phenotyping of minimal residual disease in bone marrow and lymph nodes for surgical decision making.

New methodology for defining new staging markers was the central topic of Session 4. Prof. Thomas Gress (Department of Internal Medicine, University of Ulm, Germany) gave a fascinating insight into expression profiling analysis and microarray analysis, which offer the opportunity to obtain rapid and broad information on, for example, tissue origin, proliferative/metastatic po-tential, and the susceptibility of multiple tumors to diverse therapies. A fur-ther example was given in the talk by Prof. M. Heberer (Chair, University of Basel, Switzerland), who developed a tissue array that is able to identify target tissues for immunotherapy by certain monoclonal antibodies. An earlier speech by Prof. M. Reymond (Department of Surgery, University of Magde-burg, Germany) was an overview of the current status of proteomics technolo-gy, which will become a powerful and rapid technique for identifying new tar-gets. Unresolved issues for all of the techniques mentioned include reliable procedures of normalization, negative controls, and optimal interpretation of the data. Prof. Ronald Kates (Technical University, Munich) introduced a pow-erful and innovative advanced statistical method based on neuronal networks which is able to reliably predict prognostic parameters and therapy response from learning samples. With the rapidly increasing number and complexity of and interactions among new staging parameters, such statistical methods will be indispensable in the definition of powerful staging models. Dr. Mathias Schmidt (Oncology Research Section, Byk Gulden, Konstanz, Germany) gave an interesting insight into aspects of biotech companies in searching and fo-cusing on new potential molecular targets. In addition, fascinating new tech-nologies were introduced such as the synthetic lethality screen, which allows a genome-wide search for genes that are linked to apoptosis suppression in can-cer cells. In another technique, gene expression profiling using large gene chips is used to identify tumor-specific genes and target genes responding to different chemotherapeutic agents. Dr. Nancy Colburn (Head, Gene Regula-tion Section, U.S. National Institutes of Health, Frederick, MD, USA) closed this interesting session with a description of new methodology efforts, and a newly identified tumor-suppressor, pdcd4, which potentially acts through transcriptional but also translational mechanisms and may suppress tumor progression by downregulating invasion-related genes.

Session 5, the final session of the meeting, focused on the topic *of designing new strategies of molecular targeting*. Dr. H. Lindhofer (GSF Institute of Clini-cal Molecular Biology, Munich) introduced the new concept of bispecific, tri-functional antibodies which are able to capture tumor cells (using the anti-gens EPCAM or HER2/neu) and T-cells with one arm each, and to activate ac-

cessory and APC/dendritic cells via the Fc region. First results with three patients with peritoneal carcinosis are promising regarding the elimination of
malignant ascites and peritoneal tumor cell load. A talk by Prof. M. von Kne-
bel-Döberitz (Department of Surgery, University of Heidelberg, Germany) focused on a new approach to identify coding microsatellites in cancers with
microsatellite instability, which in theory would lead to the prediction of truncated proteins as highly tumor-specific targets. Prof. M. Hallek (Department
of Oncology, LMU) introduced a new gene therapy technique which enables
modifications of the envelope of AAV vectors to a certain extent, thus enabling
an increase of specificity of the vector, a problem which has not yet been
solved in gene therapy. A transcriptional approach to target the expression of
specific genes can be performed by triplex-forming oligonucleotides, as
shown in some examples described by Prof. Klaus Degitz (Department of Der-
matology, LMU). In vivo data must be obtained to further investigate the clinical potential of this fascinating new approach. Dr. R. Kopp (Department of
Surgery, Klinikum Grosshadern, LMU) introduced clinical data suggesting
that anti-epidermal growth factor receptor (EGFR) therapeutic strategies
might be able to prevent colorectal cancer progression. The session ended
with the talk by Dr. Viktor Magdolen (Department of Gynecology, Technical
University, Munich) on the design of new small molecular inhibitors of the
u-PA-protease system, which, after the description of various x-ray structures
of u-PA/inhibitor complexes have been optimized, would be able to interrupt
the interaction of u-PA with its receptor (u-PAR, see Session 1). The promising
early in vivo data on these new protease inhibitors may open new possibilities
in the protease field.

The synopsis and conclusion of the meeting were presented by the Scientific Chairs of the congress, Dr. Heike Allgayer and Dr. Markus M. Heiss. The
meeting demonstrated several points: (1) Molecular markers which have clear
biological relevance, which have been shown to be prognostic in clinical studies, and against which innovative targeting strategies are being developed, are
at hand. (2) There are powerful methods now available to rapidly and efficiently detect new markers and targets, and to calculate reliable new staging
models for clinical applications. (3) More and more fascinating technologies
are being developed that will enable diverse strategies to target molecular
markers therapeutically. In conclusion, it only remains to continue defining
the new molecular staging models in concerted efforts with large patient populations, and to put further emphasis on the translation of new basic concepts
into future clinical therapies. Our meeting, headlined by the vision "Concepts
of Today – Therapies of Tomorrow" should thus be considered a beginning –
with the larger goal of opening up a new forum for scientific exchange and in-
tensified and fruitful crosstalk in this fascinating field of cancer research.